Praise for *On the Nature of Food Allergy*

Review by Michael Young, M.D.
Assistant Clinical Professor of Pediatrics,
Harvard Medical School
Assistant in Medicine,
Children's Hospital, Boston
Author of the *Peanut Allergy Answer Book*

On the Nature of Food Allergy is a unique book that combines important medical information from the most current studies with valuable advice and recommendations from the vast clinical experience of the author, Dr. Paul Hannaway. Even more, the book is a fascinating mélange of history, culture, human interest and personal anecdotes, all told in a breezy comfortable and reassuring style. As an allergist with a special interest in food allergy, I find this work to be very important not only for patients, their families and caretakers, but equally important for physicians and allergy specialists as well. It is the only work on food allergy I am aware of that is organized by the specific foods, which is particularly useful. The chapter on uncommon food allergies is worth the read alone. I also enjoyed Dr. Hannaway's opinions and discussion on why he thinks the current food allergy epidemic may be a direct result of the current medical recommendations on maternal and infant diets. *On the Nature of Food Allergy* is another winner from Dr. Hannaway and I recommend this book not only to all my patients with food allergies but to my colleagues as well.

Review by Michael H. Mellon, M.D.
Associate Clinical Professor of Pediatrics,
University of California San Diego School of Medicine

This is a remarkable book. Claiming to be intended for patients, parents, health-care providers, emergency care staff, restaurant owners, chefs, school nurses, teachers, and child-care providers, it delivers on this promise by being a unique single source on all aspects of food allergy. The book outlines the history of the current food allergy epidemic we are observing in North America and developed countries worldwide. It then goes on to detail the basic science of the food allergens involved as well as the sources of these food allergens, an area little known even to many allergists. Strategies for prevention and treatment are provided in language intended for patients. In addition, there are chapters describing other self-help books, patient support organizations, Web sites, and medical centers that specialize in food allergy treatment and research.

As a practicing pediatric allergist, I especially enjoyed the mix of basic science, food information, case reports, and theories on the possible causes and needed interventions for the current food allergy epidemic. Dr. Hannaway directly answers many of the most frequently asked questions about food allergy (e.g. peanut and tree nut cross reactivity; are seafood allergic people allergic to iodine? which patients outgrow allergies?). Providing language suitable for counseling patients is another benefit for health-care providers.

Always a keen observer of the passing medical scene, Dr. Hannaway encompasses the experience, credibility, and iconoclastic critical eye that may be necessary to solve the mystery of the food allergy dilemma. To this end, he examines and questions the current trends in feeding practices and the American Academy of Pediatrics recommendations for infant feeding in one of the most engaging sections of the book.

The manual is written in an extremely readable style for different levels of understanding. It is the right book about the right subject and certainly appears at the right time. For anyone involved with food allergy, it is a must read.

Review by Phillip E. Korenblat, M.D., C.C.I.
Professor of Clinical Medicine,
Washington University School of Medicine

This food allergy handbook serves a major need at a time of increasing incidence of food allergy. Dr Hannaway has included information about some less well-understood non-allergic adverse food reactions, as well as information concerning reactions to food additives. Sections explaining anaphylaxis and preventive measures that can be taken to avoid accidental exposure of ingested allergens are included. This excellent handbook, authored by an expert in the field, will be helpful to those living with food allergies, as well as to many disciplines of medicine that are concerned about this issue.

Review by Frank J. Twarog, M.D., Ph.D
Associate Clinical Professor of Pediatrics, Harvard Medical School

This book is a must-read for anyone interested in food allergy, especially for parents of children or patients who have food allergy! It is an A-to-Z compendium of information regarding food allergies. An easy read is guaranteed by the mixture of interesting anecdotes, case reports, basic science, and solid recommendations regarding the increasing problem of food allergy and the real risk for severe, life-threatening reactions.

The volume is full of useful information that can inform even the physician reader regarding little-known facts related to food allergy. In particular, for those wishing to explore specific food sensitivities, the text is arranged in a simple, easily accessible fashion. In contrast to some sources which create undue anxiety, Dr. Hannaway has provided a balanced discussion of how to deal with food allergy, when to really be concerned, and what strategies may be undertaken to minimize risks. The author should be congratulated on producing yet another valuable resource for individuals afflicted with food allergies or for family members wishing to understand this problem.

Review by Phillip L. Lieberman, M.D.
Clinical Professor of Medicine and Pediatrics,
University of Tennessee

After 35 years of practicing allergy and reviewing several patient-oriented books on allergy, I must admit that I have become somewhat jaded and approached the *On the Nature of Food Allergy* by Dr. Paul J. Hannaway with a sense of obligation rather than enthusiasm. However, upon opening the handbook and scanning its pages, I quickly realized that this text was not only educational for patients, but for me, and I suspect the vast majority of allergists, as well. It is a unique and valuable resource not only for patients who suffer from food allergy but also for physicians who treat such patients. I have never seen information on food allergy presented in this way and also never before encountered such a complete compilation of applicable and useful facts about food allergy. I could list endless examples of facts I have never seen recorded elsewhere, but in the interest of time and space, I will only mention a few, such as: the helpful discussion of glucosamine and chondroitin, various tables pointing out species and cross-reacting relationships between foods and the entire chapter on "Less Common Allergic and Adverse Food Reactions." Such examples are valuable not only to patients but also to physicians, especially allergists.

In addition to its wonderful and unique contents, the book is written in clear, plain, and expressive English. It is not only easy to read but also fun to read. There are interesting anecdotes from Dr. Hannaway's practice which spice (pardon the pun) the text and hold our interest, and there are tantalizing bits of history about the foods discussed which compel the reader to continue the exploration of the book. The text is, as expected, a rich source of helpful addresses (contained in the appendix) and a very helpful tool to aid the patient in evaluating alternative therapies and controversial treatments.

In summary, the text is a must for any patient suffering from food allergy, and I personally found it a valuable resource to help guide my advice to patients suffering from allergic reactions to foods. I believe it is a superb example of a text which will enrich the knowledge of patients and physicians alike—one that I will add to my library as a reference source, and one which I will also read through just because it is enjoyable.

Review by J. Brian McCarthy
President and CEO,
Kelly's Roast Beef, Inc.

Any restaurateur who truly loves his profession and his customers as well will find this book fascinating and useful in the day-to-day operations of any restaurant. Serving over 2.3 million meals a year, we view the health and well-being of our customers as more important than ever. Dr. Hannaway's book *On the Nature of Food Allergy* gives us laymen the basic understanding of the science involved in allergies and how it directly affects our industry. This book has opened my eyes to the realization that, as an owner, I should be fully aware of the ingredients of all menu items and strive to become a peanut-free restaurant. This book is a must for any and all restaurant owners and managers who want to be ahead of the curve and take food safety to a different level.

Review by Jean Marcoux, M.D.
Associate Clinical Professor of Pediatrics and Internal Medicine,
University of Texas Health Science Center at Houston

Let me congratulate Dr. Hannaway on the quality of this book. The amount of information is phenomenal. I can't imagine where he found the time to research and process all the information on food allergy and put it on paper. Now I understand why his golf handicap is going up! His style of writing with all the historical facts and anecdotes made the reading so pleasant that I read the whole thing over a weekend.

Review by Gary N. Gross, M.D. Clinical Professor of Medicine, University of Texas Southwestern Medical School

Dr. Hannaway has blended the correct proportions of science, history, story-telling and he sprinkled in a dash of humor to create the perfect recipe for this educational and informational book. This book contains up-to-date science presented in a readable way that will help the reader understand why food allergy exists. The history of foods and drinks provides a new dimension to food allergy literature and the personal anecdotes bring the field of food allergy to life. This is a well-researched and well-written work that should be in every allergist's office. If restaurant owners, managers and chefs read this book, it will save them time and trouble in the future and save lives in their restaurants.

Review by Richard F. Lockey, M.D.
Professor of Medicine, Pediatrics and Public Health,
University of South Florida
Joy McCann Culverhouse Chair of Allergy and Immunology

Precise, concise, to the point and easy reading are words that come to mind when reviewing *On the Nature of Food Allergy*. Dr. Hannaway has summarized the "nuts and bolts" about this subject. The questions that need to be answered about food allergy are immense, however, this book, in a practical way, summarizes the useful and helpful take-away points to treat and prevent food-induced allergic reactions. The book should be easily understood by the more sophisticated lay reader. More importantly, it is an excellent reference and practical discussion of how food allergy should be approached by any physician, even an allergist/immunologist. Congratulations, Dr. Hannaway, job well done.

Review by Ron and Christina Adams
Parents of two food allergic children

On the Nature of Food Allergy is a must read for anyone interested in understanding the current food allergy epidemic and its impact on our daily lives. As Dr. Hannaway states, when his children were young, peanut butter was the sandwich *du jour*. Today many schools are peanut-free zones. In my own family of six, three suffer from food allergies. My son's peanut allergy is very severe and has caused us a lot of anxiety. After reading Dr. Hannaway's book, we feel we can make intelligent decisions and follow a flexible and prudent action plan. All told this book is informative and thorough, provides a clear and concise explanation of a complex and often misunderstood topic. It is a must read for all parents of food allergic children.

Review by Nancy Sander
President, Allergy & Asthma Network-Mothers of Asthmatics

I love this book! It would have been so helpful years ago when I was struggling to feed my food-allergic daughter who also had asthma and eczema. Back then, food allergies were not considered real or possible causes of her symptoms. *On the Nature of Food Allergy* makes tedious information timely and interesting. It's organized for quick reference and for those of us who want to understand the subject from the inside out. Brilliant!

Review by William E. Berger, M.D., M.B.A.
Clinical Professor, Department of Pediatrics,
University of California, Irvine
Author of *Asthma for Dummies*

When I first started practice over 25 years ago, true food allergy patients were rarely encountered, and there was very little information available to practitioners and patients suffering from these conditions. My, have things changed! Now, not a day goes by that I do not see at least one or two patients with severe food allergy or read about new discoveries concerning these disorders in my medical journals. What a perfect time for Dr. Paul Hannaway to write this outstanding and comprehensive handbook for those who suffer from food allergies, and also for those who provide care and service to these patients. This manual is truly a smorgasbord of tasty morsels of information that should be slowly and carefully digested by all those interested in the field of food allergy.

Review by Anne Muñoz-Furlong
Founder and CEO, The Food Allergy & Anaphylaxis Network

Dr. Paul Hannaway has written a book that is chock-full of the latest information about food allergy. This book is rich in background information about foods that is not found in other food allergy books. His extensive research about the processing of foods and the history of some of the ingredients makes this a unique and tremendously interesting book for those with and without food allergies.

Review by Harris A. Steinman, M.D.
Founder and Head of FACTS
Food and Allergy Consulting and Testing Services
Capetown, South Africa

This is a terrific book. It is rare to find a work on allergy so packed full of science yet written in such an engaging and readable style. Although the book is aimed primarily at the layperson, it contains a wealth of information that will be educational for every health professional, even allergists. In fact, there is no other allergy-related book that addresses food allergens in such an encompassing and interesting way. The information is current and very relevant and will assist allergic individuals as well as health practitioners to achieve improved compliance and management of a debilitating disease.

On the
Nature
of Food
Allergy

A Complete Handbook on
Food Allergy for Patients, Parents,
Restaurant Personnel, Child-Care
Providers, Educators, School Nurses,
Dieticians and Health-Care Providers

Paul J. Hannaway, M.D.

Author of the American Medical Writers
Association Book Award Winner,
The Asthma Self-Help Book and
Asthma—An Emerging Epidemic

Foreword by
Albert L. Sheffer, M.D.

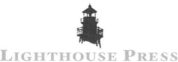

LIGHTHOUSE PRESS
MARBLEHEAD, MASSACHUSETTS

Illustrations by Tim McDonough, McDonough+Company
Edited by Rachel Butler
Cover and book design and production by Arrow Graphics, Inc.
www.arrow1.com • info@arrow1.com
Printed in China
Address all inquiries to:
Lighthouse Press
P.O. Box 602
Marblehead, MA 01945
Phone: 1-800-794-0744 or 978-745-0512
Fax: 978-745-6208 or 781-631-2225
E-mail: Lhtpress@aol.com
Web site: www.onthenatureoffoodallergy.com

Publisher's Cataloging-in-Publication
(Provided by Quality Books, Inc.)

Hannaway, Paul J.
    On the nature of food allergy : a complete handbook
on food allergy for patients, parents, restaurant
personnel, child-care providers, educators, school
nurses and all health-care providers / Paul J. Hannaway;
foreword by Albert L. Sheffer.
    p. cm.
    Includes bibliographical references and index.
    LCCN 2006905340
    ISBN 13: 978-0-9621799-3-8
    ISBN 10: 0-9621799-3-0

    1. Food allergy.   I. Title.

RC596.H36 2007   616.97'5
                           QBI06-600421

*To my patients and families
afflicted with food allergies*

◆

Acknowledgements

I thank the following individuals for their contributions to this manuscript: Ron and Christina Adams; Alvart Badalian; Kate Bandos; William Berger, M.D.; Carlos Camergo, M.D.; Sharon Castlen; Jean Conwell; Anne Muñoz Furlong; Gary N. Gross, M.D.; Holly Hannaway; Phil Korenblatt, M.D.; Phil Lieberman, M.D.; Richard F. Lockey, M.D.; Jean Marcoux, M.D.; Brian McCarthy; Tim McDonough; Michael Mellon, M.D.; Marilyn Nagle; Katie Reilly; Carlene Roundy; Nancy Sander; Al Sheffer, M.D.; Carol Sikora; Harris Steinman, M.D.; Frank Twarog, M.D.; Michael Young, M.D.; and my dear wife Bunny. ●

Contents

Foreword

Albert L. Sheffer, M.D.
Clinical Professor of Medicine
Harvard Medical School

Dr. Paul Hannaway is an astute allergist dedicated to the education of his patients suffering from allergic diseases. An allergy practitioner for nearly 35 years, he has focused his care on the transfer of knowledge regarding the nature and treatment of allergic disorders. The ability to reflect upon the current research observations pertinent to this specialty and integrate such facts into his extensive practice experience requires a unique ability.

This text, his fourth publication, is devoted to the education in regard to food allergy. Dr. Hannaway has a unique capacity to review the causes and treatment of food allergic disorders and clearly explain the most complicated medical situation in simple, understandable vernacular for most allergic sufferers. Food allergic symptoms present with several clinical scenarios, ranging from mild skin rashes to the life-threatening symptoms of deadly anaphylaxis.

Often explosive in onset, anaphylaxis is the most severe manifestation of an allergic disease—the result of an allergen-induced release of potent chemical mediators, such as histamine from previously sensitized bodily cells called mast cells. As explained by Dr. Hannaway, an allergic or IgE antibody, attaches to the mast cell and, upon re-exposure to the sensitizing allergen, the mast cell releases the mediators of the acute allergic reaction. Such substances, such as histamine, trigger the symptoms of an anaphylaxis, such as swelling, hives, vomiting, diarrhea, wheezing or bronchospasm, and cardiovascular collapse or shock.

This text describes the treatment of adverse food reactions, ranging from prevention to the reversal of symptoms of life-threatening anaphylaxis. These writings of Dr. Hannaway are accurate, up-to-date and provocative. For instance, he includes the necessity for affected individuals (and any one affected by food allergy) to always carry and know how to administer auto-injectable epinephrine. The text also describes newer modalities of therapy that may lower the concentration of the patient's allergic antibody and reducing the risk for life-threatening or even minor allergic events. He illustrates such occurrences with instructive case reports and reviews the historical aspects of food allergic disorders in great detail.

Thus, Dr. Hannaway has added to his previously well-received texts on asthma. This lucidly written, comprehensive compendium on food allergy is not only germane to food allergy sufferers and their families, but provides valuable instruction and information for health-care professionals, school nurses and schoolteachers, and food handlers and restaurateurs. With such a valuable educational resource, the allergy professional community is hopeful that food allergies will become more readily recognized, and more promptly and appropriately treated, with fewer life-threatening consequences. ●

"*What is food for some may be fierce poison for others.*"

Titus Lucretius Carus, first century AD
De Rerum Natura
On the Nature of Things

Introduction

In the late 1960s, I elected to specialize in the field of allergy and immunology. This decision was undoubtedly brought about by my encounters with asthma and hay fever, both as a patient and as a parent. While I was serving as a medical officer in the Air Force, my four-year-old son developed difficult-to-control asthma. These personal experiences prompted me to spend two additional years training in this field. When I finally settled into private practice and a part-time teaching position, there were about 1,500 fully trained allergy specialists in the United States. I went to annual meetings of allergy specialists that were attended by only 300 doctors. Thirty years later, more than 5,000 doctors travel the globe to attend these same meetings.

While research in allergy and immunology has lead to tremendous improvements in the understanding and treatment of allergic diseases, something strange has happened. The prevalence of the "Big Four" allergic diseases (asthma, allergic rhinitis or hay fever, eczema or atopic dermatitis, and food allergy) has nearly tripled during the past three decades. In the late 1970s and early 1980s, many medical publications reported a dramatic rise in asthma cases and asthma deaths. The number of people with asthma in the United States increased from 6.7 million in 1980 to an estimated 26 million in 2006.

This asthma epidemic was not confined to the United States—it occurred worldwide. Epidemiologists (experts on health care statistics) call it a pandemic. The most striking rise in asthma was reported in Aus-

tralia, where approximately one in every four children is now diagnosed with asthma. This asthma epidemic has been observed in all levels of society, from affluent white suburbanites to inner-city black Americans and Hispanics. This phenomenon prompted me to write several books on asthma and the asthma epidemic.[1]

The food allergy story is an entirely different one. When I started practice in the 1970s, there was scant interest in food allergy. It was essentially an orphan disease that received little or no attention. Most of the cases of food allergy that I encountered in those days were infants and children with mild reactions to cow's milk or eggs. On rare occasions I would see a child or adult who reacted to peanuts, tree nuts or seafood that qualified as "an interesting or unusual case."

At that time, my family consisted of six young children who attended various schools in Marblehead, Massachusetts, a seacoast town of approximately 20,000 people. Their hungry friends who visited our busy household often feasted on easy-to-prepare peanut or peanut butter snacks. In fact, our first family lobster boat was named, the "Fluffernutter," a famous sandwich combination of peanut butter and

---

[1] *The Asthma Self-Help Book* (*Marblehead, Mass*: Lighthouse Press, 1989.)
The Asthma Self-Help Book—How to Live a Normal Life in Spite of Your Condition (Rocklin, Calif.: Prima Publishers, 1992.)
Asthma—An Emerging Epidemic (*Marblehead, Mass*: Lighthouse Press, 2002.)
What To Do When the Doctor Says Its Asthma (Gloucester, Mass.: Fair Winds Press, 2004.)

Marshmallow Fluff. At that time, I cannot recall any child in Marblehead who had a significant food allergy to peanuts or tree nuts. No parents or schools had to carry or have auto-injectable epinephrine devices on hand or worry about snacks, cookies, Halloween candies or birthday cakes that might contain a hidden food allergen, such as a peanut or tree nut.

How things have changed! I now have seven grandchildren (none with food allergy, thank goodness) living in this same town with the same population. Scores of their friends have food allergies, especially to peanuts and tree nuts. Most town schools and even our public library are now designated as nut-free facilities. In my practice, I often see two new patients a day with a food allergy. I recently conducted a study of the incidence of food allergy in the Marblehead Schools.

Nearly 3 percent of children enrolled in kindergarten through grade five had been prescribed an auto-injector epinephrine device for a peanut or tree nut allergy. Many of these children are prone to a severe allergic reaction or what doctors call anaphylaxis. Thus, great care must be taken when serving foods at home and, more importantly, away from home in schools, summer camps or restaurants. A peanut butter snack is no longer a quick fix for a hungry youngster. This food allergy epidemic has led to a great deal of concern in affected patients, parents, caretakers, and school, camp and restaurant personnel.

■ History of Food Allergy

The term allergy was coined more than 100 years ago by Clemens von Pirquet after he observed that some patients who received a horse-derived antiserum for diseases like diphtheria and tetanus developed fever, skin rashes and joint and lymph gland swelling that he called serum sickness. Von Pirquet realized that the antiserum had produced a changed or altered reactivity for which he proposed the term allergy from *allos* or other and *ergon* or work. He also suggested the word allergen to describe the agent that induced this altered reactivity after one or more exposures. This was the foundation of modern immunology—that a second and subsequent exposure to a foreign substance could sensitize the recipient.

While ancient medical historians lacked a basic understanding of allergic diseases, many described adverse reactions to foods. Hippocrates stated that many were intolerant of milk and cheeses. "Cheese does not harm all men alike, some can eat their full of it, while others come off badly. If cheese were bad for human consumption, it would have hurt all." In the first century the distinguished Latin philosopher Titus Lucretius Carus stated, "What is food for some may be fierce poison for others."

In other words, one man's meat is another man's poison. In 1808, Dr. Robert Willan vividly depicted a tree nut reaction in his patient, Dr. Thomas Winterbottom, who had eaten a small serving of almonds: "Symptoms were soon followed by an edematous swelling of the face, especially of the lips and nose, which were very hot and itchy. There was at the same time an uneasy tickling sensation in the throat … the tongue likewise became enlarged … soon after going to bed an eruption (hives) took place over the whole body of spots nearly as large as a sixpence." In 1906, food allergy research intensified after Alfred Wolff-Eisner's description of severe allergic or anaphylactic reactions. Once the concept of food allergy was accepted, many case reports described allergic reactions to legumes, cow's milk, eggs and nuts.

The Food Allergy Epidemic

The low incidence of food allergy in the 1950s and 1960s is reflected by the fact that the first large series of food allergy cases was not published until 1969. In the late 1980s, additional reports depicted an increase in food allergy in both children and adults. Doctors from The Isle of Wight in England were first to describe a twofold increase in food allergies in the 1990s—especially peanut- and tree nut-allergy. Also in the 1990s, Dr. Hugh Sampson reported that the incidence of peanut- and tree nut-allergy doubled in the United States from 1985 to 1996. Investigators in Montreal, Canada, described similar findings. A study of schoolchildren in Toulouse, France, found that nearly 7 percent had a food allergy. The average age of onset was 3.4 years. The most common allergenic foods were cow's milk, eggs and peanuts, with an upswing in allergies to exotic fruits like kiwi and to shellfish. A Germany survey reported that more than 4 percent of German schoolchildren had a food allergy.

It is now estimated that 11 million Americans have a food allergy. Current statistics suggest that food allergies strike 8 percent of children under age three, 6 percent to 8 percent of school-age children and nearly 4 percent of adults. Food allergies are more common if a child is breast-fed or if their parents have a higher income and educational background. Mothers of food-allergic children are three times more likely to be over age thirty, and their offspring are more likely to have hay fever and eczema. In some studies, premature infants have fewer food allergies than full-term infants, and children delivered by Caesarean section are more prone to food allergy. About 3 million people have a peanut or tree nut allergy. In one adult study of forty-five patients, the average age of onset of a food allergy was thirty-two years, and nearly 90 percent reported they had an allergy to at least three foods. While peanut allergy gets all the press, seafood allergy is actually the most common food allergy as it affects nearly 7 million Americans. Milk, eggs, wheat, fruits, vegetables, and soybean products account for other common food allergies. Food allergy is now the leading cause for emergency room visits for an allergic reaction in the United States, Great Britain, Canada, France and Australia.

Anaphylaxis—The Killer Allergy

Nearly 50 percent of people with food allergy may experience a severe allergic reaction known as anaphylaxis. While there are many medical definitions for anaphylaxis, one of the newest definitions describes it as "a serious allergic reaction that is rapid in onset and may cause death." Anaphylaxis triggers about 1 million emergency room visits in the United States every year. Studies in the United States and the United Kingdom looking at the triggers of allergic reactions that required an emergency room visit found that the leading cause, by far, was a food allergy which accounted for one in every three emergency room visits for allergic reactions.

Food-induced anaphylaxis is believed to trigger 30,000 trips to the emergency room each year in the United States and between 150 and 200 deaths a year. The prevalence of anaphylaxis is probably not as rare as believed. There may be more than 90,000 victims a year who go to a clinic or a doctor's office or simply do nothing and stay at home. Several symptoms, such as itching, hives, flushing, difficulty breathing, vomiting, diarrhea, dizziness, confusion, or shock may occur at the same time. It can happen at home, in restaurants, schools, child-care and sports facilities, summer camps, cars, buses and airplanes.

All first responders to a victim of an acute allergic reaction or anaphylaxis (including the patient) should be thoroughly familiar with the signs and symptoms of anaphylaxis. They should know when and how to administer auto-injectable epinephrine and initiate other life-saving first aid measures. This responsibility applies to everyone, including the patient, family members, and school, restaurant, and camp personnel. As most anaphylactic deaths occur suddenly and unexpectedly outside of the hospital, many lives could be saved by the prompt administration of auto-injectable epinephrine by responsible individuals capable of recognizing the signs and symptoms of anaphylaxis and treating an anaphylactic reaction. Very few, if any, victims of anaphylaxis die once they get to an emergency room. Thus, non-medical personnel—including the patient, family, friends, school, camp and restaurant personnel—have the best chance to save the life of a victim experiencing a life-threatening anaphylactic reaction.

The auto-injectable epinephrine device is a great first aid tool, especially for patients, families, and school and camp personnel involved in remote outdoor activities, such as camping, hiking, boating, and golfing. As will be discussed in the chapter "Risky Restaurants," I feel all food establishments should train their staff how to use these life-saving devices. I wholeheartedly agree with Dr. Estelle Simons, past president of the American Academy of Allergy, Asthma and Immunology, who has stated, "auto-injector epinephrine devices should be readily available anywhere where anaphylaxis is likely to occur."

Economic Impact

If you add up the direct and indirect costs of food allergy and food anaphylaxis, it is a billion dollar disease. Such costs include medications, doctor visits, allergy skin and blood tests, emergency room care, and hospitalizations. Indirect costs generated by patients and families afflicted by food allergy include loss of days at work and implementation of preventive programs in day-care settings, schools, colleges, and summer camps. Enactment of laws at the local, state, and federal levels; stricter labeling requirements, lawsuits and costly educational programs for food service providers and the restaurant industry further add to this economic burden.

Quality of Life

Patients and families with food allergy must enact significant lifestyle changes to prevent potentially life-threatening episodes of anaphylaxis and maintain health and safety. These changes are often a source of tremendous anxiety and stress for patients and their families. In a United Kingdom survey, 20 children with peanut allergy were compared to 20 children with insulin-dependent diabetes. Children with peanut allergy felt more restricted and threatened than the diabetic children. Nearly 50 percent of children and teenagers surveyed at educational conferences on food allergy stated that their peers harassed them, they felt socially isolated, and feared being away from home.

Another study compared patients and their families with a peanut allergy with those who had chronic diseases, such as lupus and rheumatoid arthritis. Peanut-allergic children and their families experienced more stress and impairment in their quality of life and family relations than the victims of lupus and rheumatoid arthritis.

The Allergy Clinic at the University of Maryland Medical Center surveyed the patients and families of 101 children. The study group included patients from diverse racial and socioeconomic backgrounds. One of the most important findings was the negative impact of food allergy on meal preparation activities. Of even greater interest was the finding that nearly 60 percent reported that the family's social activities were significantly altered. Children's activities that were modified or eliminated included participation in sleepovers, camp and birthday parties, sports, and school field trips. Family behaviors that were altered included eating at restaurants and children's participation in play activities at a friend's home. Forty-one percent of the parents felt they were stressed by their child's food allergy. Food allergy had a negative influence on family activities, the child's psychosocial development, and the psychological well-being of the entire family. Education and specialty care seems to be a key factor in reducing such stress.

A survey at Children's Hospital Medical Center in Boston found that most parents of food-allergic children who had attended group support meetings or had seen an allergy specialist did not feel that their children were negatively impacted by food allergy.

A Wake-Up Call

In response to this impressive food allergy epidemic, proactive organizations, such as the Food Allergy and Anaphylaxis Network (FAAN), The Food Allergy Initiative (FAI),[2] and food allergy research programs at the Jaffe Institute in Mount Sinai Hospital in New York City, Duke University, Johns Hopkins University and several European centers have greatly expanded the knowledge and understanding of food allergy over the past decade. In my practice, we now offer a food allergy education program that includes videotapes, hands-on-teaching and handouts for food allergy sufferers and their families. With the exception of publications by FAAN and several books reviewed in the appendix, there are few comprehensive manuals for patients, parents and laypersons interested in learning more about food allergy. Many publications on bookstore shelves or listed on the Internet focus on controversial or unproven theories that would have you believe that food allergies trigger all sorts of conditions, such as arthritis, migraine headaches, chronic fatigue, gastrointestinal problems, hyperactivity disorders, and psychological disturbances. Many of these publications are simply fronts for authors or organizations that promote self-serving junk science based on unproven homeopathic remedies. Such publications also

---

[2] The Food Allergy and Anaphylaxis Network will be referred to as FAAN and the Food Allergy Initiative as FAI throughout the book.

blur the lines between serious and some-times life-threatening food allergies and food intolerances. This is a great disservice to all those affected by food allergies, as it causes confusion and misunderstanding in the general public.

In an effort to improve upon my personal efforts in food allergy education, I started to write a brief handout (or a *Reader's Digest* version) for my patients and families impacted by food allergies. The purpose of such a handbook was to try to condense all the educational points of food allergy into one manual. The worldwide explosion in food allergy research and educational programs made this an impossible project.

Unlike many well-written books that focus on peanut or tree nut allergy, the goal of *On the Nature of Food Allergy* is to provide patients, parents, health-care professionals, dieticians, school and camp personnel, and food service providers with a comprehensive guide to all forms of food allergy. In the early chapters, I explain the impact of the ongoing allergy epidemic, especially as it relates to food allergy. You will learn why exposures (or non-exposures) to allergens during pregnancy, while breast-feeding or in early infancy or childhood may program your immune system to trigger allergic problems for a lifetime. I will discuss the important role of our largest organ the gastrointestinal tract.

What has caused the allergy epidemic? I will explore in detail proposed theories and hypotheses that attempt to solve this mystery. Readers will learn how patients; parents; and school, camp, and restaurant personnel, who are often the first responders to a severe allergic reaction, can recognize and actually treat a severe allergic or anaphylactic reaction. Those involved in the food service industry, restaurants, schools, camps, and colleges can reduce the risks of devastating food reactions. In the middle section of the book, I will review both common and uncommon food allergies focusing on the "Big Eight" foods, which account for 90 percent of all food allergy reactions. I will also present what I have found to be interesting historical and nutritional facts on various foods and beverages. The dangers posed by peanut, tree nut, fruit, vegetable, and seafood allergy will be detailed in separate chapters. I will present cases of near-fatal and fatal food allergy reactions reported from around the world in both the lay press and medical literature. Many of these preventable deaths have occurred in children and young adults outside the hospital in schools, school buses, camps, restaurants, shopping malls, and home. Lessons learned from these tragic cases could undoubtedly save many lives down the road.

I will also review the pros and cons of total peanut and tree nut bans in schools and public places. In later chapters, I will concentrate on crossover reactions with various foods and how to travel safely and

> *Unlike many well-written books that focus on peanut or tree nut allergy, the goal of On the Nature of Food Allergy is to provide patients, parents, health-care professionals, dieticians, school and camp personnel and food service providers with a comprehensive guide to all forms of food allergy.*

avoid hidden allergens on a day-to-day basis. You will learn why a westernized diet and breast-feeding may be triggering this food allergy epidemic and why today's approach to delaying feeding solid foods in infancy may be totally wrong. I will review the findings of cutting-edge food allergy research and discuss potential preventive treatments and cures that may be forthcoming for food allergy. Lastly, it is my hope that *On the Nature of Food Allergy* will be a comprehensive resource for all who must cope with this extraordinary food allergy epidemic.[3] ⬤

---

[3] As this book is not intended to be a medical text, scientific articles published in the medical literature are usually not referenced. Most cited manuscripts can be found from Internet searches of authors and subjects. The appendix contains references of what I consider to be the more important scientific papers on food allergy published in the past two decades.

Chapter 1

Why Food Allergy?

Before discussing the nuts and bolts of food allergy, I will review why some individuals acquire an allergic disease like a food allergy and some do not.[1] Take pity on the unfortunate newborn who starts out in life by developing an itchy skin condition called eczema, or atopic dermatitis. Next, this infant experiences red skin welts, or hives after ingesting hen's eggs or cow's milk. A few months later, the child begins to wheeze with respiratory infections or allergen exposure, and, in later childhood, starts to sneeze in the early spring or summer. This poor child has now "hit for the cycle"[2] and has developed all the Big Four allergic diseases, which are eczema, food allergy, asthma, and allergic rhinitis, also known as "hay fever." Allergy specialists like to refer to this scenario as the "atopic march." What has propelled this child down this allergic or atopic[3] highway? Medical detectives, also called epidemiologists, have proposed many intriguing answers to this complex question.

The Elusive Allergy Genes

Every living organism, including all plant and animal life, contains a substance called deoxyribonucleic acid, commonly known as DNA. Human DNA is composed of approximately 30,000 genes that act like computer chips that program your body to develop individual characteristics, such as baldness, brown hair, or blue eyes. DNA, passed down from one generation to the next, determines what ailments you may or may not develop during your life-

time. Most genetic studies in the field of allergy have focused on asthma, and several asthma genes have been identified. When one parent has an allergy, the risk of allergy in his or her offspring doubles. If both parents are allergic, the risk increases four- to six-fold. While there is no doubt that most allergic diseases are inherited, to date no specific gene or genes have been linked to food allergy.

The Immune System

Human beings are equipped with a powerful biological defense network called the immune system that is composed of organs, cells, and glands that protect us against, or make us immune, to all types of foreign invaders. The four major organs of the immune system are the thymus gland, lymph nodes or glands, spleen, and bone marrow.

These organs produce a vast array of cells, chemicals, and protective proteins, or, antibodies, that ward off outside invaders. Such invaders include viruses, bacteria, parasites, allergens, and a host of other stimuli, including cancer-inducing substances. When the immune system fails to work properly, we can get very sick. Failure of our immune system to protect us from outside invaders ranges from a virus

---

[1] The next two chapters discuss the basic science and immunology of allergy and possible reasons for the allergy epidemic. Readers who are not interested in such science may want to skip to chapter 3.

[2] A baseball expression where a batter has four hits in one game—a single, double, triple, and a home run.

[3] Atopy from the Greek *atopos*, meaning out of place, is the medical term for allergy.

that triggers a common cold to the Acquired Immune Deficiency Syndrome or AIDS. To fully understand how our immune system works, we must review the two basic components of the immune system—the humoral system and the cell-mediated immune system.

■ The Humoral Immune System —Antigens and Antibodies

Any foreign substance, such as a virus, bacteria, or allergen, that enters the body is called an antigen. When the body's immune system encounters an antigen, certain white blood cells called B-cells make a protective protein, or antibody, against the antigen. The next time the body encounters this antigen, the antibody neutralizes it. When the immune system functions normally, we develop resistance, or immunity, to invading antigens that may last for years or even a lifetime. This is the basis of all vaccinations or immunizations. During our lifetime, the immune system produces tens of thousands of antibodies that protect us from all types of viral and bacterial infections, parasites, and other diseases, thereby allowing us to lead a healthy life. However, sometimes our immune system overreacts to antigens, and we may develop an autoimmune disease, such as

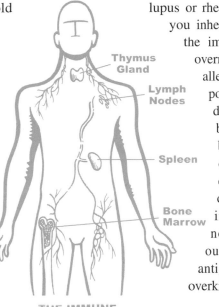

THE IMMUNE SYSTEM

Thymus Gland

Lymph Nodes

Spleen

Bone Marrow

lupus or rheumatoid arthritis. If you inherit an allergy gene, the immune system may overreact to a harmless allergen like a food or pollen grain and produce an allergic antibody called IgE antibody. All allergic diseases are the direct result of an overreaction of our immune system to normally harmless outside invaders, or antigens. Picture it as overkill by friendly fire.

■ Cell-Mediated Immunity

The second component of our immune response is called cell-mediated immunity, where antigens are processed by a series of cells called T-cells. They are called T-cells because they are derived from the thymus gland. These T-cells are present in our bone marrow and lymph nodes, or glands. Once an antigen reaches a lymph gland, several types of T-cells come into play. Some T-cells kill the antigen (killer T-cells), some suppress the antigen (suppressor T-cells), and some actually help the antigen (helper T-cells). The T-cells are more important than the antibody-producing cells as they determine whether or not you will develop any of the Big Four allergic diseases. A new type of T-cell, called the regulatory, or T-reg, cell has recently been discovered. As we shall see, this T-cell may

All allergic diseases are the direct result of an overreaction of our immune system to normally harmless outside invaders, or antigens. Picture it as overkill by friendly fire.

be the big-boss T-cell that tells all the other T-cells how to behave.

■ The Allergic or IgE Antibody

As we discussed, our immune system produces many thousands of antibodies to viruses, bacteria, parasites, or allergens over the course of our lifetime. The antibody that plays the major role in allergic diseases is called immunoglobulin E, or IgE antibody for short. The concept that man had a certain protein in his body that could trigger an allergic reaction was advanced by an astute observation in 1919 by Dr. M.A. Ramirez, who was treating a patient for aplastic anemia, a rare blood disease that required frequent blood transfusions. Several days after a transfusion, while riding in a horse-drawn carriage through New York's Central Park, Ramirez's patient experienced an attack of asthma for the first time in his life. Ramirez traced the recent blood transfusion to a horse-allergic donor who had asthma. Ramirez concluded that something in the donor's blood was transferred to his patient that made him allergic to horses.

The 40 million Americans who inherit the tendency to make IgE antibodies have a higher risk of developing an allergic disease.

Nearly forty years later, the search for this elusive protein led to the discovery of the allergic antibody by two groups working independently of one another. Doctors Teruko and Kimishige Ishzaka identified IgE antibody in their laboratory in Denver, Colorado. Concurrently, a Swedish group led by Doctors Hans Bennich and S.G.O. Johansson isolated a strange protein from a multiple myeloma patient. In 1968, the World Health Organization decided that the two new proteins were indeed the same allergic or IgE antibody.

Approximately one in every five individuals inherits a gene (or genes) that primes the immune system to overproduce this IgE antibody. The fascinating aspect of IgE antibody is that it once protected man against common tropical and parasitic diseases. Through the process of evolution and diminished exposure to such diseases, this once-friendly antibody has turned on mankind. It is now a "bad antibody" that overreacts to common environmental allergens like dust mites, molds, animal parts, drugs, latex, insect stings, pollen grains, and foods. The 40 million Americans who inherit the tendency to make IgE antibodies have a higher risk of developing an allergic disease.

■ The Mast Cell and IgE Antibody

What makes IgE antibody so influential in food allergy and other allergic diseases? This antibody has a special affinity for one of the more powerful cells in the human body—the mast cell. Millions of mast cells line our skin, nose, intestines and bronchial tubes. Each mast cell contains more than a thousand tiny granules that are loaded with dozens of potent chemicals, or mediators, including histamine. In essence, when the IgE antibody attaches itself to the mast cell, the mast cell becomes a chemically laden bomb just waiting to explode.

When you inherit the capacity to become allergic and make IgE antibodies, the first time you are exposed to a potential food allergen such as a peanut, you do not react to it. However, once your body starts to produce IgE antibody to the peanut, the antibody attaches itself to the surface of the mast cell. The next time you eat a peanut, the peanut protein (the antigen) binds to the IgE (the antibody) on the

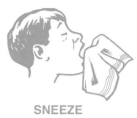

SNEEZE

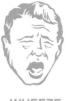

WHEEZE

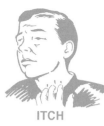

ITCH

surface of the mast cell. The mast cell then erupts and releases powerful chemicals, like histamine, into the surrounding tissues. The surrounding tissues then become inflamed and swollen. When the mast cell erupts in your nose, you sneeze; when the lungs are targeted, you wheeze. If the skin is the site of the reaction, you itch, swell, or get hives. If the intestinal tract is attacked, you develop cramps, nausea, vomiting, or diarrhea. The end result of this mast cell eruption is the classical SWI, or "sneeze, wheeze and itch" reaction. As a former baseball-softball player, I sponsor a town softball team called the SWISOX. Unlike my beloved Boston Red Sox, they have yet to win it all.

Common allergens that trigger allergic reactions are dust mites, molds, animal dander, pollens, stinging insects, drugs, latex and foods. When doctors first discovered that allergens could induce attacks of hay fever, asthma, or hives, they set out to develop ways to determine if a person was allergic, or sensitive, to these substances. Thus, the medical specialty of allergy was born. The allergist became the doctor who could identify allergens that caused people to sneeze, wheeze, or itch. Over the past three decades, advances in immunology have produced a greater understanding of our immune system.

As a former baseball-softball player, I sponsor a town softball team called the SWISOX. Unlike my beloved Boston Red Sox, they have yet to win it all.

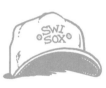

Such discoveries are beginning to explain some of the potential reasons for the allergy epidemic and define why allergen exposures (or non-exposures) during pregnancy, while breast-feeding, or in infancy or childhood may alter the way our immune system handles allergens for the rest of our lives.

■ Anatomy 101— The Digestive Tract

The human body is equipped with an incredible array of organs. The healthy heart that beats 72 times a minute pumps over 14,000 quarts of blood a day. That equates to 5 million quarts a year. Our lungs inhale and exhale about one-half quart of air 20 times a minute and move about 600 quarts of air every hour. Despite these impressive numbers, the largest and the most underrated organ in our body is our gastrointestinal, or GI tract.

In order to understand food allergy, we must review how the intestinal tract functions. In our lifetime, the average human consumes between 700 to 1,000 tons of food—that averages out to 550 chickens, thirty-six pigs, thirty sheep, eight cows, 10,000 eggs, and eighteen tons of milk! No wonder obesity is a big problem. Most of the time, nutrients from these foods are absorbed and waste products are eliminated in an efficient manner. Our intestinal tract is essentially a conduit that begins at the mouth and ends at the anus. Its sole purpose is to transport and digest food. Along the way, the conduit changes character, as different functions are required at different points. Food is broken apart in the mouth and stomach, nutrients are then absorbed by the small intestine, and waste products are transported to the large intestine and rectum for removal.

The three essential foods for the human body are carbohydrates, fats and proteins. There are two types of carbohydrates, simple and complex. Simple carbohydrates are sugars, such as table sugar, molasses, honey, lactose (in milk) and fructose (in fruits). These sugars break down quickly during digestion and provide an immediate source of energy. Complex carbohydrates are starches that are found in grain products and some vegetables, such as potatoes and corn.

> *Complex carbohydrates break down slowly during digestion, giving the body a time-release source of energy.*

Complex carbohydrates break down slowly during digestion, giving the body a time-release source of energy. Proteins consist of amino acids that are essential for tissue maintenance and growth. Some essential amino acids must be obtained from foods because the body cannot make them or convert them from nutrients. Fat is the third essential food nutrient that provides calories and helps to absorb vitamins.

■ Take Me Out to the Ball Game!

What happens when you eat a bag of peanuts at "The Old Ball Game?" Peanuts are placed in the mouth where they are ground up by the teeth and moistened by saliva from your salivary glands that lubricates and binds food, enabling easy transport to the stomach. Peanut proteins can be rapidly absorbed from the mouth, which is often the first source of allergen uptake. Peanut particles then enter the esophagus and are propelled to the stomach. A sphincter, or muscle, at the end of the esophagus works like the drawstring of a purse, relaxes and allows the peanuts to enter the stomach and then tightens up to keep them from going back up the esophagus. When this sphincter does not close properly, acidic stomach contents repeatedly reflux back up into the esophagus, giving you heartburn, what is called gastroesophageal reflux disease (GERD).

■ The Stomach

The stomach is a muscular organ that further breaks down the peanuts. The wall of the stomach is lined by millions of gastric glands that secrete one to two pints of gastric juice at each meal. Gastric juice is a mixture of mucous, hydrochloric acid, pepsin, and bicarbonate. Gastric juices are a barrier to ingested bacteria. The stomach is essentially a reservoir where very little food absorption takes place. However, water, aspirin, and alcohol are rapidly absorbed from the stomach, accounting for the quick relief of thirst and headaches and the rapid appearance of ethanol in the bloodstream after imbibing alcohol. After the stomach breaks down and liquefies the peanuts, they enter the duodenum, the first part of the small intestine.

■ The Small Intestine

The small intestine is so named due to its small (about one inch) diameter. The term small is misleading, as it is not small at all—when stretched out it is about twenty feet long. The small intestine's job is to digest carbohydrates, proteins, and fats in the peanuts and allow passage of essential vitamins and nutrients into the blood stream for distribution to the rest of the body. Two important digestive organs, the liver and the pancreas, secrete their products into the duodenum, or upper end of the small intestine. The liver makes bile that helps to digest fats. Bile is then stored in the gall bladder before it flows down the bile duct and enters the duodenum.

The secretions from the pancreas include sodium bicarbonate and several powerful enzymes that neutralize stomach acids and break down the carbohydrates and proteins in the peanuts. Partially digested peanut particles arc thcn transported to the second part of the small intestine, the jejunum. Here peanut particles are broken down even further and absorbed through the villi that line the wall or mucosa of the small intestine.

Under the microscope, these villi look like steep mountain ranges that greatly increase the surface area of the wall of the small intestine. If you lay these villi end-to-end, the total surface area of the entire intestinal tract is about the size of a tennis court that is 200 times larger than the surface of our skin.

Just below the surface of these villi is the largest collection of lymphoid tissue in the body. As we shall see in the next chapter, this area of lymphoid tissue is where all the action takes place as these lymphoid tissues determine whether or not the peanuts you have just eaten will or will not trigger an allergic reaction. The third section of the small intestine, the ileum, has a thinner wall with shorter villi and ends with another valve or sphincter that separates the small intestine from the large intestine or colon. This valve regulates the movement of fluids from the small intestine into the colon or large intestine.

■ The Large Intestine

The large intestine, or colon, is so named because it is wider than the small intestine, not because it is larger. It is much shorter than the small intestine, measuring about five feet in length. It begins in the lower right side of the abdomen and travels up and across the midline and back down the left side, much like a square picture frame. These three segments are called the ascending, transverse and descending colon. The last parts of the large intestine are the sigmoid colon (so named because it is shaped like an "S"), the rectum, and the anus. Stool is stored in the rectum before being excreted through the anus, which has two muscular sphincters that are crucial in keeping the stool in your rectum. Expulsion of the waste fecal material is usually under voluntary control and is undertaken when socially convenient.

By the time the peanuts reach the large intestine, most of their nutritional value has been extracted, leaving behind a watery waste product. The main function of the

Esophogus

Liver

Gall Bladder

Small Intestine

Stomach

Pancreas

Large Intestine

GI Tract

large intestine is to prevent dehydration by reabsorbing water and to deliver food waste, or residue, to the rectum for removal, or defecation. Excess water promotes diarrhea. Too little water causes constipation. The large intestine also makes mucous to help the stool slide through the colon. The stool that slowly forms as it goes through the colon starts out as a runny mixture and ends up as soft well-formed stool in the rectum. Ingested peanuts may take up to forty-eight hours to complete their journey through the intestinal tract. Most of that time is spent in the colon. At this point, what's left in the colon? Most of the essential nutrients, carbohydrates, fats, and protein from the peanuts have been digested and absorbed in the small intestine. What remains in the colon are undigested peanut particles, fiber, bile, mucus, and an incredible amount of bacteria.

Half of the average bowel movement of 100 grams (a quarter-pounder) is composed of bacteria.

■ The Critical Role of Bacteria

"Beans, beans the musical fruit, the more you eat, the more you toot." While we all learned this rhyme in childhood, I always wondered what makes man (and my dog) toot? The answer is bacteria. A healthy large intestine nourishes an enormous population of bacteria that accounts for the foul odor of flatulence and feces. Where do these bacteria come from? The unborn fetus has a sterile intestinal tract. Bacteria from the mother's birth canal colonize the infant's intestinal tract during delivery. It starts with less friendly bacteria such as E. coli, streptococcal and staphylococcal bacteria, and later colonizes with more friendly bacteria, like the lactobacillus group present in foods like breast milk. By adulthood, the number of bacteria in the large intestine is astounding—about three and one-half pounds or several billion bacteria from 400 different species. There are ten times as many bacteria in the intestinal tract as there are cells in the rest of the entire body! Half of the average bowel movement of 100 grams (a quarter-pounder) is composed of bacteria.

When undigested food makes its way into the large intestine, hungry bacteria digest these foods and produce a variety of intestinal gases, such as nitrogen, carbon dioxide, oxygen and the smelly hydrogen sulfide, which is the main source of the foul odor of flatulence—the exhaust fume of digestion. The large volume of gas produced by bacteria in one's large intestine results in an average of fifteen emissions a day. Certain foods, like beans, produce more flatulence than others because they contain more indigestible carbohydrates.

A proper balance of diet and intestinal bacteria protects us from excess intestinal gas or flatulence, as well as many gastrointestinal diseases. Recent and exciting research studies suggest that an imbalance of friendly and unfriendly intestinal bacteria in infancy and early childhood may play a major role in the allergy epidemic. This has led to the concept that one might prevent the development of allergic disease by administering live, friendly bacteria called probiotics in pregnancy, while breast-feeding or in early infancy. The pros and cons of preventive probiotic therapy will be fully discussed in chapter 16.

■ The Intestinal Immune System

The small intestine is critical for the proper digestion of carbohydrates and proteins and fats and absorption of essential minerals and vitamins. Once a food or beverage enters the small intestine, fats are converted to lipids and fatty acids by secretions from the bile duct. Carbohydrates are reduced to smaller sugars, and food proteins are broken down into peptides and amino acids by enzymes secreted from the pancreas. An elaborate defense system prevents undesirable bacteria and toxins from reaching the systemic circulation. This intestinal defense system produces mucous and antibodies that culls out safe and unsafe proteins, toxins and bacteria.

Basically, there are three responses to ingested peanuts once they reach the small intestine. Some are coated by mucous and transported to the large intestine. This is why you often see undigested peanuts in your stool. Secondly, nutrients from peanuts are absorbed without any difficulty, indicating that the host has a tolerance of the peanut proteins. Lastly, if the body has previously made an IgE antibody to a peanut protein, an allergic reaction may occur. Once a peanut protein passes through the mucosal trap, it is broken down into smaller particles called peptides.

> *This intestinal defense system produces mucous and antibodies that culls out safe and unsafe proteins, toxins and bacteria.*

After these peptides cross through the intestinal wall, they encounter special cells called the DC, or dendritic cells, which are white blood cells with fine branches called dendrites. Former biology students will remember them as the macrophages that are stationed at parts of the body most likely to come into contact with foreign proteins, particularly the skin and mucous membranes. These DC cells capture foreign proteins and act like a taxicab that transports them to nearby lymph nodes or glands where the critical phase of the immune response occurs.

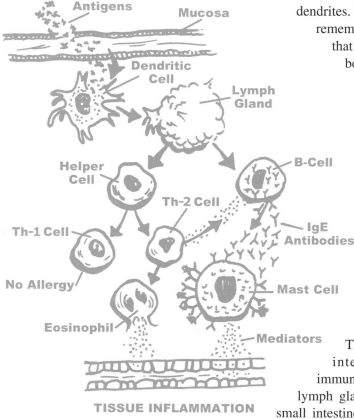

TISSUE INFLAMMATION

■ The Lymph Gland Reaction

The major component of the intestinal tract's defensive immune system is a network of lymph glands located throughout the small intestine. The typical lymph gland has a center composed of B-cell lymphocytes surrounded by T-cell lymphocytes. These glands act as filters against invading agents. They mount an immune response to neutralize invading antigens while, at the same time, avoiding local tissue injury. These lymph tissues determine how a food protein is processed before it reaches the systemic circulation and why we usually tolerate the vast array of foods and beverages we ingest throughout our lifetime.

The lymph glands lining the intestinal tract are the same type of tissue as the tonsil and adenoid tissues in your throat. However, there is one major difference. The lymphoid tissue in the intestinal tract is the largest lymphoid tissue in the body. There are 10 trillion lymphoid cells for every foot of small intestine! Think of it as having your entire small intestine lined by tonsil-like lymphoid tissue.

All unborn babies are a mass of foreign protein living in their mother's womb.

Before continuing on, we must again review the role of the B-cells and T-cells. The B-cells make antibodies, such as IgE antibody and gammaglobulin, or IgG antibody. The T-cells are more complicated and more important in allergic diseases. T-cells that kill the invader are called killer T-cells. T-cells that suppress invaders are labeled suppressor T-cells. Lastly, helper T-cells program various pathways in the immune system. Helper T-cells send out signals that bring other cells into the area to combat the invader. These helper T-cells labeled Th (h is for helper) are very influential T-cells that determine the path the immune system follows after being exposed to an outside invader, like a food antigen. Immunology research has found that helper or Th cells can be divided into two major cell types labeled Th-1 and Th-2 cells. These critical cells determine if you will develop a food allergy, eczema, asthma, hay fever, or other allergic diseases. Lastly, a newly discovered T-cell, may regulate or control these Th-1 and Th-2 cells, hence this cell is called the regularity or T-reg cell for short.

When the Th-1 cells are activated, they release chemicals that drive the immune system away from an allergic response to an invading allergen. Too much Th-1 cell activity may lead to an autoimmune disease. On the other hand, the Th-2 cells are pro-allergic cells. They produce chemicals that signal the B-cells to manufacture IgE antibody. The Th-2 cells also send out signals to attract allergy blood cells, like eosinophils and mast cells from other parts of the body. These potent cells heed the call of the Th-2 cells and migrate into the local area of antigen invasion and secrete mediators like histamine into the surrounding tissues. Once these chemicals reach the local tissues, they cause swelling and inflammation, or the sneeze-wheeze-itch response. Thus, an allergic disease is the end result of the all-important Th-2 cells driving the immune response in the direction of an inflammatory, or pro-allergic response.

■ Th-1 Versus Th-2 Cells

What makes our immune system go in either of these two directions? Allergy genes may send the immune system down the Th-2 allergy highway. People who do not carry an allergy gene are more likely to mount a Th-1, or non-allergic response, to an invading allergen. The second factor that determines what road your immune system follows is environmental exposure. The reason some individuals who inherit allergy genes never develop allergic diseases is because they had little or no exposure to allergy-triggering antigens, such as foods, animal allergens, dust mites, molds, and pollens, at key periods of their lives. On the other hand, those who have inherited the allergy gene may have no chance if they are exposed to an offending allergen at the crucial time of their life.

What is the crucial time? Immunologists now believe that allergen exposures during pregnancy, infancy, and early childhood are the key factors in the development of allergic diseases, such as eczema, asthma, hay fever, and food allergy. The most fascinating aspect of this immune scenario is that a pro-allergy, or Th-2 response, may be determined by what your mother eats during pregnancy or while breast-feeding, or by what you are exposed to or injected with in infancy or early childhood. As we shall see, whether or not your immune system travels down the Th-2 allergy highway may be determined by your family size, month of birth, attending a day-care center, being raised on a farm or keeping (or not keeping) pets in your home at an early age.

The developing fetus has markedly different blood and tissue types from the mother. All unborn babies are a mass of foreign protein living in their mother's womb. Transplant immunology has taught us that when you try to graft or unite different types of organs or blood types, the host, or recipient, promptly rejects the graft, or organ transplant. This is called the graft-versus-host reaction. One of the greatest miracles of the animal kingdom is that unborn mammals are rarely rejected by the mother's immune system. The reason for the mother's acceptance of this foreign fetus organism is that the unborn baby mounts a strong Th-2 immune response that prevents rejection by the host mother. Thus, all healthy infants are born with the pro-allergic Th-2 immune system in con-

trol. Why don't all newborns then follow the Th-2 allergy highway? Here's where Mother Nature (or our genes) takes over. In newborns destined to be non-allergic, the immune system shifts over to the non-allergic Th-1 pathway shortly after birth. Just the opposite occurs in infants born with an allergy-prone genetic makeup. When the fetus or newborn carrying the allergy genes is exposed to a variety of antigens or allergens in pregnancy or early in life, the end result is that the pro-allergic, or Th-2, system remains in control.

■ A New Boss on the Block?

For every complicated question, there is often a simple answer that is usually wrong! Just when immunologists thought they had it all figured out, it appears the Th-1–Th-2 concept may be an over simplification. If you accept the Th-1–Th-2 theory, the incidence of Th-1-driven diseases, like diabetes and rheumatoid arthritis, should have decreased with an increase of allergic Th-2 driven diseases. This is not the case. Over the past twenty years, the incidence of diabetes and rheumatoid arthritis has followed the same path as allergic diseases.

For every complicated question, there is often a simple answer that is usually wrong!

Such observations prompted scientists to look for cells that might suppress or regulate inflammation and promote tolerance to allergens. A new line of T-cells, called the regulatory T-cells, or T-reg cells, has been discovered. These T-reg cells appear to be capable of turning off both the Th-1 and the Th-2 inflammation response. It appears these cells are critical for a healthy immune response to allergens and play a

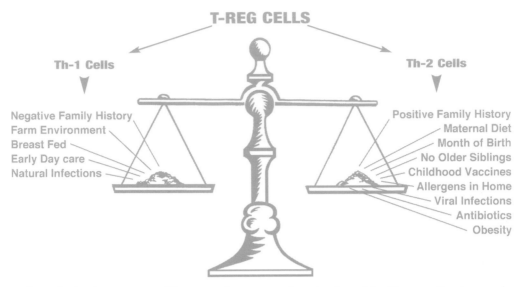

T-REG CELLS

Th-1 Cells

Th-2 Cells

Negative Family History
Farm Environment
Breast Fed
Early Day care
Natural Infections

Positive Family History
Maternal Diet
Month of Birth
No Older Siblings
Childhood Vaccines
Allergens in Home
Viral Infections
Antibiotics
Obesity

major role in the success of immunotherapy or allergy injections. T-reg cells apparently talk to the B-cells and shut down the production of IgE antibody and the triggering cells of inflammation, like mast cells and eosinophils. Simply stated, T-reg cell dysfunction may lead to unchecked Th-1 and Th-2 cell activation.

Nature has provided a fascinating model for studying T-reg cell deficiency. There is an inherited disease called the IPEX-XLAAD syndrome (you don't want to know what that stands for) that only strikes infant males. Victims of this rare disease develop neonatal diabetes; multiple blood, intestinal and endocrine diseases; severe allergic inflammation; eczema; food allergies; and very high IgE levels. Despite aggressive immunosuppressive therapy, most victims die in early childhood. These unfortunate children have poorly functioning T-reg cells. T-reg cell dysfunction has been found in other diseases, such as multiple

If a way is found to manipulate these T-reg cells, a potential cure for many autoimmune and allergic diseases may not be all that far away.

sclerosis, hepatitis C, myasthenia gravis, and rheumatoid arthritis.

Preliminary studies have found that children who outgrow cow's milk allergy have more T-reg cell activity, suggesting that these cells induce a tolerance to cow's milk. Cortisone drugs may up-regulate T-reg cell activity, explaining why these drugs are so effective in treating allergic diseases. T-reg cells may prevent excess activation of the immune system by intestinal bacteria. Injected and oral immunotherapy (ingestion or injection of small amounts of an antigen) may also modify the T-reg cell response. If I were a young researcher dreaming of winning a Nobel prize, I would intensively study these T-reg cells that may be capable of inducing the all-important state of immune tolerance.

If a way is found to manipulate these T-reg cells, a potential cure for many autoimmune and allergic diseases may not be all that far away. ●

Chapter

2

Eat a Pound of Dirt Before You Die

What has triggered man's immune system over the last 20 years to promote the allergic Th-2 pathway and the allergy epidemic? The allergy epidemic has taken place in less than a generation—too short a time to be blamed on genetic or evolutionary factors. The answer may lie in changes in the environment and lifestyle in developed countries. Alterations in maternal and infant eating habits, environmental exposures (or lack thereof), and the expanded use of childhood vaccines, antibiotics, and other drugs may be propelling the immune system down this allergic highway.

During my childhood, when I came home in a dirty and disheveled state, my mother was fond of quoting the old Irish proverb, "If you want to live a long and healthy life, you should eat a pound of dirt before you die." Mother may have been right on the money. There is mounting evidence that a lower incidence of bacterial infections, combined with the increased use of drugs, antibiotics, and vaccines in infancy and early childhood, being disconnected from the soil and reared in too clean an environment may all favor the pro-allergic pathway. Many theories have been proposed to explain the allergy epidemic. The most widely popularized theory is called the "hygiene hypothesis."

■ The Hygiene Hypothesis

The hygiene hypothesis was first proposed by Dr. D.P. Strachan in 1989, when he reported that younger siblings in large families had fewer allergy problems than the older siblings in the same family. Strachan theorized that younger children who experienced more infections that were brought home by older siblings were protected against allergic diseases later on in childhood. We can thank the fall of the Berlin Wall for yielding more clues that a hygienic or an overly clean environment may be one reason for the allergy epidemic. Investigators looked at the incidence of allergy and asthma in East German and West German citizens—two ethnic populations with similar genetic backgrounds who lived under totally different conditions after World War II.

At the outset of the study, investigators proposed that the residents of the less hygienic, more industrialized, and heavily polluted East Germany would have more allergy and asthma than the citizens of the more hygienic West Germany. Much to their surprise, they found just the opposite.

West Germans had three times more asthma and other allergic disorders than the East Germans. This study suggested that infants and young children reared in the more hygienic environment of West Germany with clean air, sophisticated childhood immunization programs, and easier access to antibiotics experienced fewer

> *The allergy epidemic has taken place in less than a generation—too short a time to be blamed on genetic or evolutionary factors.*

respiratory infections in early life. A follow-up study by Dr. Erika von Mutius found that the incidence of hay fever rose in East Germany after the unification, suggesting that East Germans were more likely to develop allergic diseases once they became westernized. Proponents of the hygiene hypothesis believe that a lack of exposure to naturally acquired infections and soil or air pollutants produce a lazy or lightly challenged immune system that is more likely to follow a pro-allergic pathway.

■ Down on the Farm

Additional support for the hygiene hypothesis came from an unlikely source—the farm. Studies in Austria, Canada, Germany, and Finland found that farm-reared children had less asthma and allergic diseases. The Austrian study arose out of a local doctor's observation that children in his practice who lived on farms had less asthma and allergy than children brought up in the local villages. Indeed, when epidemiologists investigated his shrewd observation, they found that children reared on farms did have fewer allergy-asthma problems than their classmates who lived in local villages. As neither group was exposed to outdoor air pollutants, the thought was that exposure to soil organisms and farm animals somehow protected farm-reared children from developing allergic disorders and asthma.

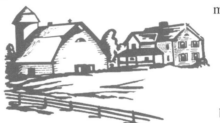

Additional studies in Canada and elsewhere confirmed these findings. Canadian investigators studied 1,199 children in fourteen elementary schools in rural Quebec. They divided the children and their families into two groups—subjects reared on farms and those who lived in local towns with no farm exposure. The children in both groups underwent allergy skin tests, breathing tests, and inhalation challenges. They found less asthma and allergy in the children who lived on farms. Children reared on dairy farms in eastern Finland had less asthma and allergy, especially if they housed dogs or cats. Farm-reared children may also eat differently than children reared in towns and villages. They are more likely to drink non-pasteurized milk and cream and eat more butter and fresh vegetables grown in bacteria-laden farmland.

Children reared on farms are exposed to a vast array of potential toxins and allergens, including dairy barns, pigsties, and chickens that provide a constant source of airborne bacteria, molds, animal dander, and irritant chemicals. One farm exposure that may be protective is contact with animal dung that harbors a form of bacteria called gram-negative bacteria. The cell walls of these bacteria produce endotoxin, a potentially toxic compound found in the cell wall of certain bacteria that may drive the immune system down the non-allergic Th-1 pathway.

Day-care settings may also be protective. American and German children enrolled in day-care centers at an early age have less asthma and wheezing than children kept at home. Working mothers take notice. These findings should relieve some of your guilt when you drop your child at a day-care center infested with all sorts of respiratory infections. You may prevent your child from developing asthma, hay fever, or a food allergy later on in life. Less-than-ideal housekeeping may also prevent asthma and allergy.

Excess dust or dirt in the home may produce more endotoxin. Most homes contain small amounts of endotoxin. When researchers looked at the homes of a group of wheezy-allergic infants, they found their homes had less endotoxin than the homes of a control group who did not have any allergies or asthma.

Additional observations lent credence to the hygiene hypothesis. Second and subsequent children have a lower incidence of asthma than firstborn children (Both my son and I are firstborns.) The reasoning is that younger siblings experience more respiratory infections at an early age than older siblings, as viral infections are brought home by older siblings attending germ-infested day-care centers or schools.

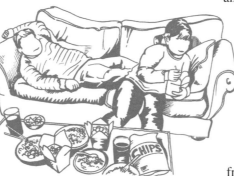

Investigators in Tucson, Arizona, have tracked the respiratory status of 1,035 children from birth to age thirteen. Children with more than one older sibling at home and those who attended day care at an early age had more wheezing in early childhood than children with no older siblings or less exposure to day-care centers. However, by age six, the younger siblings and children who attended day care at an early age had less wheezing. This study suggests exposure to common viral respiratory infections at an early age, either in or out of the home, protected against wheezing and asthma later on in childhood. The hygiene hypothesis may explain why pre-

In that bygone era, we had no coaches, umpires, referees or uniforms, and, even more importantly, no parents were involved in our athletic activities.

mature infants tend to have less allergy and eczema. Premature infants who enter the world before their immune systems are fully primed are more susceptible to infections, especially intestinal infections.

■ The Couch Potato Theory

Allergies and asthma are rare diseases in undeveloped lands like New Guinea, China and rural Africa where there is no television, electricity or motorized transport. Children in these countries play outdoors a great deal, and they walk or run ten to twenty miles a day to and from school. No wonder the Kenyans continue to dominate the Boston Marathon! Prior to 1960, most American children played outdoors after school for several hours a day, or from dawn till dusk in the summer months.

I recall my own school days when, depending on the season, my friends and I would gather after school or during the summer months for unsupervised games, including pickup baseball, football, basketball, or hockey. In that bygone era, we had no coaches, umpires, referees, or uniforms, and, even more importantly, no parents were involved in our athletic activities. We organized our own games that lasted for hours. As many families of that era only had one automobile, we walked or cycled several miles a day to and from school or athletic fields. Nowadays, SUV-driven children rarely walk or cycle to and from their schools or playing fields, even if they play a relatively short distance from home. You rarely see children participating in an athletic event without uniforms, coaches, or referees. Most of today's children would not be capable of organizing any type of pickup game like "rolly at the bat."

Is this pattern of childhood activity playing a role in the asthma-allergy epidemic? Dr. Thomas Platts-Mills has proposed an intriguing theory that could be labeled the "couch potato theory." Platts-Mills feels that the sedentary after-school habits of modern children (no outdoor play, lying on carpets or rugs, and watching television or computer screens) allows children to spend more time indoors in poorly ventilated homes or apartments. Inner-city children often stay indoors after school due to the threat of violence in their neighborhood. Such homes may be loaded with indoor allergens, like house dust mites, molds, household pets, and cockroaches, which in turn lead to increased allergy sensitization and asthma. This lifestyle has concomitantly led to a new generation of obese children.

The couch potato theory is supported by several studies on asthma and obesity. Obesity has been found to be a definite risk factor for both children and adults with asthma. One study of over 80,000 female nurses found that overweight nurses were three times more likely to develop asthma than their thinner colleagues. A British study of 8,000 people found that heavier adults were more likely to have asthma.

Dr. Carlos Camargo studied 16,862 children between nine and fourteen years of age and found that asthma was more prevalent in overweight children. He suggested being overweight compresses the airways and makes obese people more reactive to common asthma triggers. Over the past twenty-five years, the number of overweight children and adults who have allergies and asthma has impressed me. I assumed that obesity was related to inactivity or lack of regular exercise due to asthma. One group of obese children especially prone to asthma is overweight adolescent females who develop a severe form of non-allergic asthma or late-onset childhood asthma. While the obesity theory has validity for asthma, it is difficult to tie it to food allergy as so many infants and young children experience their first food reaction at a younger age when obesity has not yet developed.

■ Early Allergen Exposure

Can unborn infants be sensitized to food or inhalant allergens while in the mother's womb? Blood from an infant's umbilical cord has been found to contain allergic antibodies to egg, milk, dust mites, cats, and birch pollen. One interesting study showed that infants born before their mothers were exposed to grass pollen had no antibody to grass pollen in their umbilical cord blood, while infants born to mothers exposed to grass pollen during pregnancy did have grass pollen antibody in their umbilical cord blood.

Scandinavian infants born in late winter before the spring birch pollen season have more birch pollen allergy than infants born after the birch pollen season. The mother's placenta allows antigens from her body to cross over to the fetus, possibly triggering an allergic immune response in the fetus. Such a response may start as early as the twenty-fourth week of pregnancy, when the fetus adopts a Th-2 posture to prevent rejection by the mother.[1] A higher maternal age may be another risk factor for food allergy. One American survey reports that infants born to mothers over age thirty had

---

[1] The concept that food allergy may be prevented by maternal and infant diet manipulation is discussed in detail in chapter 20.

three times more food allergy and a higher incidence of eczema and hay fever.

■ Antacids and Acetaminophen

Some studies suggest the widespread use of antacid-like medications for gastroesophageal reflux disease (GERD) in infants and using acetaminophen to lower fevers in young children may increase the risk of allergy. Researchers who fed caviar and fish protein to two different groups of mice found that mice who were pretreated with antacids developed allergic antibodies to fish protein; whereas mice not given antacids did not produce allergic fish antibodies. The proposed mechanism is that antacids lower stomach acidity, alter digestion of food proteins and promote food allergy. Is the use of antacids by pregnant women a risk? There are no studies on this intriguing question, despite the fact the 50 percent of pregnant women take antacids during pregnancy.

Is acetaminophen a factor? Due to the risks of Reye's Syndrome[2] in infancy and early childhood, acetaminophen, not aspirin, is often used to lower fevers in sick children. During the past several years, there have been a number of studies suggesting that regular use of acetaminophen, both during pregnancy or early childhood, may be a risk factor for childhood allergy and asthma. Interestingly, the recommendation to switch from aspirin to acetaminophen was made in the early 1980s, approximately the same time we began to see the dramatic rise in asthma and other allergic diseases. So far, acetaminophen has not been linked to food allergy. Both the antacid and acetaminophen theories need more study before one can recommend avoiding antacids and acetaminophen in "at-risk" pregnant mothers, infants and children. [3]

■ Is Early Use of Multivitamins Harmful?

According to a study by Dr. Joshua Milner, early use of vitamins may boost the risk of asthma and allergy. Milner and his colleagues at the National Institute of Allergy and Infectious Disease collected data from the National Center for Health Statistics in Hyattsville, Maryland, that evaluated more than 8,000 children. The mothers reported whether or not they had given their children vitamins at an early age, and if their children developed a food allergy or asthma. Formula-fed children who took supplemental vitamins before six months of age had a 70 percent greater risk for a food allergy compared to formula-fed children not given a multivitamin supplement. There was a 30 percent increased risk of developing asthma by age three in black infants, regardless of having been formula-fed or breast-fed. There was no increased risk of food allergies in children who were solely breast-fed, regardless of their ethnicity. Milner speculated that the increased risk of food allergies among formula-fed infants was due to the higher amount of vitamin D found in formulas.

Many experts have mixed feelings about this study. Prospective studies with more accurate accounting of the type, timing, and dose of multivitamins, as well as longer follow-up with validated methods of diagnosing allergy and asthma are necessary to confirm these results. Parents

---

[2] Reye's syndrome is believed to be caused by the ingestion of medicines that contain aspirin-like drugs. It occurs when abnormal accumulations of fat develop in the liver and other organs of the body, along with a severe increase of pressure in the brain. It affects mostly young children and teenagers and occurs after a flu-like infection or the chicken pox.

[3] Throughout the text, the term "at-risk," is defined as having one or more immediate family members (a parent or a sibling) with an allergic disease.

should still follow their doctor's recommendations regarding the use of multivitamins in infants and children.

■ A New Theory— The Microflora Hypothesis

Many researchers believe the hygiene hypothesis has some holes. For example, it does not explain why inner city children living under poor hygienic conditions have the highest rates of asthma in the world. Nor does it explain why residents of clean air mountain climates have experienced the asthma and allergy epidemic as well. Residents of industrialized cities where air pollution has been lowered have not experienced a decrease in asthma or allergic diseases. These observations have given birth to a new theory called the "microflora hypothesis." This theory proposes that the allergy epidemic may be due to a combination of overuse of antibiotics in infancy and early childhood, eradication of friendly bacteria in the intestinal tract, and a dramatic change in maternal and infant diet in westernized societies.

■ Too Many Antibiotics?

Several studies suggest that the use of antibiotics in infancy may increase the risk of allergic diseases. Researchers from the University of Michigan believe that changes in the composition of bacteria in the intestinal tract may intensify the immune response to common allergens, such as molds, pollens, animal dander, and foods and increase the risk of developing allergies and asthma. They tested their theory in mice by killing all the bacteria in their intestines by administering a five-day course of antibiotics. They then fed the mice egg protein and mold allergens. Later, mice challenged with the egg and mold protein demonstrated an increased reactiv-

ity in their airways compared to the control mice not given antibiotics. These investigators proposed that the change in the bacterial composition of the gut caused by widespread use of antibiotics and a modern high-fat, high-sugar, low-fiber diet, might be the reason for the ongoing allergy epidemic. Instead of developing a normal response or tolerance to inhaled or ingested allergens, an intestinal tract with altered bacteria sets up the T-cell response that favors the atopic march.

A New Zealand survey found that children who received an antibiotic in infancy had a fourfold risk of having asthma in their teens. Infants treated with antibiotics before twelve months of age were nearly twice as likely to develop asthma in childhood, according to a study by researchers in Vancouver, Canada. A review of seven studies of 12,082 children compared exposure to at least one antibiotic to no antibiotic exposure in the first year of life. The report concluded that for each extra course of antibiotics during the first year of life, a child was 1.16 times more likely to develop asthma. Similar results were found in Germany and United Kingdom surveys.

Yet, other studies looking at the use of antibiotics in the first six months of life have yielded mixed results. In Boston, a prospective study of 498 children born to parents with a history of allergy did not support the theory that the use of antibiotics in early childhood was associated with the development of asthma or allergy by five years of age. Persistent wheezing was more commonly linked to male sex and a maternal history of asthma. This was the first prospective study on this issue. The Boston researchers concluded that antibiotic use in the first year of life was not associated with the development of asthma, allergic rhinitis, or eczema. Personally, I think the overuse of antibiotics started long before the rise in the incidence of allergic diseases, especially food allergy.

■ The Westernized Diet

The last part of the microflora hypothesis proposes that a westernized diet may promote allergen sensitization. Numerous studies have found less allergy and asthma in rural countries where local diet favors the consumption of unsaturated fatty acids; vegetable oils; oily fish like tuna, herring, mackerel, trout; and salmon, and fresh fruits and vegetables that contain vitamin C and vitamin E. Once an allergy starts, dietary changes may not be effective; intervention studies with diets high in vitamins C and E and antioxidant-rich fruits have not halted the progression of allergic diseases.[4]

They Paved Paradise and Put Up a Parking Lot!

They paved paradise
And put up a parking lot
With a pink hotel, a boutique
And a swinging hot spot.
Don't it always seem to go
That you don't know what you've got
Till it's gone
They paved paradise
And put up a parking lot.

They took all the trees
And put them in a tree museum
And they charged all the people
A dollar and a half just to see 'em.
Don't it always seem to go
That you don't know what you've got
Till it's gone
They paved paradise
And put up a parking lot.

Hey farmer, farmer
Put away that DDT now.
Give me

Spots on my apples,
But leave me the birds and the bees
Please!
Don't it always seem to go
That you don't know what you've got
Till it's gone
They paved paradise
And put up a parking lot.

The lyrics from this great song, "Big Yellow Taxi," popularized by Joni Mitchell, may have been prophetic. Doctors Leena von Hertzen and Tari Haahtela from Helsinki, Finland, have proposed a brilliant spin to the microflora hypothesis. They propose that the allergy epidemic may be due to the "disconnection of man from the soil." They cleverly studied the asphalt index that tracks the use of paved asphalt in Finland on a yearly basis. They found that asphalt production in Finland rose tenfold in three decades—from 1966 to 2000.

The lyrics from this great song, "Big Yellow Taxi," popularized by Joni Mitchell, may have been prophetic.

During this period, the number of farmers declined from 17 percent to 5 percent of the Finish population, while the incidence of asthma and allergic rhinitis increased nearly tenfold. In support of their theory, they cite the more than thirty studies published in the past six years that show that living on a farm and contact with farm animals protected against allergic diseases. They also cited the higher rate of allergic diseases in Finland versus the Russian Karelia region, a neighboring country with an almost identical climate and geography. The major difference between these two

---

[4] More on the westernized diet in chapter 17.

regions is that surface water in Karelia is rarely treated with chemicals, and the Russians drink water that runs off from bacteria-laden soil. This soil-disconnect thesis may also explain why consumption of non-pasteurized milk may protect against allergy. Studies in Mongolia depict far less allergy in rural villages compared to Mongolian towns and cities.

This thesis is based on the premise that exposure to friendly soil bacteria induces a state of immune tolerance by properly programming the regulatory, or T-reg cells. The concept makes good sense. Before paradise was paved into a parking lot, humans had much more exposure to soil bacteria that was ever-present in our air, food, and non-chlorinated water. Increasing coverage of the earth by concrete and asphalt has resulted in less exposure to soil microorganisms that may, in turn, have produced a dysfunctional T-cell system.

Should we turn the clock back and return to the less hygienic living conditions of the past? Certainly not—improvement in public health and childhood vaccines are two of the major reasons for the increase in our life span. However, my mother was probably right—eating a little dirt may be beneficial to one's health. One hundred years ago man was constantly exposed to common infectious diseases, worms, and parasites that repeatedly stimulated the immune system. These infections probably protected humans against allergy and asthma by triggering the immune system to favor the Th-1 non-allergic pathway. The low incidence of food allergy and other allergic diseases in Third World countries where parasitic infections are still common suggests that our immune system is not as tough or as well conditioned as it was decades ago. Such countries also introduce potent food allergens, such as peanuts and seafood, at a much earlier age, perhaps inducing a state of immune tolerance that prevents food allergy.

The improvements in public health and hygiene and the overuse of antibiotics mean people are no longer exposed to strong immune stimulants. In essence, the trade-off for living a longer, healthier life may be a higher incidence of allergic diseases like eczema, asthma, hay fever, and food allergy. It is exciting to speculate that, if indeed a lazy immune system is responsible for the ongoing asthma and food allergy epidemic, some type of vaccine strategy that stimulates a lethargic immune system in infancy or early childhood may prevent allergic diseases. An interesting approach may be injecting high-risk infants and young children with bacterial vaccines to prevent allergic diseases. One bacterial vaccine currently under study is *Mycobacterium vaccaea*, a harmless soil bacteria that evokes a strong Th-1 or non-allergic response in mice.

Early human clinical trials with this vaccine in subjects with allergic rhinitis and asthma appear promising. To date there are no similar studies in food allergy prone infants or children.

The low incidence of food allergy and other allergic diseases in Third World countries where parasitic infections are still common suggests that our immune system is not as tough or as well conditioned as it was decades ago.

■ The Bottom Line

What is the "take-home" message of all these different theories? Concepts from the hygiene hypothesis, the couch potato theory, the microflora hypothesis, and soil-disconnect theory all help to explain the allergy epidemic. They explain why some countries like rural Africa and China have one-tenth the incidence of allergy, asthma, and food allergies as compared to more developed westernized societies. Exposure to allergens in infancy or early childhood may trigger the pro-allergic pathway in at-risk children. Early exposure to animals, large families, farms, day-care centers, lazy housekeeping, nuts, and seafood may be protective by inducing immune tolerance to common inhalant and food allergens. All these theories need more study. In all likelihood, there are many reasons for this emerging allergy epidemic. ●

Chapter

3

Is It Really Food Allergy?

In many surveys, nearly 25 percent of individuals perceive they or their children have a food allergy. Yet, when these people are subjected to an allergy skin or blood test or an oral challenge to a suspected food, only one in every ten or twenty will actually be found to have a true food allergy. Most abnormal responses to foods or beverages can be classified into a broad category called an adverse, or non-allergic, food reaction. While I mainly focus on food allergy throughout this book, it is important to review the common types of non-allergic or adverse food reactions that can be mistaken for food allergy. Such reactions include food intolerances, chemical reactions, idiosyncratic reactions, pharmacologic responses, and toxic or food-poisoning reactions.

> *Another common example of food intolerance is gluten intolerance, where the intestinal tract does not process the gluten protein in wheat in a normal manner resulting in gluten intolerance, also known as celiac disease.*

■ Food Intolerance Reactions

Most adverse food reactions can be lumped into the food intolerance group. For example, many victims of lactose intolerance think they are allergic to milk. They are not. Milk and dairy products contain lactose, a sugar that is broken down into glucose by an enzyme called lactase. When you do not produce enough lactase, undigested lactose causes nausea, cramps, bloating, or diarrhea. You do not experience typical allergic symptoms, such as hives, swelling, low blood pressure, or difficulty breathing. Thus, lactose intolerance is really an enzyme or lactase deficiency. Another common example of food intolerance is gluten intolerance, where the intestinal tract does not process the gluten protein in wheat in a normal manner resulting in gluten intolerance, also known as celiac disease.

Many people suffer from chronic, unexplained health problems, ranging from migraine headaches, inflammatory bowel diseases, depression, and arthritis to chronic fatigue syndrome. The common belief that such ailments are due to food intolerances has fostered a multitude of publications that focus on theses controversial issues. Due to space constraints, I have elected to concentrate on true food allergies and common adverse food and beverage reactions in this book. If you want to learn more about food intolerances, like lactose and gluten intolerance, I highly recommend *Food Allergies and Food Intolerance* by Dr. Jonathan Brostoff and Linda Gamlin, and *Dealing With Food Allergies* by Janice Vickerstaff Joneja. Both these books present sound discussions on food intolerances and food allergy.

■ Chemical Reactions

Thousands of chemicals and additives, including food dyes, binders, colorings, preservatives, and flavor enhancers, are added to foods and beverages. The next time you go to a supermarket, spend some time reading the labels on packaged foods. The number of listed ingredients is mind-boggling. Many food additives are capable of causing adverse non-allergic reactions. Reactions to food dyes and additives— including the two most common examples of food additive reactions, MSG (mono-sodium glutamate) and sulfite sensitivity, will be thoroughly reviewed in chapter 15.

■ Pharmacologic Reactions

Reactions caused by naturally occurring chemicals present in foods or beverages are classified as pharmacologic reactions. Typical examples would be insomnia from caffeine present in tea or coffee or an itch or a hive-like reaction induced by hista-mine that is often present in high levels in fresh strawberries, certain fish, and processed meats. Many migraine sufferers experience headaches after eating natural-ly occurring chemicals in wine, aged cheese, chocolate, and processed meats, such as hot dogs and sausages.

■ Food Poisoning and Food Toxicity

A food poisoning or toxic food reaction is the result of ingesting foods contaminated by a virus, bacteria, or toxin. Most food poisoning is caused by food spoilage and bacterial contamination of food. Typical examples of food poisoning would be out-breaks of viral hepatitis A, and nausea, vomiting, and diarrhea caused by over-growth of staphylococcal and E. coli bac-teria. While seafood spoilage is the most common form of food poisoning, fruits and vegetables are now responsible for more food-borne illness than meat, poultry, or eggs.[1] The two reasons for this are the rise

in popularity of fresh fruits and veggies and the long food chain from the farm to the fork. The most risky fruits and vegeta-bles are tomatoes, melons (especially can-taloupes), lettuce, and green onions. Pre-packaged and pre-washed vegeta-bles are prime cul-prits. In 2003, Mex-ican-grown green onions triggered food-borne illness in over 500 Ameri-cans, and three vic-tims died. In July 2005, salmonella-tainted tomatoes sickened 561 peo-ple in the United States and Canada. Sources of bacterial contamination are irrigation water and waste products from wildlife. One study estimated that 65 mil-lion to 81 million Americans become sick each year from eating food prepared in their own homes. Meticulous preparation, refrigeration, washing, and discarding damaged fruits and vegetables are the best ways to minimize the chances of a food-borne illness. Not all food-borne illnesses are due to viruses or bacteria.

Many migraine sufferers experience headaches after eating naturally occurring chemicals in wine, aged cheese, chocolate, and processed meats, such as hot dogs and sausages.

Typical examples of toxic food reactions include diarrhea, triggered by lectins in castor, red kidney and jack beans; liver and kidney failure from poisonous mushrooms; and headache and bloating after excess salt consumption. Several forms of toxic reac-tions to seafood are reviewed in chapter 12.

■ Food Allergy Symptoms

Unlike hay fever and asthma, which only affect our respiratory system, food allergy symptoms are quite varied and can strike

---

[1] *Wall Street Journal*, November 30, 2005.

several organs at once. In the mildest form, food allergy victims develop an itch, hives, or mild swelling at the point of contact with the food. Young infants and toddlers who cannot verbalize their symptoms may cry, rub their mouths or faces, or spit out the offending food. More subtle symptoms include hoarseness, throat tightness, hiccups, and fullness in the ears. The terms oral allergy syndrome or pollen-food syndrome are used when symptoms are limited to the lips, tongue, or mouth. When the skin is affected, symptoms include acute hives (urticaria), swelling (angioedema), itching and flushing, or paleness. Chronic hives that last for weeks or months are rarely due to a food allergy.

When the intestinal tract is targeted, victims develop abdominal cramps, nausea, vomiting, or diarrhea. In more life-threatening reactions, the cardiovascular and respiratory organs are affected.

In such cases, low blood pressure may induce collapse and shock, or the victim may experience airway swelling or a severe asthma attack. When two or more body systems are involved, doctors use the term anaphylaxis to describe the allergic food reaction.

> *When two or more body systems are involved, doctors use the term anaphylaxis to describe the allergic food reaction.*

■ How Doctors Diagnose Food Allergy

A food allergy reaction usually first comes to the attention of emergency room doctors, family practitioners, pediatricians, and internists. While these health-care providers are capable of diagnosing and treating food allergy reactions, in many cases the expertise of an allergy specialist may be needed to confirm the diagnosis, pinpoint the offending food, and develop a treatment and education plan for victims and their families. Allergists are doctors who complete a three-year residency in either pediatrics or internal medicine followed by a two- to three-year fellowship program in allergy and immunology. Such training qualifies them to handle all types of allergic and immune diseases, such as asthma, hay fever, eczema or atopic dermatitis, and drug and food allergy.

At the first visit, the allergy specialist will take a detailed history, as this is the best way to differentiate between an allergic and an adverse food reaction. The timing and symptoms of the reaction are important clues. The doctor will want to know what foods and how much were ingested before the reaction. The clinical history can be challenging. The allergist must consider what was eaten, confusing labels on packaged foods, how a food was prepared, and what were the chances of a cross-contamination reaction.

Once you make an appointment with an allergist, come prepared. If the cause of a reaction is unclear, prepare a list of ingredients from packaged foods you have eaten. If the reaction took place in a food-service establishment, obtain the ingredients of the meal from the restaurant manager or chef. If you were treated in an emergency room, obtain the emergency room records. Compile a list of questions and obtain copies of any allergy-related tests done prior to your first visit.

During the physical examination, the doctor will focus on your skin, eyes, ears, nose, throat, and chest looking for signs of other diseases frequently associated with food allergy, like eczema or hives. Inflammation in your eyes may signify an underlying eye allergy or allergic conjunctivitis.

Dark circles under the eyes, called "allergic shiners," or swelling in the nose are both telltale signs of allergic rhinitis, or hay fever, often associated with food allergy. The doctor will rely on the stethoscope and breathing tests to detect wheezing or asthma. The physical examination in a food-allergic patient is usually normal, with the exception of infants and young children with eczema. After completing the medical history and physical exam, the allergy specialist may use three methods to diagnose food allergy—allergy skin tests, allergy blood tests, and, in special instances, an oral challenge to the suspected food. The typical allergy evaluation may require one to three visits. At the last visit, the allergy specialist should review the results of the allergy consultation with the patient or family and outline a treatment and education program in a written report. This report can be shared with primary care providers as well as other caretakers, including school, college, or summer camp personnel. The doctor may then request follow-up visits—usually once a year to determine the status of your food allergy.

■ Allergy Skin Tests

The scratch or prick skin test is a relatively painless procedure that produces no more discomfort than scratching your skin with a fingernail. Despite some popular

Despite some popular misconceptions, allergy skin tests can be done in any age group, including infants and young children.

misconceptions, allergy skin tests can be done in any age group, including infants and young children. The number of tests performed varies between allergy specialists. Our practice usually applies sixty skin tests to older children and adults. In infants and toddlers, you can usually get by with sixteen to twenty tests. Intradermal (under the skin) food skin tests are not recommended because they are potentially dangerous, overly sensitive, and associated with an unacceptable rate of false-positive reactions.

When your body has an allergic or IgE antibody to an allergen, the test antigen combines with IgE antibody in your skin and produces a wheal and flare, or a small hive, at the test site within five to twenty minutes. The flare refers to the redness, and the wheal is the white center in the middle of the redness. The size of the wheal, measured in millimeters (mm), often reflects your level of sensitivity to the test allergen.[2]

Skin tests are very helpful in identifying allergies to inhaled substances, such as dust mites, molds, pollens and animals. Unfortunately food skin tests are not as reliable as inhalant skin tests. Sometimes the food skin test is falsely positive (about one in twenty), as many foods simply irritate the skin. Also skin tests may remain

---

[2] A millimeter, or mm, is 1/1000th of a meter. For example, a 10-mm sized skin test equals four-tenths of an inch.

positive for several years after a food allergy is outgrown. Food skin tests also have a high rate of false negative reactions, as food extracts lose their potency when processed in a commercial allergy lab. However, allergists have now developed very accurate diagnostic cutoff levels based on the size of the skin test in children with cow's milk, egg, and peanut allergy that allows one to predict their chances of having a reaction to these foods.

In some situations, especially when the suspected food is a fruit or vegetable, it is necessary to test with a fresh food. In most cases, if the skin test is negative and there is no history of an allergic reaction to the tested food, there is usually no reason to avoid this food, as there is a 95 percent chance you will not react to that food. Lastly, in patients who have experienced a severe allergic reaction to a food, especially a peanut or tree nut, it may be necessary to do a blood test first, as skin testing to the suspect food may be unwise due to a small risk of triggering an allergic reaction.

> *Although a high serum IgE level is often seen in an allergic or food allergy patient, a normal IgE level does not rule out food allergy. Likewise, a high IgE level does not always signify a food allergy.*

■ Allergy Blood Tests

Three blood tests help the doctor diagnose food allergy. The first test measures the level of eosinophils in the blood. These are blood cells that can signify an ongoing allergy. A high eosinophil count often parallels the severity of a food allergy and may point to some rare food hypersensi-

tivity diseases. The second important allergy blood test is the serum IgE test, which measures the amount of IgE antibody in your body. A high IgE level indicates that allergies may be playing an important role in your food reactions. This test often helps to predict if an infant or a young child with a food allergy will develop other allergies, such as eczema, hay fever, or asthma. Although a high serum IgE level is often seen in an allergic or food allergy patient, a normal IgE level does not rule out food allergy. Likewise, a high IgE level does not always signify a food allergy.

The third and most important blood test for diagnosing food allergy is called the RAST test. In the RAST test, a blood sample is processed through an analyzer to determine if your serum contains an allergic antibody to a specific food allergen. Refinement of this RAST test has led to a new test called the CAP RAST test.[3] This test measures the precise amount of IgE antibody to foods like eggs, cow's milk, peanuts, tree nuts, and seafood.

This test is reported in units called k/U/L, ranging from a low of 0.35 units to over 100 units. The big advantage of the CAP RAST test is that doctors can precisely track the levels of an IgE antibody to a specific food over several years. When the results of the CAP RAST tests are combined with skin tests, the doctor can predict the odds of having a reaction to foods like cow's milk, eggs, peanuts, and fish. For example, individuals with a peanut CAP RAST level over fifteen units have a 95 percent chance of reacting to peanuts. Just like the skin test, the CAP RAST test may be falsely negative or falsely positive and does not always predict the severity of a reaction. When both the skin and the CAP RAST tests decline

---

[3] Throughout the text the specific IgE RAST test will be referred to as the CAP RAST test.

to acceptable levels, allergists may consider conducting an oral food challenge.

Many homeopathic practitioners and commercial labs promote blocking antibody tests, called IgG or IgG4 antibody, to identify foods that trigger non-allergic diseases, such as the chronic fatigue syndrome, inflammatory bowel disease, migraine headaches, arthritis, and hyperactivity disorders. Other worthless junk science tests include hair analysis and cytotoxic tests. Scientific studies have conclusively found that these tests have no validity whatsoever in linking food allergy to these common conditions.

In July 2006, researchers led by M. Cecilia Berin at Mount Sinai School of Medicine in New York City showed for the first time that CD23, a protein normally present in a person's intestinal tract, acts as a receptor for the IgE antibody. This protein was found in the stool samples of nine food-allergic children. Larger clinical trials are planned to determine if analyzing stool samples may be a new non-invasive way to diagnose food allergies.

The Atopy Patch Test

A new test for food allergy has gained a foothold, especially in Europe. In the atopy patch test, a food allergen is applied to the skin, covered and left on for twenty-four to seventy-two hours. This atopy patch test is the same test allergist and dermatologists use to diagnose contact dermatitis to substances like nickel. Some studies have found the atopy patch test to be more helpful than the skin test in identifying food allergies in children with eczema.

Other reviews found that the atopy patch test did not offer any advantages over skin and CAP RAST blood tests. A study looking at the clinical relevance of the atopy patch test in predicting hypersensi-

tivity to cow's milk and hen's eggs in 486 children concluded that the atopy patch test did not detect food hypersensitivity not predicted by skin tests or CAP RAST tests. Therefore, the atopy patch test could not be recommended in daily practice for the diagnosis of hypersensitivity to cow's milk and hen's eggs in young children.

Oral Food Challenges

The proof is in the pudding! Every food allergy publication states that the oral food challenge is the "gold standard," or best way to diagnose a food allergy. Oral challenges are conducted in several ways. In a labial challenge, the suspect food is placed on the lower lip for about two minutes and the patient is observed for twenty to thirty minutes. When this test is negative, doctors follow it with a taste challenge where the food is chewed for thirty seconds and spit out. When there is no reaction to the taste test, you can perform a thirty-minute open food challenge with a regular serving.

Doctors can blind the challenge by disguising the food. For example, you can hide the food in tuna fish, grape juice or a chocolate mint. The best oral challenge test is the double-blind-placebo-controlled food challenge or the DBPCFC test. In this test, both the food and a placebo, like sugar, is hidden, or blinded. Neither the patient nor the doctor knows what the test substance contains. The DBPCFC challenge is an expensive, time-consuming procedure that may be beyond the capability of many allergy specialists. Thus, DBPCFC challenges are most often done at allergy centers that specialize in food allergy.

Why conduct an oral challenge? A negative oral challenge offers the patient or family the opportunity to lead a more normal life by eliminating needless dietary restrictions at home, in restaurants, schools, or the workplace. On the other hand, a positive food challenge reinforces the need for strict dietary precautions and continued vigilance. Allergists can combine the clinical history with the results of skin and CAP RAST tests to determine when and if an oral challenge is indicated. Oral challenges are not risk-free and should be performed under close medical supervision by allergy specialists trained in conducting oral challenges. A review of approximately 1,000 food-sensitive children who underwent food challenges at Philadelphia's Children's Hospital found a positive food-challenge in 413 of 998 children, or 42 percent of all oral challenges. The most common foods associated with a positive oral challenge were cow's milk, eggs, and peanut. Most patients had an initial skin reaction followed by multi-organ involvement. Peanuts, milk, and eggs were more likely to cause severe reactions than wheat or other foods. The key finding from this study was that milk, eggs, and peanuts are common foods used in food challenges, and patients tend to experience challenge reactions similar to their real-life reaction.

A similar study at Johns Hopkins Food Allergy Center reviewed its experiences with 605 challenges in children. The average age of challenged subjects was five years, and 57 percent of the challenged children passed the test. Children with smaller skin test reactions and low CAP RAST levels (less than five units) were more likely to have a negative challenge, whereas, children with eczema, asthma or other food allergies were less likely to pass the oral challenge test. London children and young adults who had high CAP RAST levels (>15 units) and large skin tests (>8mm wheal) who underwent a nut challenge were found to be unlikely to pass the oral challenge. Thirty-six percent of 718 orally challenged at the Jaffe Institute in New York City had a positive reaction to an oral challenge. Most were mild reactions, involving only the skin or intestinal tract. Ninety-three percent were treated with an antihistamine, and only one patient required epinephrine. Passing an oral challenge test does not mean you are home free.

Four of eighteen patients with negative skin and CAP RAST tests who passed their oral egg challenge test in Manitoba, Canada, subsequently reacted to raw or undercooked eggs. The take-home message: once you pass an oral challenge test, you should eat the food on a regular basis and maintain access to auto-injectable epinephrine until the tested food has been repeatedly and safely consumed.

■ The Food Elimination Diet

In my early years of practice, I frequently recommended a four- to six-week allergy-elimination diet in patients with suspected food allergies or food intolerances. A typical elimination diet removes the more allergenic foods, dyes, colorings, and preservatives, while allowing less allergenic foods, such as beef, pork, lamb, and most fruits and cooked vegetables. After a specified period, foods and food additives are gradually reintroduced one at a time. The availability of skin and CAP RAST tests has

> *Thirty-six percent of 718 orally challenged at the Jaffe Institute in New York City had a positive reaction to an oral challenge. Most were mild reactions, involving only the skin or intestinal tract. Ninety-three percent were treated with an antihistamine and only one patient required epinephrine.*

reduced the need for such tedious elimination diets. It is best to avoid prolonged eliminations diets as restrictive food intake may lead to eating disorders, personality changes or prompt patients to seek out unscientific and costly alternative therapies.

The elimination diet may be very helpful in tracking down foods and beverages that trigger eczema and non-IgE-triggered diseases, such as celiac disease, protein-induced gastrointestinal diseases, migraine headaches, and irritable bowel syndrome. Due to space constraints (and a total lack of culinary skills), I have elected not to include extensive elimination diets, recipes, and meal plans in this book. Health-care providers dealing with food allergy should be able to provide or refer you to sources of information on elimination diets. The best sources I found for elimination diets, recipes, and meal plans are the many publications of FAAN, and Dr. Janice Vickerstaff Joneja's book, *Dealing With Food Allergies.*

■ The Multiple Food Allergy Patient

One of the more difficult situations I now encounter in my practice is patients who present with a history of multiple food allergies. Adults who complain of multiple food allergies are more likely to have non-allergic or food intolerance reactions. On the other hand, an increasing number of young children, especially those with severe eczema, may present with many food allergies. Approximately half of the patients with multiple food allergies have more than one food allergy; however, few have more than four food allergies.

Many patients or families falsely attribute their symptoms to multiple foods when only one allergen may be involved. For example, a milk-allergic child who reacts to soy, canned tuna, wheat crackers, and steamed shrimp may be labeled as being allergic to milk, soy, finfish, wheat, and shrimp. Smart detective work may uncover the fact that soy and canned tuna contain the milk protein casein; the wheat crackers contained milk—perhaps listed as "a natural flavoring"—and shrimp was dipped in milk to eliminate its fishy odor. Thus, this patient may only be allergic to milk. Taking a careful history, performing skin tests and CAP RAST blood tests, combined with oral food challenges can help sort out food allergies in such complicated cases and eliminate needless dietary restrictions.

Some children with severe eczema and high IgE levels who are difficult to skin test have positive CAP RAST tests to nearly every tested food and need special consideration. Their bodies are simply oversaturated with IgE antibody. All too often, they are placed on strict elimination diets that impinge on their lifestyle, psyche, nutrition, and growth rate.

Adults who complain of multiple food allergies are more likely to have non-allergic or food intolerance reactions. On the other hand, an increasing number of young children, especially those with severe eczema, may present with many food allergies.

Many private allergy practices may not be able to provide comprehensive care for such patients who require the expertise of a dietician, psychological counseling, and lengthy oral challenges. Most private allergy practices do not house all these services under one roof. Fortunately, our practice is close to Children's Hospital Medical Center in Boston, where an outstanding food allergy center is available for the evaluation of these complicated cases.

Why Are Some Foods More Allergenic than Others?

Our intestinal tract is exposed to carbohydrates, proteins, fats, minerals, and food additives on a daily basis, yet relatively few individuals experience allergic reactions to foods or beverages. Most people develop an oral tolerance to potential food allergens. The key factors in developing tolerance are your genes, your age, the bacterial flora in your intestinal tract, your immune system, and the dose and nature of a potential food allergen. Food allergens are almost always proteins, but not all food proteins are allergens. Allergenic food proteins must survive the extremes of food processing, escape the digestive enzymes of the gastrointestinal tract, and interact with our immune system. For example, of the twenty proteins in cow's milk and a hen's egg,

> *For example, of the twenty proteins in cow's milk and a hen's egg, only a few can actually trigger an allergic reaction.*

only a few can actually trigger an allergic reaction. The typical food allergen has small proteins that stimulate the production of IgE antibody, and re-exposure to these proteins triggers an allergic reaction.

Food proteins are composed of eight to ten amino acids called epitopes that resemble a series of linked chains. When present, the IgE antibody combines with these epitopes, and an allergic reaction ensues. These epitopes have important functions in nature. Seed storage proteins allow plants to grow, structural proteins allow plants to keep their shape, and regulatory proteins are vital for plant fertilization.

Cooking may denature some protein epitopes and render a food less allergenic.

This explains why some milk-allergic or egg-allergic children tolerate baked goods containing milk and eggs or why fruit-allergic and vegetable-allergic adults usually tolerate cooked fruits and vegetables. Unfortunately, the protein epitopes of many foods, such as peanuts, tree nuts, and seafood, are not altered when processed. Some foods become more allergenic when heated. Isolation and identification of food protein epitopes may someday lead to tests that will predict who will or will not outgrow their food allergy and vaccines that may prevent food allergy.

Cross-Reactivity of Food Allergens

As previously noted, relatively few foods are capable of triggering an allergic reaction. Foods can be classified into food families based on their botanical structure. Table 3.1 lists the more common allergenic foods and their food families. One would think that an allergy to one member of a food family would mean you would be likely to be allergic to all members of this family. Sometimes this is the case, sometimes not. For example, if you are allergic to cashews, you are likely to react to pistachios and mangoes—members of the cashew family. Likewise, if you are allergic to a finfish like cod or a crustacean like shrimp, you may react to many other finfish and crustaceans. The same holds true for the parsley family. If you are allergic to celery, you are quite likely to react to carrots.

On the other hand, if you are allergic to peanuts (a legume) you only have a 5 percent chance of being allergic to other legumes, such as soybeans, peas, and beans, as legumes have very different protein structures. Wheat-allergic patients often tolerate other members of the grain family. Thus, elimination of all grains is often unwarranted.

Mother Nature has played all kinds of tricks on mankind. For instance, the tropomyosin allergen found in crustaceans, such as shrimp, crab and lobster, is also present in house dust mites and cockroaches. The profilin protein is found in birch tree pollen as well as many fruits and vegetables, explaining why many victims of birch pollen hay fever are allergic to apples and celery. This is called the oral allergy syndrome. The latex rubber tree contains the protein, chitinase which protects it from insects. Chitinase, also present in several foods like avocado, banana, chestnut and kiwi, is responsible for the latex-fruit-allergy syndrome. Important examples of cross-reacting and non-cross reacting food allergens will be discussed throughout the book. ●

Table 3.1 Classification of Animal and Plant Food Families

Banana family
Banana
Plantain

Beech family
Beechnut
Chestnut

Birch family
Hazelnut

Birds
Chicken-turkey
Duck-goose
Pheasant
Partridge-Grouse

Buckwheat family
Buckwheat
Rhubarb

Cashew family
Cashew
Pistachio
Mango

Citrus family
Orange
Grapefruit
Lemon
Lime
Tangerine
Kumquat

Compositae
Lettuce
Endive
Artichoke
Dandelion
Chicory
Guava

Crustaceans
Shrimp
Crab
Lobster
Crawfish

Fish*
Cod
Haddock
Anchovy
Sardine
Hake
Salmon
Pollock
Tuna
Trout
Flounder
Swordfish

Gourd family
Casaba
Pumpkin
Squash
Cucumber
Cantaloupe
Muskmelon
Honeydew
Watermelon

Goosefoot family
Beets
Spinach
Swiss chard

Grains
Wheat/ Gluten
Bran
Rye
Barley
Corn
Oats
Rice

Grape family
Grape
Raisin

Heath family
Cranberry
Blueberry

Laurel family
Avocado
Cinnamon
Bay leaf

Legume family
Navy bean
Kidney bean
Lima bean
Soybean
String bean
Lentil
Pea
Peanut
Licorice
Acacia
Senna

Lily family
Asparagus
Onions
Garlic
Leek
Chive
Aloe

Mammals
Beef
Pork
Lamb
Goat
Horse
Deer
Whales/seals

Nightshade family
Potato
Tomato
Eggplant
Peppers

Nutmeg family
Nutmeg

Olive family
Olives
Peppers
Chili
Tabasco
Pimento

Palm family
Coconut
Date
Sago

Parsley family
Carrot
Celery
Parsley
Parsnip
Celeriac
Caraway
Anise
Dill
Coriander
Fennel
Cumin

Papaw family
Papaya

Pedalium family
Sesame seed

Pineapple family
Pineapple

Pine family
Juniper
Pine nut

Rosaceae family
Apple
Apricot
Almond
Nectarine
Pear
Peach
Plum
Prune
Cherry
Quince

Rose family
Raspberry
Blackberry
Loganberry
Strawberry

Sterculia family
Cocoa
Chocolate

Sunflower family
Jerusalem artichokes
Sunflower seed

Walnut family
English walnut
Black walnut
Butternut
Hickory nut
Pecan

* Includes any fish with a vertebrae or backbone.

Chapter

4

Diseases Associated with Food Allergy

Several other diseases often closely associated with food allergy that merit discussion include allergic rhinitis or hay fever, atopic dermatitis or eczema, asthma, and food protein-induced gastrointestinal diseases, such as eosinophilic gastroenteritis, food-induced enterocolitis, food protein-induced enteropathy and food protein-induced proctocolitis.

■ Allergic Rhinitis

Allergic rhinitis, or hay fever, is a relative newcomer to the allergy stage. While the ancient Greeks described asthma and food allergy, there are no historical references to hay fever until the tenth century when the Persian scholar Rhazes, described cases of the coryza (nasal congestion) that took place in the spring when roses were in bloom. The first accurate report of hay fever was published in 1819 by the learned London physician John Bostock. He described his own hay fever as "an unusual train of symptoms," and for many years doctors called hay fever "Bostock's catarrh." In his second paper, Bostock claimed that after nine years of study he had only seen or heard of twenty-eight additional cases of

The term "hay fever" is a complete misnomer. Hay does not cause allergic rhinitis, nor do you develop a fever when you are having symptoms of allergic rhinitis.

hay fever. Bostock made a curious observation: "I have not heard of a single unequivocal case among the poor." The term "hay fever" is a complete misnomer. Hay does not cause allergic rhinitis, nor do you develop a fever when you are having symptoms of allergic rhinitis.

What Bostock described were farmers working with hay who probably had allergic reactions to grass pollen or mold in the hay, not to the hay itself. In 1872, a Harvard professor, Dr. Morrill Wyman, published *Autumnal Catarrah*, a series of case reports on ragweed hay fever. By the 1880s, hay fever—also known as June cold, rose fever, hay asthma, and hay cold—had become the pride of America's leisure class. In mid-August of each year, thousands of affluent sufferers of ragweed hay fever fled to the White Mountains of New Hampshire, the Adirondacks in upper New York State, the shores of the Great Lakes, or to the Colorado plateau to escape the dreaded seasonal symptoms of watery eyes, flowing nose, sneezing fits, and attacks of asthma that many regarded as the price of urban wealth and education.

In 1890, Dr. Charles Blackley, a hay fever sufferer himself, provided the first clue that pollen exposure triggered hay fever by placing grass pollen on his skin and producing a positive reaction. Blackley also dropped pollen into the eyes of patients with hay fever symptoms and triggered an allergic reaction. In the early twentieth century, hay fever was still considered to be a rare illness of the upper class. Dr. John Morrison Smith described his own hay fever while a medical student in Scotland: "I gradually recognized that it was not an ordinary cold and that the symptoms were much worse on the golf course or even during a nice day rowing on Loch Lomand. At first I did not know what I had, and neither did any other doctor I encountered in the next two or three years."

Just eighty years later, millions of people have hay fever or allergic rhinitis. While nearly 18 million Americans have asthma, more than twice as many—approximately 40 million people—suffer from allergic rhinitis. The prevalence of allergic rhinitis has followed the rise in asthma cases, as its incidence has tripled over the past thirty years in most developed countries. The impact on quality of life from allergic rhinitis is significant. Allergic rhinitis interrupts sleep and interferes with school and work performance. Sedating antihistamines contribute to diminished energy, mood disorders, learning problems, work injuries and automobile accidents. There are two forms of allergic rhinitis—seasonal and perennial. Seasonal allergic rhinitis is caused by seasonal exposure to tree, grass, or weed pollens. Perennial, or year-round allergic rhinitis, is triggered by exposure to dust mites, molds, and animals parts. Allergic rhinitis is commonly linked with asthma, as more than 50 percent of asthmatics have allergic rhinitis.

The major symptoms of allergic rhinitis are sneezing, itchy nose and eyes, and clear watery discharge. Patients with seasonal allergic rhinitis report symptoms during specific pollen seasons, while those with year-round, or perennial allergic rhinitis, complain when house dust mites, molds, and household pets precipitate or aggravate their symptoms year round. People who suffer from long-standing allergic rhinitis, especially children, can often be diagnosed just by looking at their facial characteristics and mannerisms. There is often a discoloration and swelling under the eyes called "allergic shiners." When nasal obstruction persists, the typical open-mouth, or adenoidal face is apparent. Frequent rubbing of an itchy nose results in the allergic salute, which produces a transverse "allergic crease" across the lower third of the nose. In allergic rhinitis, the mucous membranes inside the nose are often pale-bluish in color, as opposed to the typical red color seen in non-allergic rhinitis or the common cold. The treatment of allergic rhinitis includes antihistamines, decongestants, and anti-inflammatory nasal sprays similar to those used in asthma, combined with proper environmental controls. In more persistent cases, allergy injections, or immunotherapy, may be indicated. The strong connection between pollen allergy and certain forms of food allergy is thoroughly covered in chapter 9.

Seasonal allergic rhinitis is caused by seasonal exposure to tree, grass or weed pollens. Perennial, or year-round allergic rhinitis, is triggered by exposure to dust mites, molds and animals parts.

■ Eczema—The Itch That Rashes

The first sign that one has inherited a dreaded asthma-allergy gene often occurs in early infancy when infants develop an itchy skin condition known as eczema, or atopic dermatitis. This common skin disease is closely linked to asthma, allergic rhinitis and food allergies. When eczema develops before three months of age, the risk of developing asthma is significantly increased. Eczema is often accompanied by allergen sensitization and a high IgE antibody level. Population studies have found that, like asthma and allergic rhinitis, the incidence of eczema has tripled over the past three decades. In some developed countries, eczema now strikes one in every ten infants. Skin biopsies have demonstrated that eczema is a complex disorder involving many of the same inflammatory cells seen in asthma and allergic rhinitis. Major eczema triggers include foods, airborne allergens and bacterial products.

The symptoms of eczema include an itchy, patchy skin eruption on the face, arms, or legs, especially in the folds of the elbows and knees. As much of the skin eruption in eczema is self-induced by scratching, doctors have labeled eczema as, "the itch that rashes."

In a Netherlands study of 397 patients with eczema, the presence of cow's milk or egg allergy prolonged the course of eczema and predicted that the child was more likely to develop inhalant allergies later in childhood.

■ Role of Food Allergy in Eczema

The prevalence of food allergy in infants with eczema ranges from 20 to 80 percent in various studies. Studies using double-blind, placebo-controlled food challenges suggest that the true incidence is about 40 percent. Cow's milk, hen eggs, soy and wheat allergy account for about 90 percent of food allergies in children with eczema. These foods can provoke flares of eczema in sensitized infants, whereas inhaled allergens and pollen-related foods are more common triggers in older children and adults. Three types of reactions to food occur in eczema. In the first pattern, immediate-type reactions like hives and swelling occur within minutes after eating the offending food. In the second pattern, itching and subsequent scratching lead to an exacerbation of eczema. In the third pattern, called a late reaction, eczema flares six to forty-eight hours after food ingestion. Ingestion of these foods by breast-feeding mothers can also provoke eczema flare-ups in infants. Many infants (up to 67 percent) with eczema may react to food upon their first exposure to a food, especially cow's milk and eggs.

While most infants outgrow eczema, the presence of a food allergy may prolong it. In a Netherlands study of 397 patients with eczema, the presence of cow's milk or egg allergy prolonged the course of eczema and predicted that the child was more likely to develop inhalant allergies later in childhood. Japanese investigators looked at the incidence of food allergy, diagnosed by oral food challenge, in 182 children with eczema. They found food allergy in 86 percent of infants less than one year of age and 76 percent of one- to two-year-old children. They also found the incidence of food allergy declined to 14 percent by age seven years. The most common offending foods were egg, cow's milk, wheat, and fish. They concluded that food allergy was frequently associated with childhood eczema, and appropriate elimination of the offending food was necessary to avoid an acute allergic reaction, including anaphylaxis.

One of the best studies on food allergy and eczema comes from the Melbourne Australia Atopy Cohort Study that followed more than 600 newborns with a strong family history of eczema, asthma, and allergic rhinitis. Nearly 30 percent developed eczema by age one. A total of 487 children underwent skin tests to cow's milk, egg, and peanut. As eczema severity increased, so did the prevalence of food allergy for the most severely affected group—over 60 percent of the children with severe eczema had a food allergy. This study that focused on children less than one year of age supports the close association of IgE-mediated food allergy and eczema. Therefore, all infants with persistent eczema should be evaluated for food allergies.

Conventional eczema treatment includes antihistamines to relieve itching, topical cortisone creams to control inflammation, and antibiotics when secondary infection is present. Additional local measures include avoidance of irritants, dietary elimination of proven food allergens, skin hydration, and skin moisturizers. Clinical studies have found immunomodulating agents, such as tacrolimus (Protopic) and pimecrolimus (Elidel), may be beneficial when traditional eczema treatment fails. However, due to some disturbing reports of cancer in children, including lymphoma, these drugs have fallen into some disfavor.

Contact Dermatitis to Foods

Many foods can trigger an irritant or contact dermatitis. Such reactions are commonly seen in food industry workers who have wet hands due to frequent washing with soaps and detergents. Other risky occupations include cheese makers, bakers, cashew oil processors, chefs, and seafood and cannery workers. Common food triggers include onions, fruits, potatoes, garlic, celery, carrots, and lettuce. A simple patch test can determine if the reaction is simply an irritant reaction (a negative test) or due to a delayed hypersensitivity reaction (a positive skin test). The obvious treatment for contact dermatitis is wearing vinyl gloves and avoiding direct skin contact with the offending food.

Asthma

Asthma, the last of the big four allergic diseases, is a chronic lung condition that can develop at any age. It is most common in childhood and occurs in approximately 7 to 10 percent of the pediatric population. It accounts for 25 percent of lost school days. It affects twice as many boys as girls in early childhood; however, more girls than boys develop asthma as teenagers. In adulthood, females predominate. Asthma affects children in varying degrees, from mild wheezing only during vigorous exercise to very severe symptoms. Children with severe asthma may have daily symptoms that cause lifestyle restrictions. Like food allergy, the incidence of asthma has increased dramatically over the past three decades. There is a general trend of increased deaths and hospitalizations from asthma in all the industrialized countries of the world.

People with asthma have extra-sensitive or hyper-responsive airways that react by narrowing or obstructing when irritated. This makes it difficult for the air to move in and out. This narrowing causes wheezing, coughing, shortness of breath, and chest tightness. The diagnosis of asthma is made by taking a detailed medical history, physical exam, and obtaining several laboratory tests, including a chest x-ray, skin and allergy blood tests, and breathing tests. Common

Like food allergy, the incidence of asthma has increased dramatically over the past three decades. There is a general trend of increased deaths and hospitalizations from asthma in all the industrialized countries of the world.

triggers of asthma include cold air, indoor and outdoor allergens, strong fumes, irritants, stress, smoke, and respiratory infections. Asthma sufferers have a higher incidence of food allergy. In one inner city study, 45 percent of young children with asthma had a food allergy. The important link between asthma and near-fatal and fatal food reactions is fully covered in chapter 12.

■ Eosinophilic Esophagitis

Protein-induced gastrointestinal diseases, such as eosinophilic gastroenteritis, food-induced enterocolitis, food protein-induced enteropathy, and food protein-induced proctocolitis are due to an abnormal accumulation of eosinophils in the gastrointestinal tract. They can present with a wide range of symptoms.[1] Early recognition and treatment may prevent severe nutritional deficiencies often associated with these disorders. Although skin testing and measurement of food-specific IgE antibodies may provide useful clinical information, the diagnosis of a protein-induced gastrointestinal disease usually requires an intestinal biopsy or a formal food challenge.

Since its first description in 1977, eosinophilic esophagitis has evolved from a rare disease to a relatively common one in children and young adults. Dysphagia

Studies at Cincinnati Children's Hospital Medical Center have uncovered a gene called, eotaxin-3, that may be responsible for this disease. The challenge will be to develop ways to block this gene and prevent eosinophilic esophagitis.

(difficulty swallowing solid foods) is the most characteristic symptom. Additional complaints include vomiting, chest and abdominal pain, and weight loss. Although the cause of eosinophilic esophagitis is unknown, there is mounting evidence that food antigens play a role in many cases. Endoscopic biopsy is the cornerstone in the diagnosis of eosinophilic esophagitis. Food allergy is common in patients with eosinophilic esophagitis. Seventy-five percent of 146 patients in The Children's Hospital of Philadelphia with eosinophilic esophagitis were found to be allergic to several foods, including eggs, cow's milk, corn, soy and wheat. Some authorities feel, the increase in this disease may be due to the widespread use of anti-reflux medications in infants and young children.

Studies at Cincinnati Children's Hospital Medical Center have uncovered a gene called eotaxin-3 that may be responsible for this disease.[2] The challenge will be to develop ways to block this gene and prevent eosinophilic esophagitis.

■ Food-Induced Enterocolitis

This is a relatively rare syndrome. It is characterized by severe inflammation in the small intestine and colon of young infants. It starts out with profuse diarrhea, vomiting, dehydration, and failure to thrive. Severe dehydration may lead to episodes of circulatory collapse and shock in about 20 percent of patients. Patients may present with intestinal bleeding and anemia. Sensitization to multiple food proteins is common. Cow's milk and soy are considered the main causative aller-

---

[1] Adapted from Heine, Ralf G. "Pathophysiology, Diagnosis and Treatment of Food Protein-Induced Gastrointestinal Diseases;" *Current Opinion in Allergy and Clinical Immunology* (2004): 4:221–229.

[2] *Wall Street Journal*, New York City, February 14, 2006.

gens, yet other solid foods can trigger this illness. A recent paper from Spain described fourteen infants with food-induced enterocolitis who were allergic to finfish. Like most rare food-allergic disorders, the mechanisms of food-induced enterocolitis are poorly understood.

■ Food-Protein-Induced Enteropathy

This condition, characterized by chronic diarrhea and failure to thrive, is closely associated with allergy to cow's milk and soy protein. Although predominantly a disorder of infants, residual symptoms may persist into school age. Food-protein-induced proctocolitis is the most common cause of low-grade rectal bleeding in young infants. Symptoms usually develop between three and six weeks of age, but earlier presentations have been described. Infantile proctocolitis occurs in both breast-fed and formula-fed infants. Symptoms are often limited to low-grade diarrhea containing small amounts of fresh blood. As blood loss is usually minimal, anemia is relatively uncommon.

■ The Bottom Line

The diagnosis and treatment of protein-induced gastrointestinal diseases is often hampered by the fact that an allergic disorder is often not considered. Symptoms may occur forty-eight hours after allergen exposure and persist for days after the last exposure to the offending food. Treatment involves identifying and eliminating the offending food. Hypoallergenic diets include the use of extensively hydrolyzed or amino-acid-based formula and maternal elimination diets while breast-feeding. Strict elimination diets should be supervised by an experienced dietitian. Growth and nutrient levels must be carefully monitored when elimination diets are maintained for prolonged periods. Infants and younger children have a better response to elimination diets, whereas dietary therapy is less successful in older children and adults. ●

Chapter 5

Anaphylaxis—A Killer Allergy

Sometimes the symptoms of an allergic reaction may be quite mild and resolve after taking an antihistamine like Benadryl. However, in many instances, a reaction may strike several organs of the body. When more than one organ is targeted, doctors use the term anaphylaxis to describe the allergic reaction.

Anaphylaxis is a severe, life-threatening hypersensitivity reaction triggered by

exposure to the offending substance, and an allergen cannot be identified. Typical examples of anaphylactoid, or what is now called non-allergic anaphylaxis, are reactions to drugs such as Demerol or morphine or reactions to X-ray dyes in individuals with no prior exposure to the X-ray dye.

■ History of Anaphylaxis

Allegedly the first recorded victim of anaphylaxis was the Egyptian Pharaoh Menes, who succumbed from an insect sting around 2641 BC. The hieroglyphics on his tomb portrays his death after being stung by a "Kheb," or hornet. The word anaphylaxis has an interesting origin. In 1901, Monaco's Prince Alfred, an avid supporter of medical research, summoned Paul Portier and Charles Richet, two pioneer immunologists, from the University of Paris. The Prince wanted Portier and Richet to develop a protective serum for vacationing bathers who frequently experienced nasty allergic reactions to the sting of the Portuguese Man-O-War jellyfish while swimming in the Mediterranean Sea.

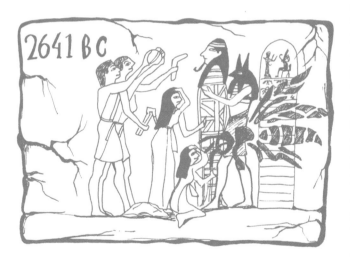

an immunologic mechanism mediated by IgE antibodies.

One of the newest definitions describes anaphylaxis as "a serious allergic reaction that is rapid in onset and may cause death." Anaphylaxis is sometimes confused with the term "anaphylactoid" reaction that produces similar symptoms but lacks a history of a prior

One of the newest definitions describes anaphylaxis as "a serious allergic reaction that is rapid in onset and may cause death."

While cruising on Prince Alfred's ship, Portier and Richet attempted to induce tolerance, or immunity, by injecting animals with the potent jellyfish toxin. Fortunately, they used dogs, not humans, in their early experiments. When the dogs received a second injection of the jellyfish toxin, many experienced a severe and often fatal reaction. Thus, instead of protecting the dogs, the second injection of toxin made them more sensitive to the toxin. Portier and Richet then coined the term anaphylaxis, a derivation of the Greek words *ana* (backward) and *phylaxis* (protection), or "against protection." In 1913, Charles Richet was awarded the Nobel Prize in Medicine for this important contribution to medicine.

The first reports of human deaths from anaphylaxis did not appear in the medical literature until 1895, when fatalities to diphtheria vaccinations with extracts derived from horse serum were described.

In 1905, the death of a child challenged with cow's milk was reported. In 1926, a similar report detailed the demise of a child challenged with peas. The next wave of anaphylactic deaths occurred after the introduction of injectable penicillin in the early 1940s. Larger series of anaphylactic cases were reported in the 1960s and 1970s. In the 1980s, articles on food allergy, exercise-induced anaphylaxis, and latex allergy surfaced. Today, the most common causes for anaphylactic reactions are foods, aspirin-like drugs, antibiotics, stinging insects, and latex products.

◼ Incidence of Anaphylaxis

According to present estimates, acute allergic reactions trigger about 1 million emergency room visits in the United States every year. About 50 percent of these are anaphylactic reactions. Studies in the United States and the United Kingdom looking at the triggers of allergic reactions that required an emergency room visit found that the leading cause by far was a food allergy, which accounted for one in every three emergency room visits for allergic reactions. Food-induced anaphylaxis is believed to trigger 30,000 trips to the emergency room each year in the United States and between 150 and 200 deaths. The prevalence of anaphylaxis is probably not as rare as believed. There may be more than 90,000 victims a year who go to a clinic or a doctor's office or simply do nothing and stay at home. Many of my patients who experience anaphylaxis exhibit total denial. They foolishly disregard their symptoms, take it no more seriously than an attack of hay fever, and rely on an over-the-counter antihistamine like Benadryl.

Anaphylactic food reactions are usually more severe in young adults with asthma, adult women, senior citizens with a drug or a stinging insect allergy, and allergic individuals who are better IgE antibody producers. In a United Kingdom survey, 75 percent of deaths from peanut or tree nut-induced anaphylaxis occurred in women. The highest rate of food-induced anaphylaxis is found in young adults in the 15- to 17-year-old age group. In a survey of 6,000 members of the Anaphylaxis Campaign-United Kingdom, 109 registrants reported 126 anaphylactic reactions, of which eighty-nine were due to foods. Seventy-five reactions occurred in children with an average age of six years. Boys outnum-

> *Many of my patients who experience anaphylaxis exhibit total denial. They foolishly disregard their symptoms, take it no more seriously than an attack of hay fever, and rely an over-the-counter antihistamine, like Benadryl.*

bered girls, and one in five reactions occurred at school. Adult women outnumbered adult men, and the average age of onset was twenty-nine years. Food reactions were more severe in patients with asthma. Thirty-five percent of victims used an auto-injectable epinephrine device. Somewhat surprisingly, 40 percent of the 126 reactions were due to uncommonly reported allergenic foods, such as exotic fruits (kiwi), peas, seeds (mustard), and food additives. The authors of this study concluded that previous surveys vastly underestimated the prevalence of severe food allergy reactions, especially in adults.

■ Symptoms of Anaphylaxis

Anaphylaxis can strike any organ, including the skin, gastrointestinal tract, and respiratory and cardiovascular systems. Amazingly, there are nearly forty signs and symptoms of anaphylaxis. No one who has experienced anaphylaxis, including myself, will ever forget it. Skin symptoms may include flushing, itchiness, excess sweating, hives and swelling. Gastrointestinal symptoms are nausea, vomiting, abdominal cramps and diarrhea. In severe cases, cardio-respiratory effects may

cause dizziness, low blood pressure or shock, swelling in the throat, shortness of breath, coughing and wheezing.

Some patients who experience anaphylaxis, about 10 to 20 percent, may not develop skin symptoms and immediately develop shock or respiratory distress. Anaphylaxis can go unrecognized in asthmatics if their only symptom is wheezing. Drugs, such as sedatives, alcohol and hypnotics, may mask anaphylaxis. The severity of one's first reaction is a poor predictor of the intensity of subsequent reactions, as only 22 percent of fatal reactions had a prior severe reaction.

Most responses to anaphylaxis are symptom driven. In other words, victims with severe symptoms are likely to seek emergency care. In milder reactions, many patients receive suboptimal care or no care whatsoever. Not all anaphylactic reactions are life-threatening. More severe reactions are often seen in patients who start out with gastrointestinal symptoms. Most anaphylactic food reactions are caused by accidental exposure to a known food allergen and cannot be prevented by taking medications before exposure. The risk of a repeated anaphylactic reaction is high. Children from Florence, Italy, who had had an

SYMPTOMS OF ANAPHYLAXIS

SKIN SYMPTOMS
Itchy Ears & Skin
Excess Sweating
Facial Flushing
Swelling (Angioedema)
Hives (Urticaria)

THROAT (LARYNGEAL) EDEMA

CARDIORESPIRATORY SYMPTOMS
Dizziness
Low Blood Pressure (Shock)
Coughing
Wheezing

GASTROINTESTINAL SYMPTOMS
Nausea, Vomiting
Cramps
Diarrhea

The severity of one's first reaction is a poor predictor of the intensity of subsequent reactions, as only 22 percent of fatal reactions had a prior severe reaction.

anaphylactic reaction were followed for seven years. One in every three children had a subsequent reaction. Children with hives, eczema and multiple food allergies were more likely to have additional reactions.

Differential Diagnosis of Anaphylaxis

Doctors use the term "differential diagnosis" when they attempt to separate out other medical conditions that may be triggering similar symptoms. The most common medical condition that can be confused with anaphylaxis is syncope, or a fainting reaction. These patients develop low blood pressure, paleness, weakness, nausea, vomiting, and sweating after a stressful situation, like drawing blood or being injected with a medication. Fainters usually do not have hives, itching or flushing, and they usually have a low pulse rate. Thus, any first responder evaluating a collapsed patient should first check the victim's pulse rate. A low pulse rate usually indicates syncope or fainting, whereas a fast, weak pulse rate is more indicative of an allergic or anaphylactic reaction.

Several medical conditions trigger the release of chemicals that produce flushing, which can be confused with anaphylaxis. Triggers of such flushing syndromes include various drugs and food additives, such as alcohol and MSG. Several forms of food poisoning, especially from spoiled scombroid fish, can be confused with anaphylaxis. Other rare diseases that mimic anaphylaxis include the carcinoid syndrome, pheochromocytoma, rare cancers, and systemic mastocytosis. Mastocytosis is a rare disorder characterized by an overabundance of unstable mast cells in the body. Laboratory tests are not very helpful in the diagnosis of anaphylaxis. The serum measurements of chemicals released during an anaphylactic reaction must be obtained in one hour for histamine and within six hours for tryptase. Also, the results of these tests are not usually immediately available for the emergency room staff. Both these tests are often normal in food-induced anaphylaxis.

Biphasic Anaphylaxis

In this dangerous form of anaphylaxis, the victim has an immediate reaction that resolves quickly with appropriate treatment, followed by a second and often more severe reaction. The interval between reactions varies from one to seventy-eight hours. Most biphasic reactions, the second reaction, occurs within four to eight hours. However, biphasic reactions have been described as late as two to three days later. Biphasic reactions occur in 2 to 20 percent of cases.

They appear to be less common in children. In a study of 103 Australian children with anaphylaxis, only 5 percent had a

In a study of 103 Australian children with anaphylaxis, only 5 percent had a biphasic reaction. It was more likely to occur when the child had needed two doses of epinephrine and IV fluids to control the initial reaction.

biphasic reaction. It was more likely to occur when the child required two doses of epinephrine and IV fluids to control the initial reaction. One study of twenty-five patients experiencing anaphylaxis found that thirteen patients had an early (or uniphasic) presentation, seven had a protracted course, and five had a biphasic presentation. Biphasic reactions are usually more severe, more difficult to treat, and, more likely to be fatal.

Dr. Phillip Lieberman has noted that predisposing factors for a biphasic reaction include:

- A delay of thirty minutes before the onset of symptoms
- A delay in the administration of epinephrine
- Failure to give epinephrine
- An inadequate dose of epinephrine
- Low blood pressure in the early phase of the reaction
- Use of beta blocking and ACE inhibitor drugs
- A delay in administering cortisone drugs

The biggest danger of biphasic anaphylaxis is that a patient may respond promptly to initial emergency room treatment and then be prematurely discharged, only to experience a biphasic reaction several hours after leaving the hospital. The ideal take-home message for emergency room doctors and nurses is that anyone who experiences a moderate-to-severe anaphylactic reaction should be observed in the emergency room for four to six hours before being sent home. As this approach is not always practical in today's overcrowded emergency rooms, advise the discharged patient (or family) to hang out in the waiting area or go to the hospital cafeteria before returning home.

■ Exercise-Induced Anaphylaxis

One unique form of anaphylaxis is called exercise-induced anaphylaxis. In 1980, Doctors Albert Sheffer and Frank Austen described a group of adolescents and young adults who, during or shortly after exercise, felt warm and itchy; developed hives or swelling, abdominal cramps, or wheezing; or experienced cardiovascular collapse. Reactions were more likely to occur in young athletes during vigorous exercise in warmer weather. In 1983, Dr. Jordan Fink reported additional exercise-induced anaphylaxis cases in which the victims experienced symptoms only when they had eaten certain foods before exercising. The most common foods that predisposed them to exercise-induced-anaphylaxis were celery and carrots.

Subsequent reports have described many other foods, such as fruits, vegetables, fish, nuts, and wheat, that trigger exercise-induced anaphylaxis. It is postulated that people with food-related, exercise-induced anaphylaxis have a subtle or unrecognized food allergy that only manifests itself when the offending food allergen is rapidly absorbed during or after intense exercise. Several factors that increase the likelihood of exercise-induced anaphylaxis include alcohol intake, aspirin-like drugs, menses, and ingestion of a large amount of the offending food. Allergy skin tests, especially with fresh foods, often help to identify the offending food. The treatment of exercise-induced anaphylaxis is quite basic.

Avoid the triggering food for up to five hours before exercising, avoid exercising in warmer weather, never exercise alone, stop exercising once symptoms begin, and always carry a cell phone and an auto-injectable epinephrine device. Unlike exercise-induced asthma that may be prevented or lessened with pre-medication and warm-up exercises, such measures are not effective in preventing food-triggered, exercise-induced anaphylaxis.

■ Do Not Jog Alone!

The following report of exercise-induced anaphylaxis, published the *La Crosse* (Wisconsin) *Tribune* in February 2006 points out why individuals prone to anaphylaxis should never exercise alone.[1]

> Taylor Williams is celebrating his 18th birthday today. He doesn't take this birthday lightly. Not after what happened when he almost died on a La Crosse (Wisconsin) sidewalk. Taylor had a food allergy reaction and went into anaphylactic shock and barely made it to the hospital in time to save his life. Taylor knew he was allergic to shellfish because he had a reaction two years ago. His tongue swelled, he said, and he broke out in hives. Tests confirmed the allergy. He stayed away from crab, lobster and shrimp. But salmon never gave him trouble.
>
> Taylor and friend Adam Heffernan went jogging at about 8 p.m. to work off some of the holiday eating before the Christmas break ended. Two hours earlier, the Central High School senior and his family had eaten a meal of a small salad, baked salmon and canned pears. The two had run about a mile when Taylor became violently ill. "I thought I was having heartburn, I hurt so in the middle of the chest, and I was light-headed," Taylor said. "I threw up, I had a bad headache and I had to sit down because I was dizzy." They tried to get passers-by and people in the neighborhood to call 911, but no one responded.
>
> Adam ran back to Taylor's house, where he tracked down Taylor's mother, Kim. "He blurted out that Taylor was in trouble," said Ron Williams, Taylor's father. He and Adam quickly drove to near 15th and State streets, where they found Taylor lying on the sidewalk, "in real trouble," Ron said. "Things got foggy when my dad arrived," Taylor said. "I couldn't lift my head, I was really wheezing bad, and I panicked because I couldn't see." Through it all, "he was able to tell me that he thought he was having an allergic reaction to something," Ron said. Ron carried Taylor to the car, and Adam drove them to Franciscan Skemp Medical Center. "I instructed Adam to slow down for traffic lights and signed intersections to check for traffic, but not stop," Ron said. "I knew we had very few minutes to spare. "Just within the few seconds we had arrived and carried Taylor to the car, he had deteriorated rapidly," Ron said. "By the time we had arrived at the hospital, Taylor had completely lost his vision and was choking and unable to breathe on his own. I was pounding on his chest to help keep him breathing."
>
> At the hospital, Ron laid Taylor on the floor in the emergency room. Staff there quickly confirmed the severe allergic reaction, Ron said. "When he arrived, they were unable to detect a blood pressure. It took about 30 minutes to get his vital signs stabilized, and was at least two hours before they moved him out of the emergency room to an intensive care unit." Quick actions might have been the difference in Taylor's survival, doctors said. "We were told that Taylor was probably within two to five minutes from an irreversible situation and possible death," Ron said. Taylor spent the night and part of the next day in intensive care, and was released from the hospital a couple of days later. They still weren't sure what caused the reaction. Now, more than a month later, they know— Taylor tested positive to salmon on a skin test, and is being tested for other

[1] Terry Rindfleisch, *La Crosse* (WI) *Tribune,* February 12, 2006.

food allergies. Taylor now carries a rescue asthma inhaler and EpiPen, with injectable epinephrine, in case he has a food allergy reaction. He also has an EpiPen available at school, home and in the family car. "I only had one food allergy reaction before, so I never expected to have a serious one like this," Taylor said. "I will be better prepared if it happens again."

Idiopathic Anaphylaxis

This term refers to repeated anaphylactic reactions where no cause can be determined after an extensive allergy evaluation. Idiopathic anaphylaxis affects individuals of all ages and is more common in adult females. Many allergy practices report that 40 to 80 percent of patients seen with anaphylaxis have idiopathic anaphylaxis. Dr. Phillip Lieberman reported that 77 percent of 593 anaphylactic patients in his clinic had idiopathic anaphylaxis. These high numbers may overestimate the incidence of idiopathic anaphylaxis, as only the toughest cases end up in an allergist's office.

> *Dr. Phillip Lieberman reported that 77 percent of 593 anaphylactic patients in his clinic had idiopathic anaphylaxis.*

As with other forms of anaphylaxis, idiopathic anaphylaxis can be life threatening. Prophylactic treatment with a combination of medications usually controls symptoms. Some patients may require long-term treatment with low doses of an oral cortisone drug like prednisone. Fortunately, most episodes of idiopathic anaphylaxis subside spontaneously after several months or years.

Near-Fatal and Fatal Food Anaphylaxis

The incidence of near-fatal and fatal anaphylactic reactions to foods has risen dramatically over the past two decades. Tragically, most fatalities occur in victims who were fully aware of their preexisting food allergy. Case studies have found that most near-fatal and fatal anaphylactic food reactions occur in asthmatics who are allergic to peanuts, tree nuts, or seafood. After accidental ingestion of the offending foods, most of these unfortunate individuals were not given the proper emergency care that could have prevented the crisis.

Dr. John Yunginger from the Mayo Clinic in Minnesota collected the first series of fatal case reports on anaphylaxis and food allergy. One case described a peanut-allergic Brown University student who died shortly after she ingested chili laced with peanuts in a local restaurant. Her needless death received national attention and led to congressional hearings that addressed the issues of menu disclosure and food labeling. The other six fatal cases occurred in children and young adults after accidental ingestion of peanuts, tree nuts, and seafood. There were several common features in these preventable deaths. All but one occurred away from the home in local restaurants. Every patient had asthma and a history of a prior allergic reaction to the offending food. Only one patient was carrying a potentially life-saving auto-injectable epinephrine device.

Dr. Hugh Sampson subsequently reported seven near-fatal and six fatal anaphylactic food reactions in children from ages two to seventeen. Once again, all near-fatal and fatal events took place in children and young adults with asthma. In thirteen cases, the victim had a history of a previous reaction to the food and all accidentally ingested the offending food. Symptoms in these patients included tingling, flushing, itching, hives and swelling, air hunger or wheezing, abdominal cramps, vomiting, and cardiovascular collapse in the fatal cases. Most of the patients with fatal reactions did not experience hives or swelling, which could have served as a warning of impending disaster. Some of the fatal cases experienced immediate oral symptoms (itchy mouth), followed by a lulling quiescent period that was followed by major cardiorespiratory collapse. None of the patients who experienced fatal reactions received epinephrine immediately after the onset of their symptoms, whereas all of the survivors received epinephrine within five minutes after developing symptoms. Once again, the most common triggers were peanuts, tree nuts, and seafood.

A Canadian survey from 1986 to 2000 collected thirty-two cases of fatal food anaphylaxis. The most encouraging finding was that there were no reports of deaths in schools or camps after 1994, as compared to four deaths in schools or camps from 1986 to 1994. Twenty of the thirty-two cases involved peanuts or tree nuts. The average age for a peanut or tree nut fatality was twenty-two years, and forty-one years of age for deaths due to other food allergies.

The largest report of fatal food reactions in the United States described thirty-two cases collected by the Food Allergy and Anaphylaxis Network. Most patients were adolescents or young adults. Only three patients were younger than ten years of age. All but one victim had asthma. Ninety percent of deaths were due to peanut or tree nut ingestion, and all but two were aware of a preexisting peanut or tree nut allergy. Two deaths related to fish and milk ingestion occurred in younger children. Most deaths occurred outside the home, including several in college settings. Sad-

ly, only three of these thirty-two victims had an auto-injectable epinephrine device available at the time of their fatal reaction.

An additional twenty-eight cases of fatal food anaphylaxis were reported at the annual meeting of the American Academy of Allergy, Asthma and Immunology in March 2006. With the exception of one fifty-year-old, the victims ranged in age from five to thirty-four years. Seventeen victims were males. Peanuts accounted for fourteen deaths—eight from tree nuts, four from milk, and two from shrimp. All of the victims apparently had asthma, and epinephrine was not available in twenty-three of twenty-five subjects where information was available. The deaths occurred at home, in schools, at friends' homes, in restaurants, and at camps.

Individuals who experienced more than one reaction were more likely to receive epinephrine or seek medical attention. The main reason for not seeking medical attention was that the reaction did not seem to be severe enough to warrant medical care.

In a recent FAAN survey of 507 food-allergic individuals, 96 percent were younger than eighteen years of age. Thirty-eight percent of these patients experienced severe, potentially life-threatening symptoms, such as throat tightness or swelling, coughing or wheezing, and cardiovascular symptoms, like shock or low blood pressure. Despite the severity of their symptoms, only 6 percent received pre-hospital epinephrine and amazingly, only 57 percent sought medical attention. Individuals who experienced more than one reaction were more likely to receive epinephrine or seek medical attention. The main reason for not seeking medical attention was that the reaction did not seem to be severe enough to warrant medical care.

One publication from the Newcastle General Hospital in the United Kingdom generated a lot of controversy. Investigators calculated that, based on the fact that in ten years there were only eight deaths from food allergy in children ages one to fifteen years in the United Kingdom, the risk of a child dying from a food allergy would only be one in 800,000 children per year. Milk caused four of the deaths, and no child under age thirteen died from peanut allergy.

Canadian researchers were not happy with this study, as their data showed the peak age for food-related deaths in Ontario was between fifteen and twenty-five, an age group that was totally excluded in the British survey. They noted (and I agree) that the United Kingdom report could lead to poor compliance and a dangerous overconfidence regarding the risks of fatal food allergy. Patients, families, doctors, schools, and child-care providers affected by severe food allergy might interpret this paper to mean that death from food allergy is very unlikely, and they might relax their vigilance.

◼ Additional Cases of Fatal Food Anaphylaxis

Many cases of fatal food anaphylaxis are not reported in the medical literature. Several unreported fatal reactions have been cited in the media and lay press.

- A thirty-seven-year-old woman banker died after eating a single spoonful of ice cream containing walnuts.

- A thirteen-year-old girl died after eating chips with curry sauce containing a tiny amount of peanut butter.
- A fourteen-year-old male with severe asthma and milk allergy died after ingesting powdered milk, which was an ingredient in a package of Crisps.
- A twenty-eight-year-old died after failing to see a peanut warning label obscured by the price sticker.
- A thirty-six-year-old woman died on an airliner after being served a meal with peanuts.
- A twenty-eight-year-old biochemist with nut allergy died after touching them in a bowl and brushing his hand across his face.
- An eighteen-year-old college student with a known nut allergy collapsed after eating in an Indian Restaurant and died after returning to her dorm to get medication.

Two additional reports highlight the dangers of inhaling food vapors.

- A twenty-nine-year-old asthmatic with severe seafood allergy finished a chicken meal in restaurant. Just as she was about to leave, a waiter carrying a hot steaming plate of shrimp passed by her table. She immediately experienced respiratory collapse and died fifty-eight minutes after the onset of her symptoms.
- A young woman with a history of a near-fatal reaction to milk reportedly died after walking through a room where milk was stored.

◼ Take-Home Messages

The take-home messages of these heart-breaking reports are:

- Waiters do not prepare your food. Food-allergic patients should speak with the restaurant manager or chef before ordering foods that may contain hidden food allergens.

- Patients and parents must learn to constantly read menus and food labels and be very vigilant in restaurants where cross-contamination or spatula carry-over may occur.
- Seafood-allergic individuals should avoid restaurants where steamed seafood is served in dining areas.
- The majority of victims were young adults with asthma.
- Most fatal reactions took place in restaurants, schools, camps, or college settings.
- Most victims knew they were allergic to the food that killed them. One exception was a two-year old child with no prior history of asthma or a food allergy who died after eating Brazil nuts. The other was a camp counselor with a known peanut allergy who had a fatal reaction to pistachios.
- Most allergens were hidden in desserts, cookies, candies, egg rolls, cakes, sauces, and ice cream.
- In most fatal cases, food labeling on packaged foods was inadequate.
- Most fatal reactions were due to peanuts, tree nuts, or seafood.
- The delayed onset of nausea, vomiting, or diarrhea, and lack of skin symptoms (hives) was an ominous sign. The first symptom was often difficulty breathing or asthma.
- Most victims did not receive or have their auto-injectable epinephrine with them at the time of their fatal reaction.

■ Risk Takers

Allergy researchers are trying to determine why young adults with asthma are more prone to near-fatal or fatal food reactions compared to younger children and older adults. One possible reason is that the typical adolescent is a big risk taker. FAAN and allergy specialists at The Jaffe Food Allergy Institute surveyed 174 teens (ranging in age from thirteen to twenty-one years) with a food allergy. While the majority (74 percent) carried their epinephrine with them most of the time, many admitted to "taking a risk" and not carrying epinephrine when they visited a friend's home, went to a dance, wore tight clothes, or participated in sports. Twenty-nine of these teens were labeled as "risk takers" in that they were less likely to carry their epinephrine and admitted that they would eat a food even though the label stated that it "may contain" an allergen to which they were allergic.

Participants in this study indicated a strong interest in having their friends educated about food allergy. This study points out that education of teenagers and their peers might reduce the consequences of risk taking in this highly vulnerable age group. The teen support programs offered by FAAN, such as PAL (Protect a Life) and their Web site for teenagers and young adults, offer valuable educational information on how educated peers can reduce the risks of life-threatening food reactions in their friends (and lovers) with food allergies. ●

Chapter 6

Treatment of Anaphylaxis

This chapter mainly deals with the diagnosis and emergency treatment of anaphylaxis outside the hospital. All first responders to a victim of an acute allergic reaction or anaphylaxis (including the patient) should be thoroughly familiar with the signs and symptoms of anaphylaxis presented in the prior chapter. They should know when and how to administer auto-injectable epinephrine and initiate other life-saving first aid measures. This responsibility applies to everyone, including the patient, family members, and school, restaurant, or camp personnel.

Most victims of fatal anaphylaxis die at home, in schools, camps, or eating establishments within minutes after their symptoms begin. Very few, if any, victims of anaphylaxis die once they get to an emergency room. Thus, non-medical personnel—including the patient, family, friends, fellow students, school, camp and restaurant personnel—have the best chance to save the life of a victim experiencing a life-threatening allergic reaction.

Non-medical personnel—including the patient, family, friends, fellow students, school, camp and restaurant personnel—have the best chance to save the life of a victim experiencing a life-threatening allergic reaction.

■ History of Epinephrine

Epinephrine, the first human hormone to be discovered, is produced in small amounts by our adrenal glands located near the kidneys. When man is confronted by anxiety, danger, or stress, the brain sends messages to the adrenal gland that increases epinephrine production. This, in turn, increases alertness, energy level, heart rate, blood pressure, and strength. This reaction is known as the "fight or flight response," in which a person's physical strength increases to combat (fight) the problem at hand or escape (flight) the stressful situation.

The British physiologist Edward Sharpey-Schäfer first described the potency of adrenal extracts in 1894, when he injected an adrenal extract into experimental animals and observed that their blood vessels were constricted, which forced a rise in blood pressure.

In 1901, based on work by American pharmacologist John Jacob Abel, the Japanese-American chemist Jokichi Takemine and Sharpey-Schäfer's colleagues isolated adrenaline. Later epinephrine became the generic name for adrenaline in the United States, Canada, and Japan. However, the term, adrenaline, is still used today in the United Kingdom. Epinephrine was soon made available to treat asthma, hemorrhage and shock, and allergic reactions. One hundred years later, the treatment of choice for an allergic reaction is still adrenaline, or epinephrine, which is now available in individual vials for hospital use and as auto-injectors devices for use outside the hospital—sold under the brand names EpiPen 2-Pak, or Twinject auto-Injector.

Thanks to the important research of Dr. Estelle Simons at the University of Manitoba, we know that epinephrine must be injected into a muscle and not subcutaneously, or just under the skin. By measuring the amount of epinephrine in the blood stream after an intramuscular (IM) versus a subcutaneous (SC) injection, Simons found the maximum blood concentration of epinephrine was achieved in approximately five minutes with an IM thigh injection, compared to approximately twenty minutes for a SC injection. (Do not administer epinephrine in the upper arm or deltoid muscle as studies have shown this is no better than a SC injection.) Unfortunately, Simons' important message has not been widely publicized. I recently gave a talk on anaphylaxis to emergency room nurses and other health-care providers.

Many attendees were surprised to learn that an IM injection was the preferred route of administration. Proper doses and indications for epinephrine administration will be covered later in this chapter.

In my earlier medical career, I moonlighted in emergency rooms two to three nights a week. Most of the lives I saved in this role were due to the use of epinephrine, one of the few life-saving drugs in medicine. Epinephrine combats anaphylaxis by raising heart rate and blood pressure, constricting blood vessels, and opening up constricted bronchial tubes. Minor side effects—such as a pounding heart, pallor, dizziness, tremors, and headache—do not last very long as epinephrine is rapidly metabolized by the body. While epinephrine has trace amounts of sulfites, this is no reason to withhold this drug in a sulfite-allergic patient as epinephrine-sulfite reactions are very rare. Dosing adjustments may have to be made with the eld-

erly, in people with heart disease, high blood pressure, abnormal heart rates, or those who are taking psychotropic drugs. Persons taking beta-blocking drugs may need repeated doses of epinephrine as beta blockers tie up the sites (the beta receptors) where epinephrine acts. In summary, there is no medical contraindication to administering epinephrine in a life-threatening situation!

Anyone who experiences symptoms of an allergic or anaphylactic reaction should administer or be administered epinephrine, take an antihistamine like Benadryl (preferably in liquid form to hasten absorption), call 911, or immediately go to the nearest emergency room. If you have asthma and experience coughing or wheezing, you should also use your quick-relief asthma inhaler. Carry extra auto-injector epinephrine devices on trips or while camping, boating, golfing, or engaging in activities where immediate medical care is not readily available.

Once you reach the emergency facility, doctors may administer additional drugs to treat anaphylaxis, including intravenous antihistamines and cortisone to hasten the recovery from an anaphylactic reaction. One new epinephrine product under development that appears promising is an under-the-tongue or sublingual tablet. In one study in rabbits, satisfactory blood levels were obtained with a 40 mg sublingual dose. Older

In my earlier medical career, I moonlighted in emergency rooms two to three nights a week. Most of the lives I saved in this role were due to the use of epinephrine, one of the few life-saving drugs in medicine.

metered-dose inhalers, like the Medihaler Epi that contain epinephrine, have not been found to be useful in treating anaphylaxis.

Auto-injector epinephrine devices are available for use in the home, school, or in public places. As many patients need more than one dose of epinephrine, the two kits available in the United States, EpiPen 2-Pak and Twinject auto-injector, contain two doses in both pediatric and adult strength doses. Proper use of these devices is depicted in their package inserts, product Web sites and the Food Allergy Action Plan (see appendix, page 271).

■ Tips: Preparing for and Treating Anaphylaxis

- Keep the epinephrine devices in a safe, accessible place.
- Check expiration dates frequently.
- Do not refrigerate or keep in hot automobiles.
- Always carry two doses of injectable epinephrine.
- If more than one dose is needed, do not delay. Give it right away!
- Always carry an oral antihistamine like Benadryl.
- If you have asthma, carry your asthma rescue inhaler.
- Only administer epinephrine in the upper outer thigh muscle.
- While epinephrine can be injected through clothing, avoid injecting it through heavy material like denim.
- If the device is outdated and no other treatment is available, give it anyway. One study found that most of thirty-two outdated EpiPens still contained some active drug.

■ When to Prescribe Epinephrine

One of the more difficult decisions for health-care providers regarding acute aller-

gic reactions to food or any other allergen is when to prescribe injectable epinephrine. I prescribe auto-injectable epinephrine to the following patients or families:

- Anyone who has experienced an acute allergic reaction to any allergen, even if the symptoms were mild
- Anyone who has reacted to a small amount of allergen
- Anyone with a skin disease that may mask the skin symptoms of an allergic reaction
- Anyone with a history of an allergic reaction and a history of alcohol or drug abuse
- Anyone who lives in a remote area or if there is a lack of telephones
- Anyone with an inability to communicate due to age, disabilities, or a language barrier
- Many allergy specialists do not prescribe epinephrine to patients with mild reactions from fruits and vegetables like those seen in the oral allergy syndrome. However, as a small percentage of these patients can progress to full-blown anaphylaxis, I prescribe epinephrine to all these patients.
- What about the sibling of patients with asthma and peanut- or tree nut-allergies who has a positive skin or blood test to peanuts or tree nuts but who has never ingested nuts before? As these children have a 50 percent chance of experiencing a reaction to a peanut or tree nut, they should be given a prescription for an auto-injectable epinephrine device.

■ When to Administer Epinephrine

The toughest question for the health-care provider, patient, family, caretaker, or first responder is when do you administer auto-injectable epinephrine. Like all decisions in medicine, it requires clinical judgment. I usually recommend administering epinephrine in the following situations:

- Any patient experiencing an allergic reaction who has a history of a prior allergic or anaphylactic reaction to food, stinging insect, or any other allergen that is documented by positive skin or CAP RAST blood tests. The one exception is that patients who have only mild skin reactions (a few hives) may not require epinephrine.
- Any patient experiencing an anaphylactic reaction who has asthma, especially uncontrolled asthma. These patients are most at risk for a severe non-fatal or fatal reaction.
- Children and adults with asthma and a history of a peanut or tree nut allergy
- Any patient experiencing an allergic reaction in remote locations where the nearest emergency room is a fair distance away—especially when hiking, camping, boating or golfing
- Anyone who has previously reacted to a small amount of allergen
- If a skin disease may mask the symptoms of an allergic reaction
- If there is history of alcohol or drug abuse
- Anyone who lives alone or in a remote area or has no telephones
- Inability to communicate due to age, disability, or a language barrier
- When there is a dysfunctional family situation

When Should You Go to the Emergency Room?

Many patients, families, and caretakers are totally confused as to when victims of anaphylaxis should go to an emergency room for treatment of their allergic reaction. Some patients stay at home. Many of my patients have foolishly gone to bed while in the midst of an acute reaction! All too many victims, especially children who experience a reaction at a day-care center or school, are taken to a local clinic or doctor's office that is not properly equipped to treat a severe allergic reaction. Such sites may not have oxygen, IV fluids, medications, cardiovascular monitoring equipment, or a health-care professional experienced in the treatment of life-threatening anaphylaxis. My guidelines for going to an emergency room are:

- Whenever epinephrine is administered
- Whenever there is more than just skin involvement
- Whenever there is a history of a previous reaction, especially a severe one
- Whenever the victim has asthma
- Whenever the patient is on heart or blood pressure drugs, like beta-blockers or ACE inhibitors
- Whenever the reaction takes place in an eating establishment
- Whenever there is a dysfunctional caretaker situation or a language barrier

Impending Doom

Whether you are a parent, school nurse, teacher, EMT, or an emergency room nurse or doctor, do not delay treating a victim experiencing an allergic reaction who says, "I feel like I am going to die!" In most instances, they are right on. A feeling of impending doom is a very ominous sign—these patients can crash very quickly. If you are the first responder to a victim of anaphylaxis, administer epinephrine immediately and call 911. If you are working in a hospital emergency department or clinic, do not let these patients sit in the waiting room or stop to fill out consent or insurance forms at a registration desk. After my discharge from the Air Force,

I worked in the emergency room at Cape Cod Hospital in Hyannis, Massachusetts, for an entire summer. On one evening when I was busy treating trauma patients, a nurse told me there was a patient in the waiting room who needed immediate attention. An elderly gentleman who had just been stung by an insect told this nurse, "I feel like I am going to die." Even though he did not appear to be in any great distress, she immediately brought him into a treatment room. Lo and behold, before we started any treatment he collapsed and went into severe shock. Thanks to the insight of this perceptive nurse, he survived.

Not all symptoms of anaphylaxis have to be present, nor do they appear in any special order. A lot depends on the timing and the amount of food ingested. The onset of symptoms varies. It is faster with drugs, X-ray dyes, and stinging insects, about fifteen minutes, compared to food reactions, about thirty minutes. In "protracted" anaphylaxis, the episode fails to resolve in a timely manner and continues on a prolonged course. These patients may require large amounts of intravenous fluids to maintain their blood pressure. A delayed onset of symptoms without skin reactions can be a bad sign, as these patients often

Co-factors which may increase the severity of an anaphylactic reaction include poorly controlled asthma, alcohol intake, exercise, use of aspirin-like drugs called non-steroidal inflammatory drugs (NSAIDs), beta blocking drugs, ACE inhibitor drugs, and general anesthesia.

experience more severe, difficult-to-treat reactions. Co-factors which may increase the severity of an anaphylactic reaction include poorly controlled asthma, alcohol intake, exercise, use of aspirin-like drugs called non-steroidal inflammatory drugs (NSAIDs), beta blocking drugs, ACE inhibitor drugs, and general anesthesia.

■ Do Not Sit Up!

One vital maneuver in treating anaphylaxis outside the hospital was pointed out by Dr. Richard Pumphrey from Manchester, England. Pumphrey studied anaphylactic deaths that occurred outside of the hospital and found that several victims died within seconds after being moved from a prone or a reclined position to an upright position.

The explanation for this is that transferring a patient in shock from a prone position to a sitting or standing position prevents blood from the lower parts of the body from returning to the heart resulting in what is called "the empty heart syndrome." All first responders who encounter victims with cardiovascular distress, such as fainting, syncope, dizziness, or collapse, need to lay the victims down and elevate their legs. Victims who have nausea or vomiting should be placed on their sides to prevent aspiration of stomach contents into the lung. Anaphylactic victims experiencing respiratory distress who appear to have normal blood pressure may be better off if kept in an upright position.

■ Need for More Education

Some authorities think epinephrine is overutilized, while others feel it is underutilized. Several papers suggest that physicians, EMTs, and emergency room doctors need more education in this area. Pediatric and internal medicine residents and staff doctors at the Mount Sinai Hospital in New York City were presented a hypothetical case of a young adult male with a history of nut allergy and asthma who came to the emergency room with hives and a cough after accidentally ingesting a snack bar that contained mixed nuts. These doctors were asked to review this case and answer four basic questions regarding treatment, observation time, prescribed medications, and risk factors for a near-fatal or fatal food reaction.

Most doctors at this major teaching hospital with a superb allergy training program flunked the quiz. Only one in three knew that epinephrine should be administered into the muscle, not subcutaneously. Less than 50 percent recommended keeping the patient in the emergency room for four to six hours to be observed for a biphasic or delayed reaction. Only one in four doctors identified the risk factors for severe reactions, such as a history of asthma and an allergy to peanuts or tree nuts. If the staff in a major teaching hospital with a world-class allergy-training program could not answer these questions correctly, it is quite likely that community-based health-care providers would do even worse.

Another study recruited 100 doctors and tested them on the use of an EpiPen device. Amazingly only two doctors knew the six steps in giving EpiPen, and only 30 percent would have given the correct dose. Ninety-five had to read the instructions, and then only 40 percent of them got it right. A survey of seventy-five primary care and ER doctors found that discharge instructions about anaphylaxis were provided by only 25 percent, and only 30 percent would refer the patient to an allergy specialist. Many professionals in this survey were not comfortable with the diagnosis and management of anaphylaxis and felt they needed more education on anaphylaxis. Simons found that only 60 per-

cent of patients in her allergy clinic at the University of Manitoba who had been prescribed an epinephrine device had it with them at their clinic visit, and only 16 percent of patients who had been advised to wear a MedicAlert device wore it at the time of a visit. Reasons for not wearing the MedicAlert device included the cost of the device, skin rashes, broken or lost devices, and the fact that a young child was always with a caregiver.

■ Keep Your Thumb Off It!

There is a natural instinct for those administering an auto-injectable epinephrine device to place a finger over the spring-loaded, uncapped end of the device. There are several reports of lay people and health-care professionals (including one of my nurses) who self-injected epinephrine into their fingers or thumb. Ouch! Such an accidental injection requires warm

> *The bottom line: keep your thumb off it; do not place your thumb or finger over the uncapped end of the auto-injectable epinephrine device.*

soaks to counteract the vasoconstrictive effects of the epinephrine. In some cases, emergency care and the administration of vasodilating drugs is needed. The bottom line: keep your thumb off it; do not place your thumb or finger over the uncapped end of the auto-injectable epinephrine device.

■ A Personal Encounter with Anaphylaxis

Does everyone experiencing an anaphylactic reaction who gets to an emergency room need epinephrine? Most allergy specialists, including myself, would answer yes to that question. Recent symposia and practice parameters state, "Injectable epinephrine is the treatment of choice for anaphylaxis and antihistamines are slow in onset and are second line drugs in anaphylaxis treatment." While there is no question that epinephrine is the preferred drug in the initial treatment of anaphylaxis occurring outside the hospital, there is some debate between emergency room physicians and allergists if epinephrine is the drug of choice for treating anaphylaxis in patients presenting to an emergency department without respiratory compromise, low blood pressure, or associated symptoms of end-organ dysfunction (e.g., collapse, fainting, or incontinence). Having had a personal encounter with anaphylaxis, I now tend to side with the emergency room doctors in this debate.

In a survey at the Beaumont Army Medical Center in Texas, only 50 percent of anaphylactic victims got epinephrine, and most of the time it was administered subcutaneously.

In July 2005, about fifteen minutes after taking two naproxen (Aleve) tabs prior to a round of golf, I experienced intense itching in my groin that was immediately followed by generalized itching, redness and swelling of my hands, feet, and tongue. Naturally, the two EpiPens I had at home were a few months outdated. (I usually carry them everywhere despite the fact I had no prior history of anaphylaxis.) As my heart was pounding and I had no obvious symptoms of respiratory or cardiovascular compromise, I elected not to self-administer Epipen—even though I was aware that the outdated device probably still contained some active drug.

My daughter then drove me to a local emergency room where a receptionist asked me to take a seat and fill out some insurance forms. Needless to say, I walked right by him and spoke to the admitting nurse and told her I was a staff allergist who was experiencing an anaphylactic reaction. Once I convinced her that this was not a joke, I was promptly put in a treatment bay and connected to an IV line and monitor. My pulse rate was 120, my BP was 160/110, and my oxygen level was normal. I did not have shortness of breath, but I looked like a boiled lobster. I also had some swelling of my tongue, palate, and uvula.

I briefly debated the merits of epinephrine treatment with the on-duty emergency physician, who was understandably reluctant to administer epinephrine in view of my age, fast pulse rate, and high blood pressure. He promptly administered IV antihistamines, diphenhydramine (Benadryl), cimetidine (Tagamet), and a cortisone (SoluMedrol) drug. The result was somewhat amazing. Within one to two minutes, I could feel (and see) the redness, swelling and itch of my hands, feet, and tongue resolving. Fifteen minutes later, I was dozing off with a pulse rate of 80 and a BP of 110/60. I did persuade the staff to keep me around for four hours, and I had a long nap in the emergency room cubicle. The emergency room did a fine job with discharge planning, in that they had up-to-date EpiPens on site and provided me with an informational printout with follow-up instructions that included a referral to an allergy specialist—me.

Recent studies by the Emergency Medicine Network suggest that epinephrine is vastly underutilized in emergency rooms.[1] In a chart review of 678 patients presenting with food allergy to twenty-one North American emergency rooms, only 16 percent received epinephrine. Another study reviewed the charts of 617 patients with insect sting allergy. In this cohort, 58 percent had local reactions, 11 percent had mild systemic reactions, and 31 percent had anaphylactic reactions as defined by multi-system organ involvement or low blood pressure. However, only 12 percent received epinephrine. In both these studies, more than 95 percent of the patients were discharged to home, suggesting (perhaps) that maybe epinephrine was not needed in many cases.

Dr. Bodo Niggemann from the University Medical Center in Berlin, Germany, collected data on German children who had experienced anaphylaxis. Boys were more commonly affected than girls. The average age of a reaction was five years. Nearly two-thirds of the reactions took place at home, and 58 percent were triggered by foods, especially peanuts and tree nuts. Only 20 percent received epinephrine. Niggemann concluded that 75 percent of these children were undertreated. In a survey at the Beaumont Army Medical Center in Texas, only 50 percent of anaphylactic victims got epinephrine, and most of the time it was administered subcutaneously.

When I was working in emergency rooms in the 1970s and 1980s, the thinking at that time was: "think epi—give epi!" Recommended doses of epinephrine (0.01 milligrams [mg] per kilogram [kg], up to a maximum of 0.50 mg) were routinely administered in this pre-auto-injector era. Patients weighing over 100 pounds, or 50 kg, who were usually given a full 0.50 mg dose of epinephrine often developed pallor,

[1] S. Clark and others, "Multicenter Study of Emergency Department Visits for Food Allergy," Emergency Medicine Network, www.emnet-usa.org (last updated August 30, 2004).

tremors and palpitations—an acceptable side effect in those days. After my own encounter with anaphylaxis, I am not so sure that the underutilization of epinephrine by emergency room physicians is as bad as we allergists perceive. (I wonder where my pulse rate and BP might have gone had I been given epinephrine.) I do not know of any case reports of fatal anaphylaxis in stable patients who have died in an emergency room.

Most reports in the lay media and medical literature describe anaphylactic fatalities occurring suddenly and unexpectedly outside the hospital. Despite the alleged expertise of allergists in treating anaphylaxis, emergency room doctors are more experienced in treating anaphylaxis. The experience of most allergists (thankfully) is limited to treating mild-to-moderate anaphylactic reactions to allergy injections in an office setting.

As an aside, now that I am no longer able to take naproxen or other non-steroidal, anti-inflammatory drugs, or NSAIDs, before teeing off, my golf handicap has gone from an eight to a fourteen—an unfortunate development that goes beyond the scope of this discussion.

I was more than impressed with the rapid onset of action of the IV antihistamines. The dogma that antihistamines are slow in onset and are second-line drugs in anaphylaxis may only apply to oral antihistamines. Clinical trials in patients presenting to an emergency room with anaphylaxis that compare IM epinephrine to IV antihistamines might be worthwhile in patients with a normal or high blood pressure, with no cardiovascular or respiratory compromise, and with no signs of end-organ dysfunction. As an aside, now that I am no longer able to take naproxen or other non-steroidal, anti-inflammatory drugs, or NSAIDs, before teeing off, my golf handicap has gone from an eight to a fourteen—an unfortunate development that goes beyond the scope of this discussion.

An Ideal World

In an ideal world, victims of anaphylaxis—especially those with delayed intestinal symptoms, low blood pressure, a history of asthma, or a prior severe reaction—should be treated in an emergency facility and observed for four to six hours before being discharged. Prolonged visits for milder allergic reactions may not be prudent in today's crowded emergency rooms. Such patients can be advised to sit in the waiting area before they are discharged to a friend or family member and given computer-generated discharge forms describing their reaction and the need for appropriate follow-up with their primary doctor and an allergy specialist.

One study found that only 8 percent of parents trained to administer epinephrine actually administered it when it was indicated.

Savvy emergency rooms will keep a supply of auto-injectable epinephrine devices on hand to demonstrate their use and give to patients or their families at the time of their discharge. Thus, if a discharged patient experiences a biphasic reaction while driving home from the emergency room, epinephrine could be self-administered, saving precious time before returning to the hospital for additional treatment.

Emergency Room Discharge Information

A patient released from a hospital after being treated for anaphylaxis should be given a printed "discharge instruction" (DI) form that advises the individual on his or her medical condition and recommends follow-up care. After reviewing DI forms from various companies that provide these instructions to hospitals, FAAN discovered that many forms contained incomplete or inaccurate information. In response, FAAN's Medical Advisory Board created its own model DI forms and has made them available to companies that provide such forms to more than a thousand hospitals.

Don't Be Timid!

Several neat studies point out that repeated educational efforts are required to ensure that parents and caretakers know when and how to administer epinephrine. Parents and caretakers frequently admit they are afraid to administer epinephrine. One study found that only 8 percent of parents trained to administer epinephrine actually administered it when it was indicated.

A survey of well-educated parents attending a food allergy support group found that only eleven of forty-one parents administered epinephrine during an allergic reaction. Most (72 percent) felt the reaction was not severe enough. Other reasons for not giving epinephrine were close proximity to a hospital and concern about pain or side effects. A study at the University of Florida tested 224 parents in the proper use of an EpiPen at repeated visits. At the first visit, only 22 percent of parents passed the test; but after three visits, 94 percent properly administered the EpiPen. The biggest mistakes were not pressing until you felt the click and not holding it for ten seconds. The most commonly cited reasons for being reluctant to administer epinephrine were:

- Failure to recognize the symptoms of anaphylaxis
- A conception that the reaction was mild
- A health-care facility was nearby
- An over-reliance on oral antihistamines
- A history of spontaneous recovery after a pervious episode
- Concerns about side effects
- A fear of a painful needle injection

Two European studies reinforce the need for more aggressive educational efforts in this area. A survey in France found that most parents had a poor knowledge regarding the use of auto-injectable epinephrine devices. Another study from an allergy center in Manchester, England, found that 69 percent of parents were unable to use an auto-injector device correctly, did not have it available, or did not know when to use it.

■ Double Up

More cases of food-allergy fatalities are being reported in victims who immediately received auto-injectable epinephrine. In 1997, the *Food Allergy News* reported the death of a college student who died after putting a peanut-laden cookie up to her mouth to see if the cookie made her mouth tingle. She died despite being administered EpiPen immediately. A lacrosse player from Massachusetts who died after eating pistachios reportedly received epinephrine right after the onset of his reaction. Such case reports have puzzled many researchers. One answer to this dilemma is that current doses administered by epinephrine devices may be too low or that

many patients do not get a much-needed second dose of epinephrine. A review of seventeen fatal reactions after allergy injections found that nine had received the recommended dose of epinephrine either immediately or within three minutes of the start of their reaction. Only one patient received the equivalent of 1 mg, or two doses of 0.50 mg.

How often is a second dose of epinephrine needed? A survey at a naval hospital in San Diego, California, found that ten of sixty-four cases (16 percent) needed a second dose. A similar study in St. Louis found thirty-eight patients of 105 (36 percent) needed a second dose. Dr. Phillip Lieberman surveyed fifty caregivers of children and fifty adults who had experienced anaphylaxis. One-third of anaphylactic victims who reacted outside the hospital required two epinephrine injections. While 50 percent of the patients treated in an in emergency facility required two injections, only 16 percent of those surveyed carried two auto-injector epinephrine doses. Lieberman appropriately concluded that the majority of persons at risk for anaphylaxis were not prepared to treat a reaction requiring more than one dose of epinephrine.

Today's auto-injector epinephrine devices come in only two strengths: a 0.15 mg and a 0.30 mg dose. The usual dose for treating anaphylaxis ranges from 0.10 mg in a small child to 0.50 mg in a full-grown adult. What should you do with children who fall between those doses? For example, if the normal dose for a 40-pound child is 0.20 mg, should you underdose or overdose with epinephrine? Simons has provided guidance to this quandary by advising treatment with the higher strength epinephrine if one or more of the following circumstances:

- The patient has asthma
- The food trigger is a peanut, a tree nut, milk, egg, or a seafood
- There is poor access to emergency medical services
- There is a dysfunctional family situation
- There is no reliable transportation available
- The patient has a past history of a life-threatening reaction

In my emergency room days before the auto-injectors were available, I always gave 0.50 mg to anyone weighing over 100 pounds. This was the dose recommended by every article and medical textbook on anaphylaxis. Many of these patients required a second dose of epinephrine. One British guideline recommends intramuscular injection of 0.50 mg in adult patients and repeating it in five minutes if indicated. Today, the first dose delivered by the auto-injector devices, EpiPen and Twinject, is only 0.30 mg—only 60 percent of the recommended 0.50 mg dose.

Thus, many first responders, doctors and EMTs administer the same dose of epinephrine to a 60-pound child as they would give to a 280-pound NFL linebacker.

Thus, many first responders, doctors, and EMTs administer the same dose of epinephrine to a 60-pound child as they would give to a 280-pound NFL linebacker. In my opinion, this may be the major reason for loss of life when epinephrine is promptly administered. These dosing shortcomings have been somewhat resolved by the availability of the EpiPen 2-Pak, which provides two syringes of 0.30 mg of epinephrine and the Twinject, which contains a second dose of 0.30 mg that has to be self-injected. I now advise all my patients and families to carry the two-dose versions of auto-injectable epinephrine devices. The manufacturers of these devices, Dey Laboratories and Verus Pharmaceuticals, are developing auto-injectors with lower doses for very young children weighing less than thirty pounds, and higher dose devices for adults weighing over 100 pounds.

What about teaching patients or parents to administer the proper dose of epinephrine the way they do it in hospitals—by drawing up the exact dose from a vial of epinephrine? Dr. Estelle Simons tested eighteen parents by giving them instructions and then asking them to rapidly draw up an exact dose of 0.09 ml and correctly administer it. Most parents failed the test. Simons concluded that it was safer to continue to rely on the preloaded auto-injectors even if some patients received more than the recommended dose.

■ Emergency Medical Technicians and Epinephrine

Most communities have three types of EMTs: EMT-Basics, EMT-Intermediates and EMT-Paramedics. In many states, some EMTs may not be authorized to carry or administer epinephrine. A FAAN survey found many states only authorize EMT-Paramedics (and sometimes EMT-Intermediates) to administer epinephrine. EMT-Basics were only permitted to "assist" a patient with the patient's own prescribed auto-injector epinephrine device. FAAN members, along with medical professionals, allergists, lawmakers, and emergency personnel, undertook an initiative to encourage laws or regulations that would make epinephrine available to EMT-Basics in all states. Thanks to this initiative, laws or regulations have been enacted in twenty-nine states and are pending in several more. FAAN hopes that EMT/epinephrine coverage will become seamless nationwide, enabling all EMTs to arrive at the scene both equipped with and authorized to administer epinephrine. FAAN advises individuals to contact their state EMT agencies or their local ambulance services to clarify the coverage in their particular area.

■ Who Should Carry Auto-injectable Epinephrine Devices?

Who, besides patients, families, and caretakers, should have access to or carry auto-injectable epinephrine devices? One answer to this question might be that every responsible person, especially health-care providers who are capable of properly recognizing the signs and symptoms of anaphylaxis and treating an anaphylactic reaction, should carry a life-saving auto-injectable epinephrine device. Consider this 2004 story by Erin Croteau from The *Eagle-Tribune* in North Andover, Massachusetts.

Mystery Nurse Saves Child's Life on Plum Island!

A perfect sunny day at the Plum Island beach turned nightmarish for Robin Farago when her three-year-old son, Anthony, nearly died after eating peanut butter given to him by a family friend. If not for the swift, skillful actions of a registered nurse on the beach, Farago and her husband, Jim, don't know if they would still have their little boy. "The whole thing happened so quickly, I never looked at the woman's face. She told me she had an EpiPen and asked if I wanted her to administer it. I watched her steady hand as she quickly injected it into his upper left thigh," said Farago,

who almost always has her own EpiPen injector handy, but had left it inside her car, 100 yards from where they were on the beach. "I honestly don't know if we would have made it back in time," said Farago. Anthony had his first allergic reaction to nuts at 18 months. "My husband's allergic to dogs, and my mom is very allergic to cashews," Farago said. Despite that family history, Farago thought nothing of giving Anthony peanut butter before his first reaction.

After eating the peanut butter at the beach, Anthony immediately went into anaphylactic shock. "First, he started throwing up. He was crying. He had hives all over his body. His eyes were swollen to the point of almost being shut, and he said his tongue was itchy," Farago said. "Somebody held up a cell phone and asked if they should call 911. Of course I should have, but all I was thinking is, 'I need to get him to the car and then to the hospital.'" Farago scooped up Anthony and two of her other children, and they ran to her friend's car before making a mad dash to a local hospital where Anthony stayed overnight and went home the next day. Farago was so frantic, she left all of the family's belongings on the beach, and she forgot to thank the mystery woman largely responsible for saving her son's life. "It's so hard to put into words, but I will never forget how she was there to help," Farago said. "I don't know if I'd have my son today if she wasn't there, and I'm eternally grateful. I would love to meet her so the whole family can thank her in person for giving us Anthony."

■ A First Responder

One of my avocations in life is golf. My wife labels it as an addiction; hence, she loves the term "golfaholic." My golf club is a nesting ground for stinging insects, especially nasty yellow jackets, which trigger allergic reactions in fellow golfers, caddies, or course employees during the golfing season. Prior to each golfing season, I make sure that EpiPen devices are readily available at the course for treating reactions to these potentially deadly insects. On one summer day after completing play, I was summoned from the nineteenth hole to evaluate a fellow member who had been stung on the golf course. Immediately after being stung, she became dizzy, collapsed, was put in a golf cart, and brought back to the Pro Shop. When I first evaluated her, she was barely conscious. She quickly responded to an EpiPen injection and was then immediately transported to a nearby hospital for additional treatment. After an allergy evaluation, she was successfully treated with venom injections, or immunotherapy.

> *The auto-injectable epinephrine device is a great first aid tool, especially for patients, families, and school and camp personnel involved in remote outdoor activities, such as camping, hiking, boating and golfing.*

This story does not end there. Shortly after being taught how to use her EpiPen device, she was shopping in a local supermarket. Lo and behold, a fellow shopper who was stung by an insect in the produce section immediately developed throat swelling and difficulty breathing. My fellow golfer immediately went to her aid and administered EpiPen to the victim, who quickly recovered and was then transported to a local emergency room. What is the risk of a layperson being sued for administering epinephrine under such circumstances? Most states cover such actions by Good Samaritan Laws. In this particular instance, the supermarket victim thanked her benefactor profusely by sending her a bouquet of flowers.

■ A Take Home Message

These personal experiences, and the fact that most anaphylactic deaths occur suddenly and unexpectedly outside of the hospital, reinforce my opinion that many lives could be saved by the prompt administration of auto-injectable epinephrine by responsible individuals capable of recognizing the signs and symptoms of anaphylaxis and treating an anaphylactic reaction. The auto-injectable epinephrine device is a great first aid tool, especially for patients, families, and school and camp personnel involved in remote outdoor activities, such as camping, hiking, boating, and golfing.

As will be discussed in the chapter entitled "Risky Restaurants," I feel all food establishments should train their staff how to use these life-saving devices. I wholeheartedly agree with Dr. Estelle Simons, past president of the American Academy of Allergy, Asthma and Immunology, who has stated, "Auto-injector epinephrine devices should be readily available anywhere where anaphylaxis is likely to occur."

■ The MedicAlert Foundation

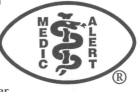

Medical practitioners agree that most vital health information for the proper diagnosis and treatment of any medical condition, especially medical emergencies, comes from the patient's medical history. Should food allergy victims wear a medical emblem that identifies their food allergy? Yes, I believe that any child or adult who has experienced an allergic or anaphylactic reaction should carry or wear such an emblem. Exceptions to this dictum include patients with mild skin reactions or young preschool children who are constantly under the wings of parents or caretakers. Adults who are resistant to wearing a warning bracelet or necklace may opt for a driver's license size card containing pertinent medical information since EMTs usually check purses or wallets to identify victims. While there are several options in the marketplace, the oldest and best service is provided by the MedicAlert Foundation.

In 1953, Linda Collins, the daughter of Dr. Marion and Mrs. Chrissie Collins, had a near-fatal reaction to a tetanus antitoxin scratch test. The realization that their daughter could have died if she had been given the full tetanus injection (that was probably derived from horse serum) made them recognize the need for her to have a personal identification device. Linda's parents then designed an emblem depicting their daughter's allergy that would stand the test of time.

Once the demand for these emblems grew, the MedicAlert Foundation was created. In 1960, it became a national presence in emergency medicine with the launch of a telephone-based service operated out of a hospital in Turlock, California. In 1978, MedicAlert was endorsed by the American College of Emergency Physicians, the Emergency Department Nurses Association, and the National Association of Emergency Medical Technicians.

In the early 1990s, the MedicAlert Foundation developed the ability to store more detailed information, including advanced directives, "do not resuscitate" orders, and medical device instructions.

The increase in international travel prompted the foundation to develop a TravelPlus program. The Internet allows MedicAlert members to update information from any location in the world through their membership number and a password. Privacy and security are never compromised.

In today's connected world, the MedicAlert Foundation provides instant access to patient-centered health information on a global basis at any time of the day or night. In 2004, President George Bush called on the federal government to work toward creating personal electronic medical records for Americans within the next ten years. The health insurance industry also is on board for creating access as long as patient privacy can be assured. In the foreseeable future, it will be possible to enter a universal health identification number that will access one's complete medical history in seconds.

In today's connected world, the MedicAlert Foundation provides instant access to patient-centered health information on a global basis at any time of the day or night.

■ The MedicAlert Foundation 24-Hour Emergency Response Service

This MedicAlert emergency service provides instant identification. The membership number on your emblem allows you to be identified with a simple phone call to a 24-hour emergency response center. MedicAlert personnel then relay key facts to emergency responders that enable members to receive faster and safer treatment. MedicAlert also calls designated family contacts so you won't be alone in an emergency situation. The twenty-four hour emergency response center provides translation in more than 140 languages. MedicAlert now serves more than 4 million members in over fifty different countries and operates out of nine international offices. For a $35 enrollment fee and a $20 annual membership fee, members receive a tag with a description of their health situation, a patient identification number, and a toll-free, twenty-four-hour telephone number for access to more detailed information. This stored information includes current medications and the phone numbers of family members and your primary physician. Medical information on file is relevant emergency information provided by the patient, but it can also include specifics provided by a physician. Members with more complicated medical conditions can carry a MedicAlert membership card next to their driver's license with their patient identification and an 800-number.

> *Remember there are no medical contraindications for administering epinephrine when treating a life-threatening allergic reaction.*

Enrollment in MedicAlert includes establishment of your MedicAlert Electronic Health Record and a MedicAlert Emergency Member Card imprinted with your emergency information, which secures online access to your MedicAlert records. The MedicAlert Emergency Response Center is on call twenty-four hours a day, seven days a week to help you at any time. Members select their choice of MedicAlert identification products from over 150 styles of bracelets and necklaces in stainless steel, silver, or gold. A new product, the MedicAlert E-HealthKEY, allows for portable storage of medical information on a USB-enabled device that members can carry on their keychain.[2]

■ The Anaphylaxis Education Tool Kit

In March 2006, the American Academy of Allergy Asthma, and Immunology (AAAAI) Anaphylaxis Public Education Task Force released its Anaphylaxis Education Tool Kit. This kit was developed in response to an AAAAI Presidential Initiative by Simons. The Tool Kit contains materials to assist health-care professionals to train those at risk for anaphylaxis in the community (and their caregivers) to recognize anaphylaxis and treat it promptly. Resources in the kit include: "Anaphylaxis, a Killer Allergy" (an informational page); "What is Anaphylaxis?" (a brochure from the AAAAI Tips to Remember series); and an Anaphylaxis Emergency Action Plan Wallet Card. Additional contents include allergy stickers; a MedicAlert and FAAN brochure; an EpiPen and Twinject trainer; and a DVD. The kit is designed for educational purposes only. It does not contain any active medications or needles and cannot be used to treat anaphylaxis. Health-care professionals who wish to order this educational kit can get information in the appendix on how to contact AAAAI.

■ EpiPen versus Twinject

Both the EpiPen and Twinject device deliver the same amount of epinephrine in pediatric and adult dosing strengths.[3] As

---

[2] The MedicAlert Foundation's informative Web site is www.medicalert.org. Some international contacts are listed in the appendix.

[3] For instructions on the use of both these devices, see appendix, page 272.

up to 36 percent of anaphylactic victims may need two doses of epinephrine, the manufacturers of these devices provide either a two-dose kit (EpiPen) or one kit (Twinject) that contains two doses in one device.

The EpiPen is a self-activated device that allows a hidden needle to enter the thigh muscle when pressed for ten seconds. When a second dose is needed, you must use a second EpiPen. With the Twinject, the first dose is administered like the EpiPen—by pressing it against the muscle. The second dose must be self-delivered into the muscle by pressing a plunger in a pre-loaded syringe with a visible needle.

The choice between these two devices depends on personal preferences. Our practice demonstrates the proper use of both devices to caretakers and patients and urges them to choose whichever they prefer. An informal poll of our patients reveals an even split between the two devices. Some people, especially health-care personnel, prefer the convenience of the Twinject. One advantage of the Twinject is that it is more compact (about the size of a large cigar) and is less cumbersome to carry. Whereas, a needle-shy individual will often choose the EpiPen, to make an informed decision ask your health care provider to show you both training devices. Which device do I recommend? As a victim of anaphylaxis, I maintain access to both devices—better safe than sorry!

■ One Final Message: Think Epi-Give Epi!

When should first responders, caretakers, parents, EMTs, nurses, and doctors administer epinephrine outside the hospital? In my opinion, it is best to err on the side of overusing injectable epinephrine. Nearly 80 to 90 percent of the victims of fatal anaphylaxis described in the medical literature and lay press did not promptly administer or receive injectable epinephrine.

In most instances, they did not carry it with them. Many patients who died had no skin symptoms or had only mild signs of anaphylaxis at the onset of the reaction. In my opinion, the time to administer injectable epinephrine outside the hospital to such patients was yesterday! There is an old dictum regarding the treatment of an acute allergic reaction or anaphylaxis: Think epi-give epi! Remember there are no medical contraindications for administering epinephrine when treating a life-threatening allergic reaction. ●

Chapter 7

Cow's Milk and Hen's Egg Allergy

Despite the fact that we consume thousands of different foods and beverages throughout our lifetimes, only about 200 foods, beverages, or food additives are capable of causing an allergic reaction. Ninety-percent of true allergic food reactions are triggered by eight foods known as the Big Eight. They are milk, eggs, wheat, soybeans, peanuts, tree nuts, fish, and shellfish. In my opinion, the Big Eight should be renamed the Big Ten, as allergic reactions to fruits and vegetables are now much more common than many foods listed in the Big Eight group. The next eight chapters will discuss the Big Ten foods. Subsequent chapters will cover less common food, beverage, and food additive reactions.

History of Dairy Products

Milk is as ancient as mankind itself, as it is the food that has sustained all mammalian infants since prehistoric times. Every female mammal, from humans to whales, produces breast milk for this purpose. Many centuries ago, perhaps as early as 6000 BC, ancient man domesticated animals to provide an alternative to breast milk. Such animals, including cows, buffalos, sheep, goats, and camels still produce milk for human consumption. While cow's milk has many detractors, without it

> *In the 8th or 9th century BC, Homer depicted the production of cheese from sheep and goat's milk in the mountain caves of Greece.*

we would have no butter, cheese, or ice cream. Egyptian murals from 2000 BC show butter and cheese being processed from milk and stored in animal skin bags suspended from poles. Only royalty, priests, and the wealthy could afford these prized dairy products. Aristotle (384–322 BC) wrote about cheese being made from the milk of mares and asses. In the 8th or 9th century BC, Homer depicted the production of cheese from sheep and goat's milk in the mountain caves of Greece.

Legend has it that cheese was discovered by "an unknown Arab nomad." The story goes that in preparation for his journey this nomad filled his saddlebag with milk in order to provide him with sustenance for the long journey across the desert. After several hours, he stopped to drink from his saddlebag only to find that the milk had separated into a pale, watery liquid with medium-sized, solid, white lumps. The desert nomad found the mixture both drinkable and edible. What the nomad did not know was "because the saddlebag, which was made from the stomach of a young animal, contained a coagulating enzyme known as rennin, the milk had been effectively separated into curds and whey (by the combination of the rennin, the hot sun and the galloping motions of the horse." As thus, cheese (perhaps not as we know it) was born.[1]

Romans were the first civilization to perfect cheesemaking into a fine art through various treatments and storage

---

[1] http://www.american.edu/ted/parmesan.htm

procedures. Wealthy Roman homes had cheese kitchens and a special area where cheese could be stored. The Romans eventually spread their cheesemaking expertise throughout the Roman Empire. While at first these skills remained with the wealthy landowners and Roman farmers, in time they spread to the local population. By 300 AD, cheese was exported throughout the Mediterranean. Trade developed to such an extent that Emperor Dioclctian had to fix prices on cheeses, including a highly popular apple-smoked cheese. One cheese, sold under the brand name of La Luna, was probably the precursor of today's Parmesan cheese. After the collapse of the Roman Empire, cheesemaking spread into southern and northern Europe. In the fertile lowlands of Europe, dairy husbandry developed at a faster pace and cheesemaking from cow's milk versus sheep's milk became the norm, leading to cheeses like Edam and Gouda in the Netherlands.

The French developed a wide range of softer cheeses in the rich agricultural areas of their country. Ancient tribes in the Swiss Alps developed their own distinctive types of "Swiss cheese." During the Middle Ages, monks developed many of the classic cheese varieties marketed today. During the Renaissance, cheese suffered a drop in popularity as it was considered to be unhealthy. Cheese regained favor in the nineteenth century, and cheesemakers ultimately moved from farm to factory production in the twentieth century.

■ The History of Ice Cream

The history of ice cream is another fascinating story. "It is dangerous to heat, cool or make a commotion all of a sudden in the body," warned the Greek doctor Hippocrates. But few citizens paid attention to the Father of Medicine. "Most men would rather run the hazard of their lives or health," he went on, "than be deprived of the pleasure of drinking out of ice." Alexander the Great, the King of Macedonia, was one such man. Tales are told of his quest to rule the world and his passion for iced drinks. Once, during an attack on the city of Petra, Alexander ordered his army to stop the battle and dig thirty trenches, then fill them with snow brought down from the mountains. Branches were laid across the trenches to keep the snow from melting so Alexander's wines, fruits, and juices would stay cold in the hot Jordanian sun.

Roman emperor Nero Claudius Caesar Drusus Germanicus (A.D. 37–68) had a love for iced drinks and desserts that was as great as his name was long. During his cruel reign as emperor of Rome, Nero often hosted tremendous feasts featuring wines cooled with snow and slushy honey-sweetened juices the world's first snow cone! Plans for these delicacies had to be made at least a month in advance. Nero would order slaves into the Apennine Mountains to gather snow. The weary servants were then forced to run a brutal relay race back to Rome, carting heavy loads of snow and ice through heat and many miles of treacherous terrain. The barbaric Nero, who thought nothing of killing his mother, his wife, and his teacher, once slaughtered the general in command for allowing the snow to melt before reaching the emperor's table. The slaves were boiled to death.

Ancient tribes in the Swiss Alps developed their own distinctive types of "Swiss cheese." During the Middle Ages, monks developed many of the classic cheese varieties marketed today.

In this case, Hippocrates was right: frozen foods and drink could be hazardous to your health! [2]

Marco Polo allegedly brought the concept of ice cream to Europe. In his travels to China, Marco Polo witnessed the staff of King T'ang of Shang lugging ice from ice-houses into his Imperial palace. Their process for making ice dishes involved taking milk from buffalos, cows, and goats, heating it, and letting it ferment with the ice. This produced a frozen product called kumiss. The result was a cool, refreshing dish that was probably a distant cousin to today's sherbet. Another popular legend has it that a French chef in the court of England's King Charles I had a secret recipe for ice cream that made it a favorite dish at Charles' royal table. Charles either paid him a handsome reward to keep it a secret, or, more likely, the chef was threatened with death if he divulged the secret recipe. Either way, after Charles I was beheaded in 1649, his chef allegedly spread his ice cream recipe throughout Europe. The Italian Catherine de Medici introduced the French court to frozen desserts in 1553 when she married Henry II of France. In 1686, Francesco Procopio dei Coltelli opened a coffee shop in Paris called *"Le Procope"* that served beverages and sherbets. The café, probably the world's first ice cream parlor, became famous for its large variety of more than eighty flavors of ice cream.

In the late seventeenth and early eighteenth centuries, long before refrigeration was available, ice cream was a rare and exotic dessert enjoyed by only the rich and, of course, the prominent politicians of that era.

In the late seventeenth and early eighteenth centuries, long before refrigeration was available, ice cream was a rare and exotic dessert enjoyed by only the rich and, of course, the prominent politicians of that era. In 1872, George Washington is said to have eaten ice cream at a party in Philadelphia. After this introduction to ice cream, Washington frequently served it to his guests at his Thursday night presidential dinners. In 1790, a New York merchant reported that President Washington spent the princely sum of $200 for ice cream in just one summer. Thomas Jefferson, who learned to make ice cream while he was visiting France, brought back an ice cream machine (a *sorbetiere*) for use in his Monticello home. Jefferson has been credited with popularizing vanilla as an ice cream flavor. His love of the vanilla flavor was so intense that, in 1791 while residing in Philadelphia as the secretary of State, he wrote to an American envoy in Paris complaining of the lack of vanilla in the United States. He requested that fifty vanilla pods be sent to him. Dolly Madison, wife of President James Madison, the fourth president of the United States, heard about this new dessert and created a national sensation by serving ice cream at her husband's second inaugural ball in 1813.

Around 1800, many owners of the great plantations in colonial Virginia built ice-houses near their riverbanks that were reached by underground passageways. Ice cut from the nearby ponds in wintertime or offloaded from New England ships was hauled by slaves, often crouched on all fours, through the narrow underground corridors to the icehouse. Layers of straw separated the blocks of ice to facilitate

---

[2] www.harpercollins.com/books/9780380802500/We_All_Scream_for_Ice_Cream/excerpt.aspx

their removal. Up to twenty tons of ice could be stored at the larger plantations. Thus, wealthy Southern plantation owners and their guests were provided with iced drinks, ice cream, and other frozen deserts during the long hot summer months.

African Americans played a dominant role in Philadelphia's ice cream business in the middle of the nineteenth century. Possibly the most influential of these tradesmen was Augustus Jackson, an African American who worked as a cook in the White House. Legend has it that he may have been the head chef at the White House. After Jackson moved to Philadelphia in the late 1820s, he started his own catering business. Jackson cleverly mixed milk with ice and salt to lower the temperature of his special mix of ingredients.

He created several ice cream flavors that he distributed in tin cans to Philadelphia's many ice cream parlors. He ran a successful business for at least thirty years and became one of Philadelphia's wealthiest African American citizens. The two ice cream parlors that were considered Philadelphia's best were Parkinson's and Isaac Newton's. At Parkinson's, ice cream was served in champagne glasses, and lemon and vanilla were the most popular flavors. Philadelphia was then (and is still) considered to be the ice cream capital of the United States because of the quantity of ice cream produced and the city's famous public ice cream houses.

One patron wrote, "In the summer season, immense quantities of the finest ice cream are sold in Philadelphia. Indeed, the city vaunts itself on producing the best ice cream in the world."

Making ice cream wasn't easy. It was done in a pewter pot kept in a bucket of ice and salt. The mixture had to be regularly stirred by hand with a "spaddle," which resembled a spade with a long handle. The revolution in ice cream production occurred in 1843, when a Philadelphia woman, Nancy Johnson, patented an invention consisting of a wooden bucket that was filled with ice and salt and had a rotating handle. In the middle was a metal container that held the ice cream.

By "churning the cream," you could produce ice cream with a smooth and even texture. From this time on, anyone could make quality ice cream at home, especially since rock salt, commonly called "ice cream salt," was a cheap commodity. Johnson's hand crank might have been fine for backyard picnics, but no one considered ice cream-making as an industry. Jacob Fussell, a milk dealer from Baltimore, Maryland, discovered how to mass-produce ice cream, and he set up the first ice cream factory in 1851. His factory utilized icehouses and a larger version of Johnson's machine. By the start of the Civil War, Fussell had opened ice cream plants in New York, Washington DC, and Boston. From then on, the popularity of ice cream skyrocketed.

Philadelphia was then (and is still) considered to be the ice cream capital of the United States because of the quantity of ice cream produced and the city's famous public ice cream houses.

The wide availability of ice cream in the late nineteenth century led to new American creations, including the soda fountain, the soda jerk, and the ice cream soda. Soda jerk (or soda jerker) is the name for the person—typically a youth—who worked the soda fountain in a drugstore. Unlike today's soda fountains that automatically mix the drink, a soda jerk had the job of measuring the syrup and then mixing it with soda water to create the drink. The term is somewhat archaic these days, as there are very few drugstores that still serve ice cream and soda.[3] In 1880, the ice cream sundae was born. There is some debate over where the ice cream sundae was invented. The most accepted story is that it started in Evanston, Illinois, where it was illegal to serve carbonated beverages on Sundays. To get around the rule, the soda jerks topped the ice cream with different syrups, peanuts, or apple cider. They called their new dessert the ice cream Sunday. In response to Puritan-like religious criticism, the name was eventually changed from Sunday to "sundae" to remove any connection with the Sabbath.

> *The United States armed forces found that ice cream was a real morale booster, and they rapidly became the world's largest ice cream manufacturer during World War II.*

In 1904, the ice cream cone was allegedly introduced at the St. Louis World's Fair by an immigrant pastry maker, Ernest A. Hamwi, who was selling a wafer-like pastry at a fairground concession. When a neighboring ice cream stand ran out of dishes, Hamwi rolled some of his wafers into cornucopias, let them cool, and sold them to the ice cream concessionaire. In 1921, the commissioner of Ellis Island issued a decree that all immigrants arriving in this country would receive a free scoop of ice cream as their first American meal. In 1927, Americans were not only eating ice cream, they started singing about it, as in the song "Ice Cream:" "I scream, you scream, we all scream for ice cream!"[4] But it wasn't until three years later that grocery stores actually sold ice cream. Even then, there was no way to keep it frozen at home until the refrigerator-freezer unit was invented in 1939. Ice cream eventually became an important symbol of democracy in twentieth-century America. During World War II, Mussolini banned ice cream in Italy because it symbolized America. The Emperor of Japan created conditions that made selling ice cream unprofitable. The United States armed forces found that ice cream was a real morale booster, and they rapidly became the world's largest ice cream manufacturer during World War II.

American fliers even designed a way to make ice cream in an aircraft bomber gunner's compartment! Like other American industries, ice cream production soared after World Was II due to technological innovations in refrigeration, packaging and shipping. Today, total frozen dairy production in the United States exceeds more than 1.6 billion gallons per year—enough for every American to eat twenty-three quarts of ice cream a year!

The History of Milk

Most dairy-producing cattle probably came from ancestors of the Brown Swiss dairy breed that existed during the Bronze Age in the area now known as Switzerland. Cattle originally served a triple purpose by providing meat, milk, and labor. By the fifth century, cows and sheep throughout Europe were prized for their milk. In the fourteenth Century, cow's milk became more popular than sheep's milk. When European dairy cows arrived in America in 1611, they helped save the starving settlers

---

[3] *Wikipedia, The Free Encyclopedia*, s.v. "Soda jerk," http://en.wikipedia.org/ (accessed July 19, 2006).

[4] Billy Moll, Howard Johnson, and Robert King, *Ice Cream Song* (1927)

of the Jamestown Colony. After the New World was settled, American farmers began importing dairy cows from Europe. The Holsteins originated in the Netherlands, and Ayrshires came from Scotland. Guernsey cows were developed on the Isle of Guernsey, and Jerseys were shipped from the Isle of Jersey, two small islands in the English Channel off the coast of France. Dairy cows were initially kept in or near American towns and cities—closer to the growing urban population. In the 1880s and 1890s, dairy cattle were taken to western parts of the United States by settlers and traders; and, in 1895, the Brown Swiss breed reached the Pacific Ocean.

Significant improvements in milk production in the first half of the twentieth century helped to control the spread of milk-borne diseases and enhance the nutritional value of milk. In the early 1900s, public health authorities promoted pasteurization and other measures to eliminate disease-producing organisms from milk. This made it possible to safely store and more broadly distribute milk. The first regular shipment of milk by rail to New York City occurred in 1841. Refrigerators replaced iceboxes. Large bulk tanks replaced the milk can. The dairy industry evolved from mom and pop dairies with only a few cows to large conglomerates.

During World War II, many food items were rationed, including meats, butter, and sugar. However, milk was not rationed, and consumption soared—shooting up from thirty-four gallons per person per year in 1941 to a peak of forty-five gallons per person in 1945. Since 1945, milk consumption has steadily fallen, reaching a record low of just under twenty-three gal-

lons per person in 2001. This decline was due to increased concern about cholesterol, saturated fats, and calories; competition from soft drinks and bottled water; and a more diverse ethnic population whose diet did not include milk.

On the other hand, cheese consumption has increased. In 2001, Americans consumed thirty pounds of cheese per person— eight times more than in 1909 and more than twice as much as in 1975. Demand for a time-saving convenience food is probably the major force behind the growth in cheese consumption.

Since 2001, milk has made a comeback in the United States, Canada, and Australia. This may be due, in part, to aggressive marketing, like the "milk-moustache" advertisements. Advocates for the dairy industry like to point out that while milk consumption declined and ingestion of high caloric soft drinks increased, obesity has sky-rocketed. Obesity currently affects more than 40 million adults in America and is a risk factor for heart disease, cancer, stroke, and diabetes.

Since 2001, milk has made a comeback in the United States, Canada and Australia. This may be due, in part, to aggressive marketing, like the "milk-moustache" advertisements.

Dietary research shows that consuming at least three servings of milk, cheese, or yogurt a day enables people to meet their vitamin D and calcium recommendations, and that may help reduce the risk of chronic health problems, such as osteoporosis and hypertension. In addition, cow's milk is a decent source of iodine, riboflavin, vitamin B12, vitamin A and potassium.

■ Cow's Milk Allergy

The first reported reaction to cow's milk was 2000 years ago when Hippocrates recorded that cow's milk caused intestinal upset and diarrhea. After World War II, the increase in cow's milk allergy was undoubtedly due to a decline in breast-feeding and the rise in the popularity of milk-based formulas. Before breast-feeding came back into vogue in the latter part of the twentieth century, the most common food allergy seen in infants and toddlers was cow's milk allergy. Even though peanut allergy gets all the attention, cow's milk allergy is still a relatively common problem in infants and young children. The older literature stated that cow's milk allergy affected nearly three in every 100 children before their first birthdays. In my opinion, these numbers may now be overinflated, and the prevalence of milk allergy has declined due to the popularity of breast-feeding and soy-based formulas.

Some milk-allergic patients tolerate well-done beef products, as high cooking temperatures may denature the milk proteins in beef. This also explains why many milk-sensitive patients may tolerate baked goods containing milk proteins.

The three major allergic milk proteins—lactoglobulin, lactalbumin and casein—are heat stable, which means that heating, or pasteurization, does not usually denature these proteins. As these proteins are also present in other animal milk, cow's milk-allergic patients should not drink buffalo, sheep, goat, camel, or ewe milk. (A ewe is a mountain goat from Europe, Asia, and Northern Africa.) Sheep's and goat's milk allergy can occur by itself. Several patients who reacted to small amounts of goat and sheep cheese had more severe reactions than those brought on by cow's milk allergy.

One report described a two-year-old boy who experienced allergic reactions after eating and touching sheep's cheese, but he tolerated cow's milk and its dairy products. He had never ingested milk or milk derivatives from a sheep or a goat. The patient was found to be allergic to sheep's and goat's milk proteins but not to cow's milk protein. Our practice has seen two similar patients who reacted to cheese made from goat's milk and sheep's milk but who tolerated cow's milk and cheese derived from cow's milk. One was a five-year-old, egg-allergic child who had ana-phylactic reactions to cheese from goat's milk and a Romano-pecorino cheese derived from sheep's milk. The second child was a three-year-old who ingested cow's milk and cheeseburgers prepared with American cheese without problems but reacted to cheese from goat's and sheep's milk. Approximately 10 to 20 percent of milk-allergic children may react to beef, as cow's milk proteins are present in beef products. Some milk-allergic patients tolerate well-done beef products, as high cooking temperatures may denature the milk proteins in beef. This also explains why many milk-sensitive patients may tolerate baked goods containing milk proteins.

■ Heiner's Syndrome

This is an older syndrome first described in 1960 by Dr. Douglas Heiner. It is primarily a disease of infancy characterized by wheezing, coughing up blood (hemopty-sis), anemia, and infiltrates in lungs. Although the etiology is unknown, a significant number of children with this disorder appear to have pulmonary bleeding related to cow's milk ingestion, and they demonstrate high titers of no-allergic antibodies to cow's milk. While I saw several of these cases in the 1970s, the incidence appears to be declining with the decreased use of cow's milk in infancy. However, it may not be as rare as perceived as Dr. Sami Bahna, chief of allergy at the State University Health Sciences Center in Shreveport, Louisiana, recently reported eight cases, all of whom responded to cow's milk elimination.

Outgrowing Cow's Milk Allergy

While milk allergy is often the first food allergy seen in infants, it is also usually the first to be outgrown, as 80 to 90 percent of milk-allergic children tolerate cow's milk by their fourth birthday. Finland researchers followed 118 children with cow's milk allergy for eight years with oral challenges. In this first study to follow patients for eight years, nearly 50 percent outgrew their milk allergy by two years of age, 81 percent by age five, and 89 percent by age eight. Milk allergy was outgrown in about one year if only the intestinal tract was involved in the allergic reaction. The outlook was less optimistic for patients with a positive family history of allergy, a severe reaction to cow's milk, eczema, and other food allergies. Cow's milk allergy is a risk predictor for developing other allergic diseases. About one in three milk-allergic infants will develop another food allergy, and nearly 80 percent may experience inhalant allergies later in childhood.

Skin and CAP RAST tests to milk can predict the development of tolerance to cow's milk. In one study, a wheal skin test size of less than 5 mm correctly identified 83 percent of infants who developed cow's milk tolerance by the age of four years; and

a wheal size of over 5 mm culled out 71 percent with persistent cow's milk allergy. A similar trend has been found in children with lower cow's milk CAP RAST blood test levels.

Treatment of Cow's Milk Allergy

The treatment of milk allergy is relatively simple—avoidance. Most milk-allergic infants do well when switched to a soy-based formula, like Isomil or Prosobee. The 5 to 15 percent of milk-allergic children who also react to soy formulas usually tolerate non-soy formulas, like Alimentum or Nutramigen.

Does the use of a soy-based formula increase risk of developing a soy or peanut allergy? Researchers in Finland followed 170 infants with cow's milk allergy who were fed a soy formula and found they had no increased risk for developing a soy or peanut allergy at age four. Thus, a soy formula is preferred over the more expensive, less palatable, hydrolyzed infant formulas in cow's milk-allergic infants.

I would not recommend using a soy-based formula as a first choice in non-milk allergic children as soy formulas do not prevent food allergy; and, once a soy allergy develops, it is less likely to be outgrown than cow's milk allergy.

I would not recommend using a soy-based formula as a first choice in non-milk allergic children as soy formulas do not prevent food allergy; and, once a soy allergy develops, it is less likely to be outgrown than cow's milk allergy. Be aware that soy formulas may contain trace amounts of milk protein. One nine-month-old boy with cow's milk allergy, eczema, and asthma experienced a severe anaphylactic reaction that required mouth-to-mouth resuscitation when he was switched to a new soy formula that was found to contain trace amounts of milk protein. As milk is a main source of calcium, do not neglect basic calcium requirements—500 mg per day for children one to three years of age, 800 mg for four to eight-year olds and 1300 mg for nine to eighteen-year olds. Consult your pediatrician, healthcare provider or dietician if you have questions regarding calcium replacement in cow's milk-allergic patients.

While most reactions to cow's milk are mild, they should not be taken lightly. Near-fatal and fatal reactions to cow's milk have been reported. In April 2002, a five-month-old, milk-allergic boy enrolled in an English nursery school was fed a cereal product containing milk that triggered a severe allergic reaction that resulted in his death. At the time of his reaction, he was suffering from a bronchitis-like illness, suggesting that asthma may have played a part in this tragic event. A legal inquiry resulted in a verdict of accidental death and neglect by the nursery school that pleaded guilty to breaching the Health and Safety at Work Act of the United Kingdom. In November 2004, British courts awarded the parents 60,000 pounds.

The newsletter of FAAN has reported several milk fatalities over the past few years. One sad case described a seventeen-year-old male with asthma and milk allergy who died after drinking a protein shake that contained whey. Whey is the watery liquid that separates from soured milk or when enzymes are added in cheesemaking. Be careful when heating milk products or milk-based formulas. One case report depicted a twenty-month-old child

with cow's milk allergy who spilled a cup of hot milk on his arm. He immediately began to vomit and then experienced respiratory arrest requiring insertion of a breathing tube and intensive care. It is likely that a small second-degree burn on his arm accelerated the absorption of large amounts of milk protein.

◼ Common Names and Hidden Sources of Milk Protein

Milk proteins are disguised by various names, including artificial butter oil, buttermilk, caramel, casein, caseinate, cheese, cream curds, whey, dried milk, high protein flavor, lactoglobulin, lactalbumin, lactose, natural flavoring, whey, and rennet (see table 7.1).

Hidden sources of milk protein include yogurt, butter, margarines, cheeses, cheese curds, creams, custards, hot dogs, meatballs, Spam, and frozen desserts. Ghee, made from simmering butter, does contain milk protein. Lactitolis, a sugar derived from lactose sweetener and a bulk agent, is less likely than lactose to contain milk protein. Pizza is frequently made from goat or sheep's milk. Non-dairy products, like coffee whiteners, are not always milk-free. Milk is commonly used to thicken Asian fruit beverages.

Kosher dietary laws prohibit the use of milk or milk products in combination with meat. The Jewish community uses a system of markings to determine if a food is kosher. The symbol "D" for the word "dairy" indicates the presence of milk protein. Thus, a product labeled D for dairy should not contain any meat, and a product labeled "pareve" should not contain milk or meat products. However, under Jewish law, a very small amount of milk may still be in a pareve-labeled product. Thus, it may be best not to rely on this symbol as

Table 7.1. Common Names and Hidden Sources of Milk

Common Names	Hidden Sources
Artificial butter oil	Yogurt
Buttermilk	Butter
Caramel	Margarine
Casein, caseinate	Cheese curds
Cheese cream curds	Creams
Whey, dried milk	Custards
High protein flavin	Hot dogs, meatballs
Lactoglobulin	Spam
Lactalbumin	Frozen desserts
Lactose	Pizza
Natural flavoring	Coffee whiteners
Rennet	Asian fruit beverages
	Canned tuna fish

several reactions to pareve-labeled products have been described.

New or Unusual Ingredients

Several new or unusual ingredients that do not contain milk protein have triggered queries by cow's milk allergic patients and their families.[5]

- Alum, a preservative used in many medications, including allergy injections, is not related to the milk protein albumin.
- Calcium phosphate, a leavening agent, dough conditioner, and anti-caking agent
- Cream of tartar, a component of baking powder and baking soda used in stabilizing egg whites
- Glucono-delta-lactonea, a crystal powder used in baked goods, deserts, fish products, pickles, and tofu
- Lactates, which refer to the chemical compound of lactic acid, like ferrous and calcium lactate

- Maltose, which increases the shelf life of meats and poultry
- Tagatose is a new food ingredient derived from lactose and galactase. It is used as a low-calorie sweetener in foods and beverages. Tagatose has approximately the same sweetness as sucrose. Although lactose often contains residual milk allergens, tagatose is much less likely to contain any milk allergens based upon the process used to produce tagatose.

Lactose in Asthma Inhalers

The milk sugar lactose, often used as filler in medications such as asthma inhalers, is usually considered to be milk protein-free. One report of a reaction to a lactose-containing inhaler described an adolescent male with asthma and milk allergy who had a severe reaction to Advair, a popular asthma medication. He had a positive skin test reaction to lactose. Other asthma inhalers that contain lactose include Serevent and Foradil. As millions of

---

[5] *FAAN Food Allergy News*, December 2004-January 2005.

patients have used these important asthma medications without reacting to their ingredients, I need to see more cases before I stop using them in cow's milk-allergic asthmatics.

The History of Eggs

Eggs are another allergenic food with an interesting historical and nutritional profile. Since birds long preceded man in evolution, no one really knows when the first bird laid the first egg. The earliest recorded egg layers were probably Chinese ducks and geese in 4000 BC. The dependability of the rooster's early morning call inspired the Chinese to describe them as "the only domestic animal who knows the time of day." The egg-laying hen that appeared 2,000 years later in India was eventually introduced to Europe around the fifth century. It is believed that Columbus carried the first egg-laying chickens to the Americas in the 1490s.

Eggs have been a symbol of fertility and religious worship since ancient Persian and Celtic cultures celebrated the vernal (spring) equinox. Gifts of red-dyed eggs were shared at a meal, and their shells were carefully crushed to drive away winter. In the ninth century, eggs were considered to be a delicacy, and thus were banned during Lent. This Lenten ban made eggs very popular at Easter when they were collected and distributed to servants and children who ate them in a huge Easter omelet. As this tradition became more popular, the nobility got into the act. In the last days of winter, they decorated eggs to give to their loved ones, their master or their king. By the sixteenth century, springtime eggs, the rage at the court of France, were decorated by the greatest artists of the day. This unique popularity of the Easter egg reached untold heights at the court of the Czar of Russia at the end of the nineteenth century when legendary Russian court jeweler Carl Fabergé created his highly detailed gold, crystal and porcelain eggs for Russian aristocrats and rulers.

Many families save their decorative eggs and pass them down through generations. Eggs laid on Good Friday and eaten on Easter Sunday are said to protect against fevers. Thrown into a hearth, eggs are thought to have the power to extinguish the fire. Buried in the garden or on the edge of a field, they guard against lightning and hail and protect beehives. An old French custom, the egg-rolling contest, consisted of rolling raw eggs (marked to identify the owner) down a gentle slope. The egg that survived the bumpy terrain and attacks by competing eggs was declared the "victory egg," symbolizing the rock that rolled away from the mouth of the Christ's tomb.

Easter-time egg fights were popular in Medieval Europe. The most famous occurred in 975 between the bishop and dean of Chester, England, and the cathedral choir. The fight broke out in the middle of Easter services and lasted a good hour with everyone having made sure to have plenty of "ammunition." Church records state that weeks later, one could still hear the crush of eggshells under one's sandals when walking through the cathedral. Today, hand-decorated eggs that are exchanged as springtime gifts in many cultures play an important role in religious ceremonies on Easter morning.

The Incredible-Edible Egg

I grew up in an Irish home that ate ham or bacon and eggs (scrambled, boiled, fried, or poached) every morning. We also ate "beans and franks" every Saturday night. Nutritional studies in the 1970s and 1980s suggested that eggs, especially the yolks, raised cholesterol levels. This prompted our family to limit egg consumption to one or two servings a week or to remove the egg yolks when consuming eggs—a big mistake. Not only have more recent studies shown that eating one to two eggs a day does not significantly alter cholesterol levels in most individuals, the latest research suggests that eating whole eggs may actually result in significant improvement in blood lipid profiles.

Eggs are unique in that they contain many essential nutrients. The reason for this is that nature designed the egg as a life-support system for a developing bird or chick. What really astounds me is that the most nutritional part of the egg is the yolk. While the egg white consists mainly of high-quality protein, the yolk provides essential vitamins and minerals, including vitamins A, D, E, B12, riboflavin, folic acid, iron, zinc, and phosphorus.

Choline in egg yolks helps to lower levels of homocysteine, a molecule that may damage blood vessels. Recent studies on eggs are even more impressive. Eggs may help lower the risk of a heart attack or stroke by helping to prevent blood clots. A study in the *Biological and Pharmaceutical Bulletin* (October 2003) demonstrated that proteins in egg yolk are not only potent inhibitors of human platelet aggregation, but they also prolong the time it takes for fibrinogen, a blood clotting protein, to be converted into fibrin. Lutein, a yellow-red pigment thought to help prevent age-related macular degeneration and cataracts, may be found in higher amounts in egg yolk than in green vegetables such as spinach, long considered to be the major dietary sources of lutein. There may be other reasons to enjoy eggs. According to Japanese researchers, a peptide found in egg white that binds to the food-borne pathogen E. coli may prevent E. coli infection.

Can eggs prevent breast cancer? Breast cancer rates more than double in Chinese women when they migrate from China to the United States. Different dietary factors between the United States Chinese women and native Chinese women may increase the risk of breast cancer. A study of 378 women with breast cancer and 1,070 age-matched controls found that two diets were strongly protective against breast cancer. Native Chinese women who ate more fruits and vegetables had a 52 percent lower risk of breast cancer compared to those eating fewer fruits and vegetables. Eating eggs—at least six a week—was also highly protective, lowering risk of breast cancer in native Chinese women by 44 percent compared to American Chinese women who ate only two eggs a week. Some nutritionists propose that the benefits of egg yolks are enhanced when they are consumed raw, as heating may destroy some essential nutrients. People who eat raw egg yolks report they have improved digestion, increased stamina, and resistance to illness. Many state raw egg yolks taste like vanilla!

Due to the risk of bacterial contamination in raw eggs, I would not recommend this approach. However, I do remember many a morning when I was late for school, my mother would quickly poach an egg in boiling water for a minute or two, drop it in a small eggcup, and I ingested the

Lutein, a yellow-red pigment thought to help prevent age-related macular degeneration and cataracts, may be found in higher amounts in egg yolk than in green vegetables such as spinach, long considered to be the major dietary sources of lutein.

egg in one quick gulp before running out the door. No one in our family ever left home without their morning egg.

■ Hen's Egg Allergy

Hen's egg allergy is the second most common allergy in infancy and early childhood. The most allergic part of the egg is the egg white, which contains two major proteins, ovomucoid and ovalbumin. The incidence of egg allergy in children is about the same as milk allergy—about 2 to 3 percent. I used to think most egg-allergic children tolerated eggs by age four or five. This may not be so. One well-done study set out to determine the likelihood of outgrowing egg allergy in children younger than two years and to identify the predictors of developing a tolerance to eggs. Fifty-two children underwent prospective evaluation with skin and CAP RAST tests and open oral egg challenges every six months up to age five. The main predictors of achieving tolerance, or outgrowing egg allergy, were milder skin symptoms, smaller skin tests and lower CAP RAST levels. Only 66 percent achieved a tolerance to eggs by age five.

Thus, egg allergy appears to be more persistent than cow's milk allergy. Egg allergy, especially in infants with eczema, is a good predictor for other allergic diseases, as many egg-allergic infants develop additional food allergies, asthma, and hay fever. The treatment of egg allergy is no different from other food allergies—avoidance and education. Egg protein can be found everywhere in the food kingdom (see table 7.2).

Eggs are often added to pretzels, bagels, and fancy coffee and bar drinks to give them a shiny or foamy look. Fresh pasta is usually egg-free, while commercially processed pas-

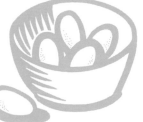

ta often contains eggs. Egg proteins are also present in bird, duck, goose, and quail eggs. Egg-allergic patients who react to chicken, turkey, or game birds suffer from what is called the "Chicken Meat-Bird-Egg Syndrome."

■ Can Egg Allergic Children Eat Cooked Egg Products?

Researchers at Hospital Sainte-Justine in Montreal, Canada, recently addressed this important question. The purpose of the study was to evaluate the proportion of children beyond the age of five, who, while allergic to eggs, were able to tolerate cooked eggs. Egg allergy was defined as a history of clinical reaction to egg with a positive skin test. Sixty children allergic to eggs performed an oral food challenge to cooked eggs (cake). The results showed that seventy-three percent of the egg allergic children tolerated egg in its cooked form. A positive skin test to egg white protein of ≥10 mm was a strong marker to predict a reaction to a cooked egg challenge. The presence of multiple food allergies increased the risk of reacting to cooked egg. Despite these encouraging numbers I would caution the parents of egg allergic children not to perform such challenges without the supervision of an allergy specialist.

■ Egg Allergy and Vaccines

Controversy exists regarding allergic reactions to measles, mumps, and rubella (MMR) vaccine in egg-allergic patients. MMR vaccine contains attenuated viruses grown in chick embryo cells, and has been shown to contain tiny amounts of egg protein. Despite this, most severe allergic reactions to MMR vaccine occur

Table 7.2. Common Names and Hidden Sources of Egg

Common Names	Hidden Sources
Albumin	Bagels, pretzels
Binder	Baked goods
Coagulant	Bouillon
Egg white	Cereals, cakes, chocolate, custard
Egg yolk	Commercial pasta
Emulsifier	Cream sauces, canned soups
Globulin	Fancy bar, coffee drinks
Lecithin	Fish in batter
Levetin	French toast, pancakes, waffles
Lysozyme	Ice creams, sherbets
Ovovitellin	Instant mashed potatoes
Powdered egg	Mayonnaise, marshmallows
Vitellin	Pasta, pies, puddings
Whole egg albumin	Processed meats
Ovalbumin	Tartar sauce
Ovomucoid	White batter-fried foods
	Wines cleared with egg

in children who are not allergic to eggs. Allergy to other vaccine components, such as gelatin or neomycin, is responsible for many reactions. To date there have been only isolated reports describing reaction to MMR in egg-allergic patients. Thus, many authorities recommend giving MMR to egg-allergic children without skin testing to the vaccine. As I have seen several anaphylactic reactions with this approach, I recommend that severe egg-allergic children be skin tested with the vaccine. When the test is negative, the vaccine can be administered in one dose. If the vaccine skin test is positive, the vaccine can be safely administered in divided doses.

Several other vaccines, such as the yellow fever and flu vaccine, are also grown in egg embryos. The reported incidence of anaphylactic reactions to vaccines is very low—less than one case per million doses. A fainting or vasovagal reaction with or without hyperventilation commonly seen with a vaccine injection is often mistaken for anaphylaxis. Correct diagnosis is important in making it possible to vaccinate those who might otherwise run the risk of a serious infection. Influenza infection, with its accompanying morbidity and mortality, represents a major public health concern to the elderly and patients with chronic respiratory disease. Egg-allergic asthmatics should not be denied flu immunization because of the risk of an adverse reactions with a vaccine derived from egg embryo tissue. Safe practical protocols that include incremental dosing with influenza vaccine can guide experienced clinicians to safely administer flu vaccine to this high-risk group. ●

Chapter

8

Wheat Allergy

■ The History of Wheat

Wheat is derived from a wild grass that first grew in Mesopotamia (Iraq) in the Tigris and Euphrates river valleys about 10,000 years ago. As early as 6700 BC, Swiss lake dwellers used wheat to make flat cakes. Wheat farming subsequently spread to Asia, Europe, and North Africa by 4000 BC. Once people learned how to grow wheat, they no longer needed to wander in search of food. Thus, villages were established as wheat provided people with a food supply that could be stored and used year round. The Egyptians discovered how to make yeast-leavened breads between 2000 and 3000 BC. Workers who built the pyramids in Egypt were paid in wheat bread. Since wheat is the only grain with enough gluten to make a raised or leavened loaf of bread, wheat was favored over other grains, such as oats, millet, rice, and barley. Roman bakers produced a variety of breads, and the first bakers' guilds were formed in Rome in 150 BC.

After the invention of the commercial bread slicer in 1928 and the automatic toaster in 1930, the consumption of wheat soared in America.

In 1202 AD, England adopted laws to regulate the price of bread and limit bakers' profits. Many bakers were prosecuted for selling loaves that did not conform to the weights required by local laws. Wheat was not grown by the early American colonists because it did not grow well in the cold climate and poor soil of New England. Wheat was first grown in the United States as early as 1839 in what is now Kansas. Between 1874 and 1884, Russian Mennonites settled in Kansas and planted Russian wheat, providing today's hard red winter wheat from the Great Plains. Cyrus Hall McCormick's invention of the mechanical reaper in 1831 allowed farmers to cut eight acres a day versus only two acres a day with hand-held scythes or sickles. After the invention of the commercial bread slicer in 1928 and the automatic toaster in 1930, the consumption of wheat soared in America.

Wheat is the second-largest worldwide cereal crop, behind Indian corn or maize. The third largest crop is rice. Today, wheat is grown on more acres in the United States than any other grain. About 63 million acres of wheat are harvested each year in the United States. If all the acres were placed side-by-side, American wheat fields would cover more than 100,000 square miles. More foods are made with wheat than any other grain.

Wheat contributes 10 to 20 percent of the daily caloric intake in over sixty countries. There are more than 1,000 varieties of wheat bread on the market. Wheat grain is used to make flour, feed livestock, and brew beer. Softer, starchy wheat varieties are used for non-fermented products, such as baby foods, pastry, biscuits, and ice cream cones that do not require dough. Hard wheat, like semolina, is used to make bread and cakes as gluten binds the flour into a more solid form.

Whole grain wheat products are an important source of dietary fiber. Four medium slices of whole wheat bread provide 7.6 grams of fiber—that is 42 percent of the recommended daily amount. Whole grain wheat contains several B vitamins, including thiamine, riboflavin, and niacin. Wheat also contains potassium, iron, magnesium, zinc, selenium, and vitamin E.

■ Powerful Pasta

Probably no food has generated more controversy in America than pasta. Many of the names given to pasta shapes are Italian, but the Italians do not have a monopoly on pasta. All types of pasta have one thing in common—they are prepared from a dough, or paste (pasta means "paste" in Italian) by mixing finely ground grain or flour with water. The Chinese ate noodles as early as 5000 BC. The history of pasta in the United States is much clearer. Thomas Jefferson brought pasta into the United States in the late 1780s after visiting Naples, Italy, while he was the American ambassador to France. The first pasta factory in the United States opened in 1848 in Brooklyn, New York. Pasta remained a relatively uncommon and unpopular food until the late nineteenth century when Italian immigrants introduced the tasty pastas that we all enjoy today.

For years, health-conscious Americans dismissed pasta as a fattening food with little or no nutritional value. Pasta is now highly regarded as rich in complex carbohydrates, high in protein, and low in fat. Why do high-performance athletes, especially marathoners, load up on pasta the night before their race? You need mucho carbos to run twenty-six miles! Simple carbohydrates, such as those found in table sugar, molasses, honey, lactose (in milk), and fructose (in fruit) break down quickly during digestion and provide an immediate source of energy. Whereas complex carbohydrates like those found in wheat and pasta (and some vegetables, such as potatoes and corn) break down more slowly, giving the body a time-release source of energy. Athletes will often eat 55 to 65 percent of their diet as complex carbohydrates to store adequate energy in their muscles before competing in endurance events. Eighty-two percent of the calories in spaghetti and other pastas come from complex carbohydrates. One cup of cooked spaghetti supplies more protein than a whole egg.

One cup of cooked spaghetti supplies more protein than a whole egg.

■ Wheat Allergy

While listed in the Big Eight, wheat allergy is relatively uncommon compared to fruit and vegetable allergy. Many reactions to wheat are adverse or autoimmune food reactions seen in patients with celiac disease or gluten intolerance. The symptoms of gluten intolerance include excess gas, bloating, foul-smelling stools, diarrhea, weight loss, and fatigue. Some patients may develop a severe skin rash called dermatitis herpetiformis. When gluten intolerance or celiac disease is suspected, you may need to consult a gastroenterologist, as an intestinal biopsy is often needed to confirm this diagnosis.

Prick skin tests and CAP RAST blood tests were studied in thirty-two wheat-allergic children. The risk of ana-phylaxis was found to be fourteen times greater in patients with a CAP RAST level of more than three units. Delayed reactions are more common in wheat allergy compared to other foods. Danish and Italian allergists studied twenty-seven adults with wheat allergy. Nearly 40 percent were also allergic to grass pollen. Cooking did not denature wheat protein. Many patients had positive wheat challenges to both raw and cooked wheat—some at very low doses. The skin and CAP RAST tests were not very helpful in predicting the outcome of a wheat challenge. Ninety cases of wheat-exercise-induced anaphylaxis have been described. One case depicted a fifty-eight-year-old male who frequently collapsed while exercising. After cardiovascular studies were negative, he recalled that most reactions occurred after eating a sandwich or pizza. An allergy evaluation found he had positive skin and CAP RAST tests to wheat protein.

Japanese allergists described a sixty-five-year-old man who first experienced hives, swelling, itching, and loss of consciousness after drinking beer at a party at the age of thirty-four years. Over the next thirty years, he frequently experienced hives and loss of consciousness while taking a walk after eating various foods—all of which contained wheat flour. His CAP RAST test to wheat flour was positive, and he had a systemic reaction during an exercise test after eating a slice of white bread.

There are a few case reports of reactions to barley hops (a major beer ingredient) in

Wheat-sensitive patients also should avoid kamut, an ancient wheat from the Middle East falsely marketed as a safe alternative to wheat. Also known as Polish wheat, kamut is frequently used in baked goods and frozen foods.

wheat-allergic patients. A fifty-nine-year-old man experienced swelling, generalized hives, and unconsciousness after ingestion of wheat beer. (Wheat beer is a specialty beer brewed from both barley and wheat malt.) He had no problems with lager beer. Skin test results with a standard series of common aeroallergens and food allergens were negative with the exception of a small reaction to wheat flour. Skin tests were positive for two brands of wheat beer and wheat malt, but negative for baker's yeast, hops, and a brand of lager beer. Oral challenges with wheat beer and wheat flour triggered a hive-like reaction.

Another report that typifies how wheat can be easily hidden described a young child who reacted to Play-Doh, a product of the Hasbro Toy Co. Wheat was not listed on the label of the Play-Doh but was found in a description of the product on the company's Web site. We have seen a similar case in our practice, suggesting that wheat-induced Play-Doh reactions may be more common than appreciated.

Can wheat-allergic patients eat other grains? Fortunately, the crossover rate of reactions to other grains is low, and most wheat-allergic patients tolerate other grains, such as corn, oats, and rice. Iran allergists studied eighteen wheat-allergic patients and found 50 percent reacted to barley and none reacted to corn and rice, probably because they belong to a different food family from wheat or barley. Wheat is undoubtedly the most difficult food to eliminate from one's diet (see table 8.1). Names to watch for in ingredient labeling

Table 8.1. Names and Sources of Wheat Protein

Names	Hidden Sources
Cereal binders and fillers	Breads
Hydrolyzed plant proteins	Baked goods
Bran	Pastries
Bulgur (cracked wheat) flour	Pasta
Farina	Cereals, crackers
Gluten	Processed meats
Modified starch proteins	Cakes, cookies
Modified vegetable proteins	Snack foods
Semolina	Polish wheat or kamut
Any flours	Spelt (an ancient wheat)

include cereal binders and fillers, hydrolyzed plant proteins, bran[1], bulgur flour, farina, gluten, modified starch, vegetable proteins, and any types of flour. Sources of wheat protein include breads, baked goods, pastries, pasta, cereal and crackers, processed meats, cakes, cookies, and snack foods. Wheat-sensitive patients should also avoid kamut, an ancient wheat from the Middle East falsely marketed as a safe alternative to wheat. Also known as Polish wheat, kamut is frequently used in baked goods and frozen foods.

■ Buckwheat Allergy

Buckwheat is commonly cultivated in Asia in poor soil as a cheap food source and often used as a wheat substitute in such dishes as served as noodles, dumplings, and buns. In 1961, Dr. A.J. Horesh identified thirty-six cases of buckwheat allergy among 514 patients in his Cleveland, Ohio, practice. A lack of case reports makes it difficult to estimate the incidence of buckwheat allergy in the United States. Most

papers come from Japan and Korea. A Japanese questionnaire collected 169 cases of buckwheat allergy, mostly among young children who reacted to small amounts of buckwheat, according to a study published in the mid-1970s. Asthma and anaphylactic shock occurred in eighteen individuals. In 2001, Japanese allergists described the tragic death of a buckwheat-allergic girl who died after consuming buckwheat noodles (zaru soba) and swimming vigorously. In 2005, a thirty-seven-year-old French woman was reported to have had two life-threatening anaphylactic reactions after eating galettes, a specialty buckwheat pancake from Brittany. The bottom line: whenever a non-wheat allergic patient suffers an unusual reaction to wheat or flour, consider buckwheat allergy.

■ Pan the Pancakes

While wheat flour is a common cause of asthma in bakers, not all such reactions are due to wheat. In one study, wheezy bakers reacted to storage mites in flour. Taiwanese allergists described an eight-year-old, mite-allergic boy who experienced a reaction after eating pancakes pre-

---

[1] Bran, one of oldest sources of dietary fiber, is the indigestible outer husk of wheat, rice, oats, and other cereal grains.

pared by his grandfather. He had no prior difficulty eating wheat or pancakes, and skin and blood tests to wheat were negative. Examination of the pancake flour bought one year earlier and left in a plastic box found storage mite contamination. Another clinic in Japan described six cases of mite-contaminated flour reactions. Two children in this group reacted to *tako-yaki* (octopus dumplings) and homemade hot cakes. In 1995, Spanish and Venezuelan allergists depicted a group of patients who reacted to foods contaminated by dust mites. Many of their patients experienced life-threatening anaphylaxis. As most of their patients reacted to mite-contaminated pancake flour, they labeled it the "pancake syndrome."

I recently saw a fifty-two-year-old mite-allergic woman who experienced eye swelling and lip tingling after eating pancakes made from a mix that had been stored in her kitchen cabinet for several months. The cause of the reaction was initially attributed to environmental allergens as she had a history of allergy to dust mites and pollen and no history of food allergy. Three months later while cooking pancakes from the same mix, she experienced wheezing, diffuse redness, and facial swelling requiring emergency care. Upon evaluation she had large positive skin tests to dust mites and the pancake mix. She had no previous problems eating wheat or flour-based products, and skin tests to wheat were negative. Microscopic examination of the pancake mix revealed that it was loaded with live house dust mites chowing down on the pancake mix.

In April 2006, a letter in the newspaper column Dear Abby described a fourteen-year-old boy who experienced difficulty breathing and cyanosis ten minutes after eating pancakes made from an outdated box of pancake mix. In 2001, doctors from Charleston, South Carolina, reported the death of a nineteen-year-old male who had a history of multiple allergies.[2] One morning, he and his friends made pancakes with a mix that had been opened and stored for approximately two years. His friends stopped eating the pancakes because they tasted like "rubbing alcohol." The decedent, an asthmatic, became short of breath and was taken to a nearby clinic where he died. Autopsy findings were consistent with an asthma death. As the pancake mix contained a high mold count, the medical examiners concluded that death was due to eating mold-contaminated pancake mix. Anaphylactic reactions to molds in fermented foods—like cheese, dried fruits, yogurt, and wine—in mold-allergic patients are quite rare. Most, if not all, of my mold-allergic patients tolerate "moldy foods." In my opinion, the "Dear Abby case" and the death of the nineteen-year-old male in Charleston were possibly due to ingestion of dust mite-contaminated pancakes.

The take home message—anaphylaxis from oral ingestion of mites is a potentially lethal condition. While most case reports come from tropical and subtropical countries, this problem may be more prevalent than recognized in temperate climates. Allergy specialists must examine implicated foodstuffs in cases of unexplained anaphylaxis. Until prospective studies determine proper methods of storage and a time frame for mite infestation in such products, at-risk patients and their families should not store such foods for prolonged periods and should discard old, damp or discolored products. ●

2 Dr. Allan T. Bennett and Dr. Kim A. Collins, "An Unusual Case of Anaphylaxis: Mold in Pancake Mix," *American Journal of Forensic Medicine and Pathology*, 22 (September 2001): 292-295.

Chapter

9

Peanut and Legume Allergy

■ Historical and Nutritional Facts

Peanuts—also known as ground nuts, goobers, pandas, monkey nuts, and Chinese nuts—have been an invaluable food source for centuries. The peanut comes from a member of the legume family that is native to South America. Excavations in Peru, where wild peanut plants still grow, date the peanut plant back to 2000-3000 BC. Once the peanut plant was domesticated, European traders spread it worldwide.

The African slave ships brought the peanut plant to America where "goobers" grew well in the Southern soil. During the Civil War, Union soldiers discovered that peanuts roasted in an open fire were an excellent food source. After the Civil War, the popularity of peanuts rose dramatically throughout the United States. The consumption of peanut products likewise increased in Europe after World War II due to the introduction of peanuts to Europe by the American Army.

George Washington Carver, a famous American agricultural researcher, was the first to describe more than 300 different uses for peanuts that, contrary to popular belief, did not include peanut butter. Carver encouraged Southern farmers to grow peanuts instead of cotton, as, unlike cotton, the peanut plant did not leach nitrogen from the soil. Carver encouraged the planting of peanuts as a viable cash crop that could provide an inexpensive source of protein for poor families.

There are many claims about the origins of peanut butter. The Chinese have crushed peanuts into creamy sauces for several centuries. Africans ground peanuts into stews as early as the fifteenth century. Civil War soldiers dined on peanut porridge. However, such use bears little resemblance to peanut butter as we now it today. In 1890, an unidentified St. Louis physician supposedly encouraged the owner of a food products company, George A. Bayle Jr., to process and package ground peanut paste as a nutritious protein substitute for people with poor teeth who couldn't chew meat. The physician apparently had experimented by grinding peanuts in his hand-cranked meat grinder. Bayle mechanized the process and began selling peanut butter out of barrels for six cents per pound.

Around the same time, Dr. John Harvey Kellogg in Battle Creek, Michigan, began using peanut butter as a vegetarian protein food for patients at his spa, the Western Health Reform Institute. His brother, Dr. William "Willie" Keith

Carver encouraged the planting of peanuts as a viable cash crop that could provide an inexpensive source of protein for poor families.

Kellogg, a former broom salesman, and now the business manager of their sanitarium, formed the Sanitas Nut Company that supplied peanut butter to local grocery stores. In 1895, the Kellogg brothers' patent for the "Process of Preparing Nut Meal" described a pasty adhesive substance that was called nut butter. However, their peanut butter was not as tasty as today's peanut butter, as the ground peanuts were steamed instead of roasted prior to grinding. William Kellogg received his M.D. from Bellevue Hospital Medical College in New York City in 1875. He was a Seventh-Day Adventist and therefore a vegetarian. In 1894, William Kellogg was trying to improve the vegetarian diet of his hospital patients. He was searching for a digestible bread substitute by boiling wheat. Kellogg accidentally left a pot of boiled wheat to stand, and the wheat became tempered or softened. When Kellogg rolled the tempered wheat and let it dry, each grain of wheat emerged as a large thin flake. The flakes turned out to be a tasty dish. Kellogg had invented cereal flakes.[1]

One pouch of Plumpy'nut packs 500 calories and costs as little as thirty-five cents a packet. Malnourished children may consume as many as three packets a day.

■ The Peanut Plant

The peanut plant is a warm season, annual plant that has yellow flowers that open in the morning. After the flower withers, the stalks, or pegs, turn to the ground and deposit a pod containing two to three (rarely one or four) peanut seeds. Peanuts grow best in light, sandy soil. They require five months of warm weather and a twenty- to forty-inch rainfall or the equivalent in irrigation water. The pods ripen in 120 to 150 days after the seeds are planted. The entire plant is removed from the soil during harvesting. If the crop is harvested too early, the pods will be unripe. If they are harvested late, the pods snap off at the stalk and remain in the soil. Improper storage of peanut plants can lead to an infection by the *Aspergillus flavus*, a mold that releases a toxin called aflatoxin.

The four major peanut crops are the Spanish peanut, runner, Virginia, and Valencia groups. Certain peanut crops are preferred over others because of differences in flavor, oil content, size, shape, and disease resistance. Most peanuts marketed in the shell are Virginia peanuts. Valencias are selected for their large size and attractive shell. Spanish peanuts are used in peanut candy, salted nuts, and peanut butter.

The United States now trails only China and India in peanut production. It is estimated that half a billion people rely on peanuts as their primary source of protein. Under the name "Plumpy'nut," 3.5 ounces, or two small bags, of peanuts are distributed by the World Health Organization to starving African children daily.

PEANUT PLANT

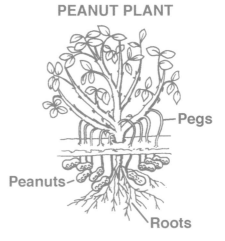

---

[1] http://inventors.about.com/library/inventors/blcereal.htm

Unlike fortified powdered-milk formulas, Plumpy'nut does not require mixing with clean water, which can be difficult to come by in war-torn and famine-stricken areas. Plumpy'nut is a ready-to-eat mixture of peanut paste, sugar, fats, minerals, and vitamins. One pouch of Plumpy'nut packs 500 calories and costs as little as thirty-five cents a packet. Malnourished children may consume as many as three packets a day.

Peanuts are grown by land-holding farmers in the United States, Africa, South America, and Southeast Asia. Forty percent of the annual 600 million-pound peanut crop grown by 25,000 American peanut farmers is now consumed as peanut butter. The principal forms of peanuts are salted or shelled nuts, peanut butter, and roasted peanuts. Despite their relatively high fat content, peanuts are a rich source of protein and unsaturated fat. The primary use of peanut butter is in the home, but large quantities are used in the commercial manufacture of sandwiches, candy, and bakery products. Raw boiled peanuts are a popular roadside snack in the southern United States. Peanut oil is popular in cooking, as it has a mild flavor and burns only at a relatively high temperature. Peanuts are often the major ingredients in mixed nuts, as they are less expensive than tree nuts.

Low-grade peanuts, unsuitable for the edible market, are used in the production of peanut oil and birdseed. Peanut byproducts are used in paints, varnishes, lubricating oils, leather dressings, furniture polishes, textile fibers, and insecticides. Many skin creams and cosmetics contain peanut oil. Peanut shells are used in the manufacture of plastic, wallboard, abrasives, cellulose, and glue.

■ The Unique Peanut Protein

Peanuts are not true nuts. They are vegetables from the legume family, which includes soybeans, peas and beans, and lentils. They grow in the ground, whereas tree nuts are the seeds of fruit-bearing trees. Just as the house dust mite and cat allergen are the most potent inhalant allergens, peanut (and tree nut) proteins are the most powerful and dangerous food allergens. The typical peanut is made up of several different proteins. One peanut contains about 200 mg of protein. Very trace amounts, as little as 2 mg of protein, or 1/250th of an average peanut, can trigger an allergic reaction.

The prevalence of peanut allergy is much higher in Chinese-Americans than in the Mainland Chinese population, despite similar consumption rates of peanuts in the United States and China. Differences in sensitization rates in the United States and China could be explained by consumption of roasted peanut in the United States, whereas in China and other Asian countries, peanuts are usually consumed boiled or fried. Thermal processing may alter

> *Just as the house dust mite and cat allergen are the most potent inhalant allergens, peanut (and tree nut) proteins are the most powerful and dangerous food allergens.*

the allergenicity of foods by changing their susceptibility to digestion, altering their allergen structure, or destroying the allergen. Recent studies have shown that roasting increases the allergen level in peanuts.

■ The Peanut Allergy Epidemic

Despite the fact that peanuts were recognized as a food allergen in the early 1920s, little attention was paid to peanut allergy until the 1970s when two pioneers in food allergy research, Doctors Charles May and Allan Bock, described allergic reactions in asthmatic children challenged with peanuts. The dramatic increase in cases of peanut- and tree nut-allergy has prompted food allergy centers throughout the world to further study peanut allergy. The most prominent of these centers, the Jaffe Food Allergy Institute at Mount Sinai Hospital in New York City headed by Dr. Hugh Sampson, is responsible for several outstanding studies in this field.

Surveys in the United States, the United Kingdom and Canada reported that the incidence of peanut- and tree nut-allergy had doubled in a ten-year span. A 2001 telephone survey conducted in the United States found that 1.2 percent of children were allergic to peanuts or tree nuts, twice the rate (0.6 percent) reported in 1999. Montreal investigators found a 1.5 percent prevalence rate of peanut allergy in 7,768 children enrolled in kindergarten through grade three. In one Australian study, nearly 5 percent of three-year-olds had a positive peanut skin test, and it was estimated that 50 percent would have a reaction if exposed to peanuts. Peanut allergy was more commonly seen in younger boys and children with egg allergy.

While the rate of peanut allergy varies from country to country in the western world, it does not appear to favor any ethnic group. For example, Jewish children in

While the rate of peanut allergy varies from country to country in the western world, it does not appear to favor any ethnic group. For example, Jewish children in the United Kingdom have fourteen times more peanut allergy than Jewish children living in Israel.

the United Kingdom have fourteen times more peanut allergy than Jewish children living in Israel. Peanut or tree nut allergy is now the most common food allergy in children after cow's milk and egg allergy. Today, peanut- and tree nut-allergy is the leading cause for emergency visits for acute allergic reactions in the United States, Great Britain, Canada, France, and Australia. It is estimated that approximately 100 Americans die per year from a peanut or a tree nut reaction.

■ Clinical Features of Peanut- and Tree Nut-Allergy

Several studies in the United States and Europe have analyzed the clinical features of peanut- and tree nut-allergy. The best survey gathered data from 4,586 registrants in FAAN's Registry for Peanut and Tree Nut Allergy. Nearly 70 percent of those surveyed had an isolated peanut allergy; only 9 percent reported tree nut allergy alone; and 23 percent had both a peanut and a tree nut allergy. Nearly one-third had other food allergies, especially to eggs.

Nearly 50 percent had asthma or eczema. Most children (82 percent) were breast-fed for an average of seven months. The average age of a first exposure was twelve months, and the first reaction to peanuts occurred at fourteen months of age. Surprisingly, 75 percent of the reactions took place on the first exposure to peanuts. The most common route of exposure was oral ingestion—91 percent of the cases. Most reactions occurred at home and started within three minutes after exposure.

Reactions to tree nuts occurred later than peanuts—the first tree nut reaction took place at an average age of thirty-six months. Sixty-eight percent reported that the first reaction to tree nuts occurred with the first exposure, and the majority of exposures (61 percent) occurred at home.

Ingestion was the most common route of exposure to tree nuts (88 percent). Most reactions involved the skin (90 percent), and nearly half had respiratory symptoms. One-third had vomiting or diarrhea, and half of the reactions involved more than one organ. A second reaction to peanuts was described by 2,226 registrants (48 percent), and 1,072 victims (23 percent) reported a third reaction. Subsequent reactions, attributable to accidental ingestion, were more severe, more commonly occurred outside the home, and were more likely to require treatment with auto-injectable epinephrine when compared with initial reactions. Ninety percent of the participants reported having epinephrine available at all times. About 5 percent of responders had never been prescribed auto-injectable epinephrine.

In another study, which followed fifty-three peanut-allergic children for five years, 58 percent of the subjects experienced subsequent reactions from accidental peanut exposure. Regardless of the nature of their initial reaction, the majority of subsequent reactions (52 percent) were potentially life-threatening reactions. In many patients, subsequent reactions often worsen, especially if the first reaction was severe and required medical care. The majority of patients reported having auto-injectable epinephrine on hand, but more than 500 patients in the FAAN survey did not have epinephrine readily available, and almost half of these 500 patients had never been given a prescription for an auto-injectable epinephrine device.

Due to improved educational programs, the rate of accidental ingestion may be declining, as recent data from Montreal, Canada, found that only 9 percent of peanut-allergic subjects experienced a subsequent accidental reaction to peanuts.

■ Proposed Reasons for the Increase in Peanut and Tree Nut Allergy

Several theories have been put forward to explain the increase in peanut- and tree nut-allergy, such as the hygiene and microflora hypothesis, an increase in the rate of breast-feeding, ingestion of highly nutritional, "quick-energy" nut products by pregnant and lactating women, varied methods of preparing peanuts (dry roasting versus frying or boiling), use of skin preparations containing peanut oil in infancy, inhalation of peanut and tree nut particles by infants, and changes in maternal and infant feeding patterns.

Several developed countries have not experienced a peanut or tree nut allergy epidemic. The low prevalence of peanut allergy in China has been linked to the early introduction of peanut products in infancy and boiling peanuts versus the dry roasting methods used in America.

In another study, which followed fifty-three peanut-allergic children for five years, 58 percent of the subjects experienced subsequent reactions from accidental peanut exposure. Regardless of the nature of their initial reaction, the majority of subsequent reactions (52 percent) were potentially life-threatening reactions.

As over 90 percent of infants and children react on their first exposure to a peanut or a tree nut, the big question is where is the necessary prior exposure coming from? The easiest answer to this question is to blame mom. Prior exposure to minute amounts of peanut or tree nut

Table 9.1. Proposed Reasons for the Increase in Peanut Allergy

The hygiene and microflora hypothesis

Increase in breast-feeding

Ingestion of high-energy, nut-containing foods in pregnant and lactating mothers

Frying and roasting peanuts

Using skin preparations containing peanut protein

Change in maternal and infant feeding habits

Inhalation or oral contact of peanut particles in infancy or early childhood

Delay in introducing peanut products in infancy and early childhood

protein can occur through the placenta or breast milk of goober-gobbling mothers. However, studies looking at this relationship are inconclusive. Most surveys have not found any solid relationship between peanut or tree nut allergy in infants or children and maternal consumption of peanuts or tree nuts during pregnancy or while breast-feeding. Later on, you will read why we may be targeting the wrong parent. In my opinion, nut-loving, football-watching dads may be responsible for exposing their at-risk infants and children to peanut protein. (see table 9.1).

Dr. Gideon Lack from St. Mary's Hospital in London suspects that modern-day infant feeding patterns might be responsible for the rise in the incidence of peanut- and tree nut-allergy. The American Academy of Pediatrics and the Department of Health in the United Kingdom now recommend that at-risk infants be exclusively breast-

Other than the use of extensively hydrolyzed formulas, there are no conclusive studies showing that dietary manipulation during pregnancy or while breastfeeding or restricting allergenic foods in infancy or early childhood prevents the development of food allergy.

fed, and that pregnant and breastfeeding mothers should not eat peanuts and tree nuts. The introduction of solid foods should be delayed until six months of age, no cow's milk until age one, no eggs until age two; and peanuts, tree nuts and seafood should not be introduced until three years of age. Other than the use of extensively hydrolyzed formulas, there are no conclusive studies showing that dietary manipulation during pregnancy or while breast-feeding or restricting allergenic foods in infancy or early childhood prevents the development of food allergy. Could these guidelines that limit exposure to allergenic foods until age three paradoxically favor IgE sensitization in a subgroup of at-risk children in a similar manner that minimal or no exposure to animal allergens promotes sensitization by preventing the development of immune tolerance? Lack suggests a delay in introducing more allergenic foods in early childhood blocks the development of immunological tolerance and favors the striking increase in peanut- and tree nut-allergy in children seen over the past five years.

I agree with Lack. What has changed in the three decades? First, unlike the 1960s and 1970s when peanut- and tree nut-allergy was rare, breast-feeding is now the norm, not the exception. The 2004 Feeding Infant and Toddlers Study found that three-fourths of American mothers now breast-feed their infants. Secondly, throughout the 1960s into the 1980s, foods like peanut butter were often an integral part of an infant's diet once solid foods were introduced at four to six months of age. Today's breast-feeding American moms are now more likely to delay the introduction of such high-risk foods and feed their infants less allergenic snacks and baked goods. Could breast-feeding or a westernized diet be detrimental in a not yet well-defined subgroup of infants at risk for eczema and food allergies? This important question will be discussed in detail in chapter 16.

■ Outgrowing Peanut Allergy

Peanut allergy is far less likely to be outgrown than other childhood food allergies, as only 10 to 20 percent of those affected ever become tolerant to peanuts. One well-done study mirrors most of the studies looking at the natural history of peanut allergy. A total of 223 patients with a diagnosis of peanut allergy was identified by chart review in two tertiary-care allergy clinics and one private practice. Patients with only skin symptoms after peanut ingestion and CAP RAST tests of less than twenty units were asked to undergo peanut challenges. One in every five of the eighty-five patients who subsequently underwent a peanut challenge had a negative challenge. Those individuals with the best shot

at outgrowing peanut allergy were children with an early onset of peanut allergy, a small skin test reaction, a low CAP RAST level, and no history of eczema or other food allergies, especially egg allergy.

What happens after outgrowing a peanut allergy? Researchers at Johns Hopkins University studied patients who had outgrown their peanut allergy. Patients were invited to undergo a double-blind, placebo-controlled food challenge (DBPCFC) unless the clinical history implied that a challenge could be dangerous. Three of fifteen patients who consumed peanuts infrequently or in limited amounts suffered a recurrence of peanut allergy, compared with no recurrences in the twenty-three patients who frequently ate peanut products. This important study concluded that some children who outgrow peanut allergy were at risk for recurrence, and that the risk was significantly higher for patients who continued to avoid peanuts after resolution of their allergy.

Repeated exposure is probably necessary to maintain a state of immune tolerance to an offending food.

Additional reports from private allergy practices have described a recurrence of peanut allergy, again, mostly in patients who did not eat the offending food on a regular basis. The bottom line: patients who outgrow their food allergy or pass an oral challenge test should eat the food on a regular basis (several times a week) and carry auto-injectable epinephrine with them even when they have demonstrated an ongoing tolerance to the food. Repeated exposure is probably necessary to maintain a state of immune tolerance to an offending food.

■ Should Peanut-Allergic Patients Eat Tree Nuts?

Should peanut-allergic patients who are able to eat tree nuts without difficulty be advised to consume tree nuts? This is a very complex question for which there is no uniform consensus amongst allergy specialists. Some food allergy experts, such as Dr. Scott Sicherer and Terry Malloy, allow responsible peanut-allergic patients to eat tree nuts, like walnuts, directly from the shell if they have no history of a reaction to walnuts. Dr. Michael Young recommends that peanut-allergic children avoid all tree nuts except for previously tolerated tree nuts or unless testing to a specific tree nut is negative. Young suggests testing for tree nuts once the child reaches age five, and if the tests are negative, consider introducing tree nuts into the child's diet. My approach to this question is somewhat more conservative. One in three peanut-allergic patients may react to tree nuts—not because they are related botanically, but because many tree nuts contain very potent allergenic proteins.

Due to the difficulty in identifying tree nuts in nut mixes and processed foods and the potential severity of a tree nut allergy, I will ask a patient or family with a peanut allergy if they have any desire to eat tree nuts. When the answer is no, I advise them that the best and safest approach is to avoid all tree nuts as there is a one-in-three chance that a peanut-allergic patient may eventually react to a tree nut.

At the present time, allergy specialists are unable to accurately predict when or what tree nut a peanut-allergic patient will react to. Older more responsible peanut-allergic patients or families who want to eat or serve tree nuts can be offered the opportunity to undergo an oral challenge when skin and CAP RAST tests are negative. I recommend that young peanut-allergic children should never experiment with tree nuts. In fact, I advise these families to maintain a peanut- tree nut-free household.

I advise all my peanut-allergic patients with asthma, regardless of their age, to avoid all tree nuts as the majority of the food fatalities reported in the lay press and medical literature are due to accidental ingestion of peanuts or tree nuts in patients with asthma. This ultra-conservative approach is undoubtedly biased by the fact that over the past decade two asthmatic patients in our practice died after accidentally ingesting a tree nut.

■ Common Names and Hidden Sources of Peanut Allergen

Many near-fatal and fatal food reactions are due to hidden peanuts and tree nuts in foods prepared outside the home. Eating out, take-away food and foreign travel can be risky ventures for those on a peanut- or tree nut-free diet. Some foreign names for peanut include: French (*pistache de terre, arachide, cacahouette*) and Spanish (*cacahuete*). Some names and hidden sources of peanut protein are listed in table 9.2.

Beware of labels that state, "may contain peanuts or nuts." Dr. Marie-Noel Primeau from the Allergy Service of Saint Justine Hospital in Montreal, Canada, described the case of a thirteen-year-old boy who had his first anaphylactic reaction

> *Older more responsible peanut-allergic patients or families who want to eat or serve tree nuts can be offered the opportunity to undergo an oral challenge when skin and CAP RAST tests are negative.*

Table 9.2. Names and Hidden Sources of Peanut Protein

Names	Hidden Sources
Artificial nuts	Cakes and pastries
Imitation nuts	Biscuits
Beer nuts	Ice cream
Goober peas	Desserts and dessert toppings
Peanut butter	Cereal bars
Emulsifiers	Confectionery and savory snacks
Nut spreads	Breakfast and muesli-type cereals
Praline	Meat products
Marzipan (usually almonds)	Vegetarian products
Frangipani	Ready-made meals
Bakewell Tarts	Stuffed bean bags and bird food
Almond essence	Arts and craft projects
Hydrolyzed vegetable protein	Amaretto products
	Macaroons
	Worcestershire and satay sauce

requiring treatment with epinephrine shortly after eating a brownie labeled, "may contain traces of nuts." Skin tests were positive to hazelnut, cashew, and pistachio and negative to peanuts. An oral challenge to hazelnut was positive. Her second case involved a five-year-old boy who developed hives fifteen minutes after eating a granola bar containing almonds, which was labeled "may contain traces of peanuts." He was a tree nut eater, but he had never eaten peanuts before. Skin tests were negative to tree nuts but positive to peanuts. One hour after an open peanut challenge, the patient developed nasal congestion and a severe cough.

Additional hidden sources of peanut allergen may include stuffed beanbags, popcorn, bird food, and arts and school crafts

Additional hidden sources of peanut allergen may include stuffed beanbags, popcorn, bird food, and arts and school crafts projects.

projects. Peanut butter is frequently used to add flavor and thickening for sauces and gravies. Its firm consistency prevents many foods like egg rolls from coming apart. Dry roasted peanuts are more allergenic than boiled or fried peanuts. New emulsifying processes used to make peanut butter may be making peanut butter more allergenic. Peanut butter and peanut oil are very popular in Asian, Indian, Thai, and Indonesian foods where sauces and salad dressings are prepared with peanuts.

■ The Peanut- Tree Nut-Oil Debate

Can patients who are allergic to peanuts and tree nuts tolerate exposure to or eat products or foods containing peanut oil or tree nut oil? Peanut and tree nut oils are widely used in pharmaceutical products, vitamins, skin creams, ointments, and orthopedic bone cement. Several studies have demonstrated that cold-pressed crude oils contained significant amounts of nut protein, whereas hot-pressed, highly refined oils do not. One study evaluated two types of peanut oil in subjects with peanut allergy. None of the sixty subjects reacted to the refined oil. Six reacted to the crude oil. The study concluded that crude peanut oil should be avoided and refined peanut oil was not a risk. Another study found that walnut, almond, hazelnut, pistachio, and macadamia oils that had undergone processing at lower temperatures posed a threat to patients with tree nut allergy. How about peanut oil in vitamin A and D preparations? A Swedish study concluded that sensitization to peanuts during childhood through consumption of vitamin A and D in peanut oil-based solutions seemed unlikely. The bottom line: production methods may vary and labels may not state how the oil was produced. Therefore, I advise patients with peanut- and tree nut-allergies and pregnant and breast-feeding mothers to avoid any product that contains peanut oil or tree nut oil.

Another study found that walnut, almond, hazelnut, pistachio, and macadamia oils that had undergone processing at lower temperatures posed a threat to patients with tree nut allergy.

A study from London by Lack's group triggered some debate. Lack reported that children who had been exposed to creams or ointments containing peanut oil (arachis) for the treatment of eczema, a diaper rash, or mother's irritated breast nipples had a higher incidence of peanut allergy. Lack suggested that peanut sensitization was occurring through skin or oral contact. Lack stated that the absence of an association with maternal consumption of peanuts during pregnancy combined with the inability to detect peanut protein in umbilical cord blood argued against the onset of sensitization during pregnancy. His study suggested a family history of peanut allergy, the occurrence of oozing skin rashes, and the topical use of peanut oil-based preparations may be causal factors in the development of peanut allergy.

This theory has some merit. Mice that had peanut protein applied to their skin were less likely to develop an oral tolerance to peanuts. Upon oral challenge, the mice were further sensitized to peanuts. Furthermore, mice with an existing tolerance to peanuts were partly sensitized following skin exposure to peanut protein.

Opponents of Lack's theory pointed out that English peanut oil is primarily a crude oil that contains peanut protein, whereas the more highly refined peanut oil used in the United States has no detectable peanut protein. In addition, most skin preparations in the United States do not contain peanut protein. One Chicago study looked for hidden food allergens in 293 pediatric skin-care products, including soaps, body washes, creams and oils. Peanut allergen was not listed in any of the skin preparations. The most common potential allergens were coconut (49 percent), herbal preparations (47 percent), soy (9 percent), and cow's milk (4 percent).

■ Can Peanut-Allergic Individuals Eat Other Legumes?

Legumes, one of man's oldest food sources, were first cultivated in Asia about 10,000 years ago. More than 1,300 species of legumes provide man with more protein than any other plant food on earth. American Indians planted legumes between rows of corn in order to replenish the soil with nitrogen. Legumes are rich in B-complex vitamins, potassium and other minerals. Legumes may lower cholesterol, and their phytochemicals may ward off cancer. Fortunately, peanut allergy does not require elimination of the entire legume family, as the chances of reacting to other legumes, such as soybeans, beans, or peas, is only about 5 percent. The one exception to this rule is lupines and lentils.

Soybean Allergy

Soybean is the most important bean in world, as it is the cheapest source of protein in many undeveloped nations where starvation and malnutrition is rampant. Soybean allergy is less common than cow's milk allergy in infants and children—about three in every 1,000. A soy-based formula is usually the best choice for the milk-allergic or lactose-intolerant child. Even though the soybean is also a legume, only 5 percent of peanut-allergic patients are soybean-allergic. Infants who react to both milk and soy formulas usually tolerate hypoallergenic formulas like Alimentum or Nutramigen.

Highly refined soybean oil is usually not a problem for soy-sensitive patients as heating denatures the soybean protein. Other beans in the legume family can cause reactions. One of the first cases of fatal food allergy reported in the literature in the 1920s depicted the death of a young child after pea ingestion. In 2005, Spanish investigators described a seven-year-old boy who developed swelling associated with inhalation of vapors from cooked white beans.

Common Names and Hidden Sources of Soy Protein

Avoiding soybean products is quite difficult as they are major ingredients in processed foods. Common foods that contain soy protein include tofu, Tamari, canned tuna, cereals, crackers, soups, baked goods, sauces, and soups. Additional hidden sources of soy protein include hamburgers, meatballs, kebab, sausages, and breads. Many farms harvest their soybean and corn crops at the same time, yet there are no reports of reactions to soybean in soy-contaminated corn products.

Highly refined soybean oil is usually not a problem for soy-sensitive patients as heating denatures the soybean protein.

Tofu is a great source of soybean protein and estrogen-like isoflavones that allegedly lower the risk of heart disease and some cancers. Tofu is often disdained by meat-loving Americans because of its bland, mushy, non-meaty taste.

Xiang F. Kong, a former molecular biologist at Boston University and Harvard Medical School, has spent more than two years developing a more palatable tofu.[2] Kong's company, Soy Foods, has developed a method to add teriyaki and other flavors to tofu. Kong calls his product, Tofettes. He plans on developing this process to produce tofu pasta. If Kong's products and others like it become more popular, the incidence of tofu-induced soy allergy will undoubtedly increase.

---

[2] *Boston Globe*, January 2, 2006.

Until I came across a report of the death of a seventeen-year-old Swedish girl who died after eating a hamburger that contained soy protein, I believed that soybean allergy was not as severe or as life-threatening as a peanut or tree nut allergy. This unfortunate death in 1992 prompted investigators to look more closely at food allergy deaths in Sweden. In the first three years of their study, they uncovered four more deaths in soy-allergic patients. All these victims had asthma and peanut allergy. Many were symptom-free for up to ninety minutes after ingesting soy products that included kebab, hamburgers, and meatballs.

Unlike other food reactions, except for wheat, the onset of a soybean reaction may be delayed several hours.

One interesting case depicts a soybean-allergic patient who developed hives and shortness of breath thirteen hours after he was challenged to fermented soybean. Another European paper described a severe reaction to soy protein that was hidden in Italian roast beef. To date there are no similar reports in the United States.

One of my patients, an eight-year-old boy with asthma and severe peanut- tree nut- and soy-nut allergy, recently had a systemic reaction to Funyuns, an onion-flavored corn chip introduced in 1969 by Frito-Lay. The chips, which are shaped like onion rings, are deep-fried in corn meal and coated with a pale yellow, onion-flavored powder. Funyuns contain three sources of soybean (soybean oil, soy flour and hydrolyzed soy protein) as well as spices, MSG, garlic and buttermilk.

The bottom line: do not underestimate soybean allergy, especially in children and young adults with peanut allergy and asthma. Furthermore, unlike other food reactions, except for wheat, the onset of a soybean reaction may be delayed several hours.

Natto Allergy

Natto is a sticky web of bacteria-fermented soybeans that has been a traditional Japanese staple for more than 1,000 years. It is usually eaten with rice and often at breakfast. Natto's touted medical benefits, which include prevention of heart disease, strokes, cancer, osteoporosis, obesity, and intestinal diseases, have led to its increased popularity. Due to its foul rotten egg-like smell and distinctive taste, Japanese natives are fond of the saying, "Only real Japanese eat natto!"

One interesting report described a thirty-six-year-old man who experienced hives, chest tightness, abdominal cramps, palpitations, vomiting, dizziness, and headaches about two to three days a week. He often ate dinner in the early evening. Yet, his reactions did not start until the next morning. A diet diary revealed that he had ingested natto ten to twelve hours before the onset of his symptoms in all instances. Skin tests with commercial food allergens, including soybean, were negative. Skin tests with the raw ingredients in his dinners were also negative except for natto. Skin and CAP RAST tests to natto powder and manufactured natto were positive. It appears that the slow release of natto during fermentation in the intestinal tract led to a delayed food reaction. More reactions to natto may occur if natto becomes more popular in western cuisine.

ChickPea Allergy[3]

The chickpea, also called the garbanzo bean, ceci bean, bengal gram, or chana, is

[3] Compiled in part by Dr. Harris Steinman, harris@zing-solutions.com

an old member of the legume family. The name "chickpea" is derived from the Latin name, *Cicer*. It has been suggested that the chickenpox disease gets its name from chickpeas that resemble the skin lesions of chickenpox. Their origin dates as far back as 3500 BC. In classical Greece, they were called *erébinthos*, and were eaten both as a staple and as a dessert. The Romans ate several varieties of chickpeas, such as venus, ram, and punic chickpeas as a broth and in a roasted snack. Chickpeas were touted as being "less windy" and more nourishing than regular peas.

The Romans believed chickpeas increased sperm and breast milk production, provoked menstruation and urine output, and prevented kidney stones. The chickpea grows on a ten- to twenty-inch high plant that has small feathery leaves on both sides of the stem. One seedpod contains two or three peas. As chickpeas need a subtropical or tropical climate and abundant rainfall, they are mainly grown in the Mediterranean, western Asia, and India.

Chickpeas can be eaten in salads, stews, ground into a flour called gram flour or besan, shaped in balls and fried as falafel, and cooked and ground into a paste called hummus.[4] In India, where they are referred to as *"chanas,"* chickpeas provide a major source of protein in a predominantly vegetarian culture. Unripe chickpeas are also eaten as a raw snack in many parts of India. Chickpea flour is also used to make "Burmese tofu," a popular food of the Shan people of Burma. Chickpea is an important source of proteins, carbohydrates, B-group vitamins and certain minerals, particularly in developing nations. India contributes

over 75 percent of the world's chickpea production. Chickpeas are also popular in the Mediterranean, especially in Spain.

■ Clinical Reactions to Chickpeas

There are only a few reports of chickpea allergy in the North American literature. No allergens from this plant have yet been fully characterized. An extensive cross-reactivity among legumes could be expected, but, in fact, does not usually occur between most legumes. Chickpeas may induce typical symptoms of food allergy—ranging from mild oral allergy symptoms to full-blown anaphylaxis.

The largest series of cases comes from India where the majority of the population consumes a vegetarian diet made up of legumes, cereals, and vegetables. Indian allergists studied 1,400 Indian food-allergic patients and found fifty-nine individuals with chickpea allergy. As chickpea allergens are heat-stable, reactions from ingestion or inhalation of vapors from cooked chickpea (and other cooked legumes) have been described. Severe wheezing and hives one hour after the ingestion of chickpeas was reported in an eight-year-old Indian girl. She had a

> *Unfortunately, chickpea reactions can be fatal. Dr. Richard Pumphrey has surveyed every reported anaphylactic death in United Kingdom since 1992—about twenty a year. In thirteen cases of fatal food reactions that were not due to a nut allergy, two deaths were reportedly caused by chickpeas.*

---

[4] Hummus is a puree of chickpeas and tahini (sesame seed paste) that is usually seasoned with lemon juice and garlic. Originally a spread and dip in the Middle East and India, hummus is now a very popular item of American cuisine.

previous history of wheezing following inhalation of chickpea flour or its vapors. A twenty-year-old man experienced asthma after exposure to the steam from cooked chickpeas and lentils.

Unfortunately, chickpea reactions can be fatal. Dr. Richard Pumphrey has surveyed every reported anaphylactic death in the United Kingdom since 1992—about twenty a year. In thirteen cases of fatal food reactions that were not due to a nut allergy, two deaths were reportedly caused by chickpeas. In 1994, eight-year-old Nita Sekhri was playing at a friend's home where she was exposed to cooking vapors from chickpeas that exploded out of a faulty pressure cooker. She quickly experienced severe anaphylaxis and died despite receiving an auto-injectable epinephrine injection. Nita's tragic death reminds us of the dangers posed by inhaled food vapors, and that not all food allergy fatalities are triggered by foods in the Big Eight group.[5]

■ Lupine and Lentil Allergy

Lupine, a legume related to peas, beans, peanuts and soybeans, has been widely recognized in Europe as a common cause of allergic reactions and anaphylaxis. Lupines come from a pea-like plant of the lupine family. Sweet lupine or lupine flour is used in cookies, breads, and pasta. Lupine flour has been reported to produce hives, nasal congestion, and asthma in occupational settings. One forty-two-year-old woman developed abdominal pain, hives, facial swelling, cough, and shortness of breath ten to fifteen minutes after eating a bread roll. The only unusual ingredient in this bread roll was lupine bran. Skin tests with lupine

bran and the baked bread roll were strongly positive. A twenty-six-year-old woman developed hives, swelling and respiratory problems after eating lupine. She had a similar but less severe reaction to home-prepared lupine. She also reacted to imported European ginger biscuits that were found to contain lupine flour. Another twenty-five-year-old peanut-allergic woman reacted after eating a restaurant meal of chicken, French fried potatoes, and onion rings. Lupine flour was identified in the onion ring batter she had consumed.

In a French study, nearly 50 percent of peanut-allergic children had a positive skin test to lupine, and seven of eight children reacted to a lupine flour challenges. The largest study of lupine allergy describes twenty-two patients from Spain. Most cases occurred in young children (under age four) who developed hives or oral allergy symptoms. There was a high crossover reaction rate with peanut allergy.

A case from the Norwegian National Register for Severe Allergic Reactions to Food described a patient with peanut allergy who experienced a severe allergic reaction after eating a brand of hot dog bread that was fortified with lupine. Another interesting case described a two-year-old, wheat- and peanut-allergic child with eosinophilic esophagitis who was consuming large amounts of lentils. Once lentils were eliminated from his diet, all his symptoms disappeared. While there are only a few reported cases of lupine allergy in the American literature, peanut-allergic individuals should avoid lupine, lupine flour, lupine seeds, and lentils.[6] ●

---

[5] "The Nita Sekhri Story," *The MA Report-Allergy and Asthma Network-Mothers of Asthmatics,* February-March 2006.

[6] A paucity of reported cases of unusual food allergy reactions in the United States may be due to lack of national reporting registries that are available in many European countries.

Chapter

10

Tree Nut Allergy

Peanut allergy is not alone in this ongoing nut allergy epidemic. Due to an increased consumption, the incidence of tree nut allergy has dramatically increased in both children and adults. Many patients with tree nut allergy and their families are surprised to learn that tree nuts are not botanically related to peanuts or the legume family of vegetables that grow in the ground.

Tree nuts are the dried seeds of fruits from various trees. The most popular tree nuts are almonds, cashews, hazelnuts, pistachios, and walnuts. Tree nuts have been consumed since prehistoric times when Nomadic people gathered nuts growing in the wild. About 10,000 BC, settled populations began to cultivate nut-bearing trees. One of the reasons people settled in villages in early civilization was that tree nuts provided a more reliable food source than grains like wheat, as they were less susceptible to severe weather patterns and could be easily stored during long cold winters and consumed year-round.

The oil-rich kernels of tree nuts are great sources of proteins, vitamins, minerals and folate. One-third cup of tree nuts provides about five grams of protein—the equivalent of one ounce of lean meat. Essential minerals in tree nuts include magnesium, zinc, selenium, copper, potassium, phosphorous, zinc, biotin, and iron. Cholesterol-free tree nuts like walnuts are the best non-fish source of Omega-3 fatty acids. While high in fats, 85 percent are unsaturated fats that lower bad cholesterol levels. The FDA recently announced that producers of peanuts, hazelnuts, almonds, pecans, pistachios, and walnuts could claim that daily consumption of 1.5 ounces of nuts lowers bad cholesterol levels and reduces the risk of heart disease.

Tree nuts are a convenient, easy-to-eat food that are very suitable to today's fast-paced lifestyle. They require little or no preparation and are easily added to breads, muffins, pancake mixes, fruit salad, pasta, vegetable wraps, fish, and chicken dishes. Tree nuts are grown all over the world and are marketed in assorted sizes and shapes. The United States grows more than 10 percent of the world's tree nut crop and is now the world's largest exporter of tree nuts.

One-third cup of tree nuts provides about five grams of protein—the equivalent of one ounce of lean meat.

■ Incidence of Tree Nut Allergy

The incidence of tree nut allergy varies from country to country. The rise in tree nut allergy in the United States can be explained by the fact that Americans are now the world's biggest producers and consumers of tree nuts. Surveys indicate that one in every 200 Americans is allergic to a tree nut. Walnut allergy is the most common tree nut allergy in the United States. Hazelnut allergy is the most common tree nut allergy in Switzerland, and the Brazil nut allergy leads the way in the United Kingdom.

Tree nut allergy can come on at any age, but the first reaction usually occurs in children or young adults. It tends to develop later than peanut allergy. The average age of onset is between three and four years of age, whereas the average age of a first reaction to peanuts is between fourteen and sixteen months of age. The natural history of tree nut allergy is quite bleak.

Only 10 percent of victims outgrow their tree nut allergy. Once you have an allergic reaction to one tree nut, you have a one-in-three chance of reacting to another tree nut. The most distressing part of tree nut allergy is that it is a very dangerous food allergy that triggers near-fatal and fatal anaphylactic reactions. In published studies of near-fatal and fatal reactions, tree nuts are a leading cause of death. The two patients in our practice who succumbed to an accidental tree nut reaction were typical of other cases in the medical literature in that the fatal reactions occurred in an adolescent male and a young adult woman, both of whom had asthma. Thus, while tree nut reactions may be severe in younger children, this age group does not appear to be as high a risk for a fatal reaction as adolescents and young adults.

I am somewhat puzzled as to why severe peanut and tree nut reactions are rarely seen or reported in older adults, a population that is very susceptible to near-fatal and fatal anaphylactic reactions to stinging insects and drug allergy. There may be two reasons for this observation. Young victims of the nut aller-gy epidemic have not yet reached senior citizen age, or man's tolerance to potent food allergens may increase with age.

■ Ancient Almonds

Almonds are ancient ancestors of stone fruits like nectarines, peaches, plums and cherries. You can trace their origins to ancient China and central Asia. When early explorers and conquering armies carried edible almonds from Asia back to the Mediterranean, the almond seeds they dropped along the way flourished in the fertile soil of the Middle East. In the New World, Spanish monks planted almond trees along California's coastline. Later on, these settlers discovered that almonds grew better in the more Mediterranean-like climate of central California. There are more forms of almonds than any other tree nut. Natural almonds provide a more astringent taste than blanched almonds, and roasting contributes a more intense flavor. Sliced almonds improve visibility in a finished food product. Almonds are used as flavoring in drinks, ice creams, candies, baked goods, gelatins, puddings, and chewing gum.

Almond oil is also used in cosmetics. Hidden sources of almond include gourmet coffee and creamers, amaretto liquor, fried rice, and almond oil used in body massages and scented soaps. Despite their widespread use and consumption, almond allergy is relatively uncommon compared to that of other tree nuts. Almond allergy may

> *The most distressing part of tree nut allergy is that it is a very dangerous food allergy that triggers near-fatal and fatal anaphylactic reactions.*

cross react with apricots, walnuts, pine nuts, and pecans

Brazil Nut Allergy

Brazil nuts are a worldwide delicacy that come from a tree that grows in the rainforests of the Amazon basin. They grow in quantities of twelve to twenty-two nuts inside a large, woody, thick-walled fruit that can weigh up to four pounds. The Brazil trees themselves are never cultivated, but exportation of these nuts is a major Brazilian industry. Brazil nuts have a high nutritive food value, containing 60 to 70 percent oil and 17 percent protein. The Brazil nut can be well disguised in cookies and baked products.

Brazil nuts have been reported to cause near-fatal and fatal food reactions. In one series, Brazil nuts triggered the death of a two-year-old child who allegedly had never eaten a Brazil nut before. Although the reported incidence of reactions to Brazil nut is lower in the United States compared to other tree nuts, it is a troublesome allergen. One United Kingdom study found that Brazil nuts ranked second only to peanuts as a trigger of nut allergy.

Amazingly, the largest study on Brazil nut allergy comes from the David Hide Asthma and Allergy Research Centre located in the Isle of Wight (pop. about 126,000), a small island located just off the south coast of England. This center, the first to report the rising increase in peanut- and tree nut-allergy in the early 1990s, collected data on fifty-six children and adults

In one series, Brazil nuts triggered the death of a two-year-old child who allegedly had never eaten a Brazil nut before.

(age range four to eighty-three years) with Brazil nut allergy. Most subjects were highly allergic to Brazil nuts and reacted to tiny amounts of allergen, such as in taste, smell, or touch after the nuts were opened. Only three patients had eaten more than one nut when their reactions occurred. Most reactions were immediate in onset. Eighty percent had throat tightening, and 70 percent had asthma. I recall seeing two patients who experienced systemic reactions to skin testing to Brazil nuts and several others who had very large local skin test reactions to these nuts. Thus, the CAP RAST blood test may be the best and safest way to screen patients for a suspected Brazil nut allergy. I have also seen several patients whose only tree nut allergy was to Brazil nuts. Due to the risk of an unpredictable crossover reaction to other tree nuts, I advise Brazil nut-allergic patients to avoid all tree nuts, even if their skin and CAP RAST tests to other tree nuts are negative.

Cashew Nut Allergy

One of the more interesting tree nuts is the cashew nut, which grows in a double shell at the top of a small pear-like tree that is native to northeastern Brazil, India and Africa. As unprocessed cashews are poisonous, they must be removed from their shell and cooked before consumption. It is an irony of nature that two of the more delicious tree nuts, cashews and pistachios, belong to the same botanical family as poison ivy and poison oak. South American natives were the first to discover that roasting cashews removed their caustic oil and allowed the nut to be cracked open and consumed without ill effects. Medicinal uses of the cashew bark, leaves, and fermented cashew apple juice were well known prior to recorded history. Cashew teas and fruit juices are thought to have antibiotic, anti-inflammatory, and diuretic properties. Cashew tea was used to treat diarrhea, and the caustic oil was applied to skin infections and warts. Cashew oil is also used in automobile brakes, adhesives, paints, varnishes, insecticides, electrical insulation, and various antibiotics.

In the United States, cashews are more popular for snacking than for cooking. Cashews make a delicious nut butter that many people prefer over peanut butter.

Cashews may be consumed fresh, but they taste much better when roasted. Raw cashews contain high quantities of tannins that create a bitter taste and dry mouth. After India developed more efficient methods for removing the caustic oil, this country led the world in cashew production for many decades. Recently, production in Vietnam has surged about three-fold. Cashews are now the world's number one tree nut crop, passing almonds in 2003.

Cashews are a good source of iron and folic acid. They are lower in total fat than most nuts and seeds but are relatively high in saturated fat. Cashews are consumed cooked, partially dried, or candied. In India, the alcoholic drink feni is made from fermented cashew-apple juice. In the United States, cashews are more popular for snacking than for cooking. Cashews make a delicious nut butter that many people prefer over peanut butter.

■ Clinical Reactions to Cashews

In my experience, cashew nut allergy is now the leading cause of tree nut reactions in young children. The rise in production and increased consumption by pregnant and breast-feeding mothers (or nut-loving dads) may be responsible for this surge in cashew allergy. The best cashew study comes from France where researchers studied forty-five cashew-allergic children. The average age of onset of cashew allergy was twenty-four months. Affected boys outnumbered girls three-to-one. Only 20 percent had previously eaten cashews prior to their first reaction. Nearly 50 percent had another food allergy, especially to pistachios, a member of the same botanical family.

In a United Kingdom study of cashew reactions in children with no previous exposure, the average age of onset was four years. Most reactions took place at home, where unsuspecting parents kept cashews. Cashew nut allergy is associated with a high risk of anaphylaxis. One review of 213 children with peanut or tree nut allergy found anaphylaxis to cashew nut was more common than anaphylaxis to peanuts—74 percent versus 30 percent.

One of my partner's children had an anaphylactic reaction to cashews within minutes after eating only one cashew in a supermarket. He related that this was his child's first exposure, but both he and the child's mother had ingested large amounts of cashews during her pregnancy and while the infant was breast-feeding. I recently evaluated a fifteen-month-old infant whose allergic reaction to his first ingestion of cashews was confirmed by positive skin and CAP RAST tests. What was interesting about this case was that his mom neither breast-fed nor ingested cashews during pregnancy—she did not like (hated) tree nuts. However, the child's father, who fortunately was present at the time of the child's allergy evaluation, readily admitted he was a cashew aficionado who ate cashews several times a week. I recently saw another infant with a similar story; but he had his first cashew reaction at the early age of six months. This child's father also admitted to frequent consumption of cashews. Most food allergy studies have focused on the mother an as a source of occult exposure to trace amounts of food allergens in infancy. We need to look more closely at nut-loving, football-watching dads who could be transferring peanut or tree nut allergens through skin or direct oral contact with their "at risk" offspring.

Hazelnut or Filbert Allergy

Hazelnuts are grown in a strong, dense little tree that is a member of the birch family. One variety of hazelnuts, filberts, is slightly larger than regular hazelnuts. Additional names for hazelnuts include American hazelnut, Chinese filbert, Cobnut, Tibetan filbert, and Tibetan and Turkish hazel. Hazelnut consumption started in Greece and Rome and eventually spread to France and Spain. Turkey is now the world's leading grower of hazelnuts.

Oregon grows the majority of hazelnuts in the United States. As hazelnuts are very attractive to the eye, it is always tempting to eat them before they are ripe. Unfortunately, they are terribly bitter before they ripen, lending them the name, "witch hazel nuts." Shelled and unshelled hazelnuts can be eaten whole, chopped or ground up. Shelled hazelnuts quickly become rancid and should be used within a week, refrigerated for up to six months, or frozen for up to one year. For long-term storage, it's best to buy unshelled nuts. Hazelnuts can be added to salads, cookies,

cakes, and other desserts or used to make a butter to flavor entrees and side dishes. Like many other nuts, roasting brings out their flavor. As the hazelnut tree is related to the birch tree family, hazelnuts are a frequent cause of the oral allergy syndrome in countries where birch pollen allergy is a problem. One Denmark study found hazelnuts were the most frequent cause of food allergy in patients with birch, hazel, or alder pollen allergy.

Pecan Nut Allergy

Pecans, distinguished by their thin shell and sweet kernels, come from one of the largest fruit-bearing trees, which is a member of the walnut family. Pecan trees grow in the Southeastern United States along the Mississippi Delta that expands west into Texas. Pecan trees live for hundreds of years and produce thousands of nuts (about a 100 pounds) a year. They do not produce seeds until they are 20 years old. Pecans were a dietary staple of American Indians who ground pecans into flour for use in breads, stews and food seasonings. Early settlers and American Indians often bartered and traded with pecans.

One Denmark study found hazelnuts were the most frequent cause of food allergy in patients with birch, hazel, or alder pollen allergy.

The United States is the world's largest producer of pecans. Lighter-colored pecans are considered more attractive, as consumers associate a dark color with rancidity. Pecans are an excellent source of fiber, vitamins A and E, several B vitamins, folic acid, calcium, magnesium, copper, phosphorus, potassium, manganese, and zinc. Roasted or raw pecans are used in bakery products, ice cream and confections. The pecan's crunch adds texture and provides the characteristic flavor for butter pecan ice cream. The grooved surface helps hold coatings in frozen novelty applications. Raw or roasted pecan granules are ideal when combined with strong cheeses, like blue cheese. The most famous use of pecans is the tasty pecan pie. Despite their popularity, pecan allergy initially seemed to be uncommon as there were only a few reported cases in the literature. However, due to increased consumption, pecan-allergy was the fourth most common tree nut allergy reported by FAAN registrants. Pecan-allergic patients should also avoid Hicans, a combination of a pecan and a hickory nut. Pecans can cause a contact allergy.

One fifty-one-year-old Filipino woman developed a severe blistering hand rash one day after shelling one bushel of fresh pecans as preparatory work for baking pecan pies. Similar eruptions have been reported to cashew nuts.

> *One patient with the chicken-bird-egg syndrome experienced an anaphylactic reaction after snacking on some of her parrot's food that contained pine nuts.*

■ Pine Nut Allergy

Pine nuts, also known as pinon nuts, pignoles, and pignolas, grow in a pine tree in southwestern North America and the Mediterranean. American Indians ground pine nuts into flour, and Spanish explorers in the New World described eating pine nuts. These high-fat nuts grow inside a pine cone that must be heated to facilitate nut removal. This labor-intensive process makes pine nuts the most expensive of all tree nuts. Pine nuts are sold raw and intact, or ground up. They are a popular snack in salads, ethnic dishes, Spanish cuisine and Italian pesto sauces.

The literature on pine nut allergy is confusing. Spanish investigators have noted that despite their popularity, relatively few cases of pine nut allergy have been reported. They described four children, ranging in age from twelve months to six years, who suffered from allergy to pine nuts. All patients had a personal history of allergy. Two of the children had allergic reactions to other nuts. In all cases, both the skin and CAP RAST tests were positive. One patient with the chicken-bird-egg syndrome experienced an anaphylactic reaction after snacking on some of her parrot's food that contained pine nuts. A twenty-one-year-old white male developed life-threatening anaphylaxis within seconds of ingesting a small amount of a cookie containing pine nuts. In another case, a patient who was skin-tested with pine nut allergen developed shortness of breath and circulatory collapse within minutes after testing.

I have seen several patients with severe reactions to pine nuts. It has been suggested that allergy to pine nuts is related to living near or being exposed to a pine forest. This is probably a myth as significant cross-reactivity between pine pollen and pine nuts has not been reported.

■ Pistachio Nut Allergy

Originally grown in the desert regions of the Holy Land, pistachios come from the pistacia tree, a member of the cashew family. The pistachio has been considered a delicacy since the beginning of recorded history. Legend has it that lovers were promised good fortune if they sat beneath pistachio trees in the moonlight and heard them crack open. Pistachio trees are dioecious trees, meaning that there are separate male and female trees. Both trees are required for nut production, but only the female tree produces nuts. Pistachios were initially a Middle Eastern delicacy that were imported to the United States. Tannins in the pistachio shell cause discoloration if they are not processed immediately after harvesting. American importers added a red dye to pistachio nuts to hide this discoloration. This made the pistachio nuts very messy as the red dye was transferred to hands and face after eating. Today, few consumers buy red-dyed pistachio nuts.

Pistachios were introduced to California in 1854, but commercial plantings did not develop until 1970. Production from California increased in 1979 after Ayatollah Khomeni took hostages in the American embassy in Iran. Until that time, Iran was the world's leading pistachio producer.

By the 1990s, the increase in United States production eliminated the need to import pistachio nuts. Today, the evergreen trees that bear pistachio nuts are grown primarily in California. Pistachios have been reported as a remedy for sclerosis of the liver, abdominal ailments, abscesses, bruises and sores, chest ailments, and circulation problems. Powdered pistachio root oil is used for children's cough in Algeria. Pistachio leaves were used to enhance fertility in Lebanon, and Arabs consider them to be an aphrodisiac. Pistachio wood is prized for carving, cabinetwork, and firewood.

The Kerman variety, the most common pistachio nut, yields a large nut with a light green colored

shell that comes from chlorophyll. One unique feature of the pistachio nut is that the shell naturally splits open prior to maturity. The natural split in the shell is formed as the kernel grows and pushes against the shell. This allows 80 percent of the pistachio crop to be sold in the shell for fresh consumption. The remaining 20 percent is marketed as shelled nuts or processed into candies, baked goods, or ice cream. New applications of pistachios include: energy bars, trail mixes, and chocolate bars. Pistachio biscotto is a dark-chocolate pistachio bar. Chopped or diced pistachios are often sprinkled over desserts, ice cream, and salads in Indian and Mediterranean cuisine.

There are few published studies on pistachio allergy. Unfortunately, fatal reactions have been reported—usually

> *Legend has it that lovers were promised good fortune if they sat beneath pistachio trees in the moonlight and heard them crack open.*

in young adults with asthma. In one tragic case, a young Massachusetts All-Star lacrosse player and known asthmatic, ate a few pistachio nuts at a lacrosse camp where he was a counselor. Despite receiving immediate treatment with epinephrine, he collapsed, went into a coma and died several days later. This case points out the need for intense education regarding tree nut allergy, especially in young adults with asthma who have the biggest risk for a near-fatal or fatal event. Cross-reacting allergens have been found between pistachios, cashews, and the pulp of the mango fruit.

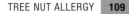

Walnut Allergy

The walnut, called the "Nut of the Gods" by the Romans, is one of the oldest known tree nuts. Centuries ago, their popularity spread from the Middle East to the ancient and New World. Spanish missionaries planted walnut trees in California, now the largest supplier of walnuts in the United States. Walnuts are second only to almonds in terms of universal appeal. They are added to snacks, appetizers, stuffing, stir-fries and salads. Chopped walnuts are found in baked foods, ice creams, brownies, and cookies. The most common walnuts are English and California nuts. Actually, walnuts do not grow in England. The name "English walnut" is due to English merchants shipping walnuts from the Middle East to the American colonies. English walnuts have a thin, easily cracked shell, and a sweet flavor with slight bitterness from its dark-brown edible skin.

Other walnut varieties include American, Chinese, Japanese, and black walnuts. Black walnuts are very hard and have a poor taste. However, the black walnut tree is one of the most valuable sources of timber in the United States.

While walnuts are higher in fat and lower in protein than most other tree nuts, the amount of Omega-3 fatty acids they contain gives them an impressive nutritional profile. A fresh walnut has a delicate, slightly astringent flavor due to the presence of phenolic acids which contribute to their antioxidant properties. In comparison to the other nuts, walnuts are higher in vitamin B6 and folic acid, and contain vitamins A, C and E, thiamine, magnesium, iron, copper, zinc, phosphorous, potassium, and calcium. Newer applications of walnuts include veggie burgers, Middle Eastern and Asian sauces, and Hispanic foods, such as chilies and nogato, are fast growing non-traditional uses of walnuts.

The prevalence of walnut allergy in children has been estimated to be as high as 4 percent of tree nut allergy, and anaphylaxis has been commonly reported. In one study based on a patient questionnaire, hypersensitivity to walnuts was more common in patients with birch pollen allergy. There is a varying degree of cross-reactivity with pecan nuts.

American Chestnuts and Acorns

This once dominant tree of the Eastern seaboard of the United States was destroyed by chestnut blight in the mid-1950s. Now most chestnut trees are the Chinese chestnuts that are more resistant to the chestnut blight. Buckeyes, also known as horse chestnuts, are the poisonous seeds of the American horse chestnut tree. Chestnut allergy and avocado and hazelnut allergy are more common in patients with the latex-food allergy syndrome.

In one study of twenty-two patients in Spain, the average age of onset of chestnut allergy was twenty-nine years, and one in three victims had a severe reaction. Water chestnuts, the edible portion of a plant root known as, corm, are not nuts but are starchy tubers that look like chestnuts. They are usually safe for tree nut-allergic individuals.

Black walnuts are very hard and have a poor taste. However, the black walnut tree is one of the most valuable sources of timber in the United States.

Acorns, the very bitter nut of the oak tree, can be quite allergenic and pose a potential risk for unknowing toddlers. Chestnuts and acorns may cross react, as they are both members of the Fagaceae family. One four-year-old boy developed ocular itching, eyelid and lip swelling, and wheezing immediately after peeling and eating an acorn. Months later he experienced similar symptoms after eating a chestnut. Skin tests were positive to acorn peel and chestnut and negative to the oak pollen.

■ Macadamia Nuts

Often called the "Queen of Nuts," macadamia nuts probably originated in Australia. Ferdinand van Mueller, a European who named the nut after the Australian naturalist John Macadam, made macadamia nuts popular in the late 1800s. Also called Queensland nuts, they have been consumed since ancient times by Australian aborigines. They are also grown in New Zealand. Their smooth, creamy texture and distinct flavor make them perfect for encrusting fish or blending with mango, papaya, and other tropical fruits. Dry roasting brings out their rich buttery flavor.

Macadamia nuts make a good addition to salads, stews, rice dishes, and desserts. While macadamias have the highest fat content, they also have one of the lowest levels of polyunsaturated fat and saturated fat of all tree nuts. There are relatively few reported cases of macadamia nut allergy in the literature.

■ Coconut Allergy

Coconuts are not typically restricted in the diet of tree nut-allergic individuals, as reactions to coconuts are rare. In my review of the literature, I found only three cases of coconut allergy. One case involved a twenty-eight-year-old man who experienced an immediate reaction after eating coconut ice cream. The reaction consisted of oral itching, vomiting, and intense swelling of the lips that subsided in twenty-four hours with symptomatic treatment in an emergency room. He had previously noticed oral itching from walnuts, but tolerated the ingestion of other nuts. The second case reported a sixty-four-year-old woman who reacted to a coconut biscuit. Another report described a patient with hazelnut allergy who experienced an anaphylactic reaction to coconut. Despite the fact that coconuts are widely used in body washes, suntan lotions and skin care products, very few cases of contact allergy have been reported. Therefore, there is usually no need to advise patients with a tree nut allergy to avoid coconuts or coconut oils.

Coconuts are not typically restricted in the diet of tree nut-allergic individuals, as reactions to coconuts are rare.

■ The Kola Nut

This nut comes from evergreen trees of the cocoa family that grow in Western Africa and tropical climates, including Central and South America, the West Indies, Sri Lanka, and Malaysia. What makes this nut so interesting is that it contains high levels of caffeine; it is one of the main "secret ingredients" of the original Coca-Cola formula. For thousands of years, Africans chewed the raw seeds to combat hunger and fatigue, indigestion, intoxication, hangovers, and diarrhea. Arabs traded gold dust for kola nuts before starting out on long treks across the Sahara Desert. The kola nut is often used in folk medicine as an aphrodisiac and to treat morning sickness and migraine headaches. It has also been applied directly to the skin to treat wounds and inflammation. The tree's bitter twig is used as well to clean the teeth and gums.

Although comprehensive safety studies have not been performed, moderate amounts of kola nut are generally regarded as safe. The Council of Europe and the FDA have approved it as a food additive. The typical caffeine-like side effects associated with kola nut are nervousness, heart irregularities, headaches, and sleeplessness. While sometimes listed a common trigger of nut allergy, I could not find any documented reports of kola nut allergy in my search of the literature.

> *Children who were allergic to more than one tree nut were less likely to outgrow their tree nut allergy.*

■ Tiger Nut Allergy

Tiger nuts, also called earth almonds, are exclusively grown in Valencia, Spain, where they are consumed raw and used to make a cool drink called tiger nut milk. Despite widespread consumption in Spain, there are only a few reported cases of tiger nut allergy.

■ Hidden Sources of Tree Nuts

Hidden sources of tree nuts include candies, cookies, cereals, desserts, donuts, sauces, pesto, suntan lotions, shampoos, bath oils, popcorn, cheese spreads, chocolates, Worcestershire sauces, ice creams, and granola bars. Gianduja is a creamy mix of chopped nuts and chocolate found in imported chocolates. Marzipan is an almond paste. Artificial nuts may be peanuts that have been flavored with a nut, like a pecan or walnut. Mandelonas are peanuts soaked in almond flavoring. Mortadella may contain pistachios. Kick sacks, hacky sacks, beanbags and draft dodgers are sometimes filled with crushed tree nut shells (see table 10.1).

■ Can You Outgrow a Tree Nut Allergy?

Less is known about the natural history of tree nut allergy compared to peanut allergy. A Johns Hopkins team studied 117 children with tree nut allergy. Twelve percent reacted to multiple tree nuts and 63 percent had a moderate-to-severe reaction. Nearly 70 percent were also allergic to peanuts. Cashews, walnuts, and pecans accounted for the vast majority of tree nut reactions. Patients allergic to cashews, walnuts, and pecans were more likely to have moderate-to-severe reactions. When these children were challenged to tree nuts, only 9 percent who had previously reacted to a tree nut passed an oral challenge test. Children who were allergic to more than one tree nut were less likely to outgrow their tree nut allergy.

While there are no similar studies in adults, it appears that adults are even less likely to outgrow a peanut or tree nut allergy. The best way to determine if one has developed a tolerance or has outgrown a peanut or tree nut allergy, is to periodically review the patient's history, repeat the skin and CAP RAST tests and, when indicated, conduct an oral challenge. I usually bring peanut- and tree nut-allergic patients back once a year for such an evaluation. When there is a history of accidental ingestion and a reaction to the offending nut within the past year, there is

Table 10.1. Hidden Sources of Tree Nuts

Candies	Cheese spreads
Cookies	Chocolates
Cereals	Worcestershire sauces
Desserts	Ice creams
Donuts	Granola bars
Sauces	Marzipan (an almond paste)
Pesto sauce	Artificial nuts
Suntan lotions	Mandelona's
Shampoos	Kick sacks or hacky sacks
Bath oils	Bean bags
Popcorn	

usually no need to repeat the skin and CAP RAST tests. When the history is negative or the patient has had no problems after an inadvertent exposure, or if the skin and CAP RAST tests decline to acceptable levels, it may be time to consider an oral tree nut challenge.

Over the past several years, I have found that very few peanut-allergic and tree nut-allergic patients qualify for an oral challenge after one year. In other words, they still have positive skin and high CAP RAST levels. I now usually recommend a two-year interval before retesting such patients. Toddlers should be reevaluated before they enter a preschool or kindergarten classroom so that appropriate educational programs can be put in place prior to entering school on a full-time basis.

Although the potential for a severe reaction exists and the ideal CAP RAST test cutoff has not been definitively established, patients four years or older with a CAP RAST level of five units or less may be candidates for an oral challenge in the proper setting with trained personnel. However, it might be more prudent to delay challenges until the CAP RAST levels are two units or less to further increase the odds of a successful challenge outcome. I would not conduct peanut or tree nut oral challenges in patients with ongoing asthma or if there was a history of a reaction in the past year, no matter what the skin and CAP RAST levels show.

■ The Bottom Line: Don't Roll the Dice!

Many allergists recommend only avoiding members of a specific tree nut family. For example, cashew-allergic and pistachio-allergic patients could possibly safely eat walnuts and pecans, members of a different tree nut family. I believe this is a dangerous approach, as crossover reactions to tree nuts are very unpredictable. The literature on this subject is confusing. I used to tell my patients there was a 35 percent chance of reacting to a tree nut if you were peanut allergic. Now it appears crossover reactions may be isolated to specific botanical families. Studies have found that with some exceptions, pistachio and walnut proteins do not cross-react with peanut protein. The strongest chance of a crossover reaction is found in similar tree nut families, such as walnuts, pecans, hazelnuts, and the cashew-pistachio family.

> **The strongest chance of a crossover reaction is found in similar tree nut families, such as walnuts, pecans, hazelnuts, and the cashew-pistachio family.**

In my opinion, until this dilemma is sorted out by more extensive studies and carefully controlled oral challenges, I will continue to advise my patients and their families (especially if the patient has asthma)—unless you want to roll the dice, if you are allergic to one tree nut you should avoid all tree nuts and peanut products.

A recent paper from Cambridge, England reinforces this recommendation. Doctors Pamela Ewan and Andrew Clark followed 784 peanut-allergic children for nine years to determine if they became allergic to more nuts as they got older. The average age of this group was five years, and the age of onset of their first reaction was two years of age. Over time these children developed more tree nut allergy—over three-fourths of teenagers were sensitized to more than one nut. Thus, it looks like younger children who may only be allergic to peanut or one tree nut can develop an allergy to other tree nuts if they continue to consume tree nuts throughout their childhood. ●

Chapter 11

Seed and Spice Allergy

Seeds and spices, which are aromatic vegetable substances used for the seasoning of food, usually come from plants, not trees. Seed and spice allergy is much less common than peanut- and tree nut-allergy. With the exception of sesame seeds, there is usually no crossover risk with peanut or tree nut proteins. Thus, mustard seeds, poppy seeds, cottonseed and sunflower seeds do not usually need to be avoided by peanut allergic patients unless they have a specific allergy to that particular seed. Many spice allergens are quite similar to pollen and vegetable proteins.

Thus, mugwort-allergic and birch pollen-allergic individuals are more likely to be sensitive to spices. Gourmet cooks know there is a wide array of seeds and spices from various worldwide cuisines. Fortunately, very few appear capable of inducing allergic reactions.

Gourmet cooks know there is a wide array of seeds and spices from various worldwide cuisines. Fortunately, very few appear capable of inducing allergic reactions.

■ Cottonseed and Sunflower Seed Allergy

Once a common ingredient of many foodstuffs, cottonseed is now mainly used to manufacture cottonseed oil for expanders in processed foods, baked goods, animal feed, and fertilizers. Cottonseed oil is usually highly processed and is not considered to be allergenic. Little is known about cottonseed allergen, but it may be a potent one. In 1950, the medical literature described a fatal reaction to an intradermal (under the skin) test with cottonseed allergen. Sunflower seed is another seed with only a few case reports of allergic reactions. In three cases depicting oral allergy symptoms after eating sunflower seeds, sensitization was thought to have occurred from inhaling sunflower seeds while feeding birds. French investigators recently described a five-year-old girl who reacted to sunflower oil. Skin tests were positive but the CAP RAST test to sunflower seed was negative. An oral challenge test with sunflower oil was positive. The patient also reacted to skin contact and inhalation of sunflower seeds.

■ Dill Allergy

Dill, a member of the parsley family native to the Mediterranean and Russia, is both an herb and a spice that is used widely in European cuisine. There are very few cases of dill allergy in the literature.

■ Cut the Mustard

The mustard seed has an important place in the history of medicine. The first medical reference to mustard is in the Hippocratic writings where mustard seeds were used to relieve muscle pain. Ancient Greeks believed that mustard was a gift to mankind from Asclepious, the god of healing. Its medicinal properties were immortalized in the Bible when Jesus spoke of the power of faith, "even if it were no larger than a mustard seed." The Chinese used mustard thousands of years ago. King Louis XI of France always traveled with his own royal mustard pot in case his hosts didn't serve it.

It was the condiment, not the plant, that was originally called mustard. Mustard got its name as it was made by grinding the seeds of the mustard plant into a paste that was mixed with *must*, an unfermented wine. The old expression, "cut the mustard," meaning to achieve the required standard, was first recorded in an O. Henry story in 1902. It reads, "So I looked around and found a proposition [a woman] that exactly cut the mustard." It may also have come from a cowboy expression, the proper mustard, meaning the genuine thing. Other linguists believe that "cut the mustard," is a corruption of the military phrase, "to pass muster," or assemble the troops for inspection.

> There are two types of mustard seeds—white and brown. The white seed is the more common ingredient of American mustards, while the brown seed is more commonly used in English, French and Chinese mustards.

Mustard belongs to the Brassica food family that includes broccoli, cabbage, cauliflower, turnips and radishes. In 1720, Mrs. Clements discovered a method for extracting the full flavor from mustard seed by grinding the seed in a mill and subjecting it to similar processes used in the making of flour from wheat. Clement's mustard gained huge popularity throughout the country, and after obtaining a patent from King George I, she traveled to all the great towns of England to collect orders for her product. There are two types of mustard seeds—white and brown. The white seed is the more common ingredient of American mustards, while the brown seed is more commonly used in English, French and Chinese mustards. One of mustard's greatest health benefits is that it provides tremendous flavor with few calories and little fat. World consumption of mustard now tops 400 million pounds a year.

Volatile mustard oil is a powerful irritant capable of blistering the skin. When diluted in liniment or a poultice, mustard creates a warm sensation, hence its use as "mustard plaster" to promote blood flow to inflamed areas. Mustard flour sprinkled in your socks is said to save your toes from frostbite. Over the years, mustard has been prescribed for scorpion stings, snake bites, epilepsy, toothaches, bruises, stiff necks, rheumatism, colic and sinus problems.

■ Clinical Reactions to Mustard

Although mustard is consumed worldwide, very few cases of mustard allergy have been reported in North America. One study from Spain described twenty-nine patients with mustard allergy. Nearly half of these patients had mugwort hay fever and other food allergies.

The most recent Spanish study of thirty-eight mustard-allergic patients found 10 percent had systemic anaphylaxis. A significant association between mustard hypersensitivity and mugwort pollen sensitization was found in most patients. Many patients were also allergic to nuts, legumes, corn, and Rosaceae fruits. The study concluded that mustard allergy is a common disorder commonly associated with mugwort allergy, suggesting a new "mustard-mugwort allergy syndrome." Additional case reports of mustard allergy come from France, the largest European producer of mustard. Surprisingly, mustard allergy is now the fourth leading cause of food allergy in French children, after milk, eggs and peanuts. In one French study, half of mustard-allergic patients had exercise-induced asthma or oral allergy symptoms. Swedish researchers described 129 cases of mustard allergy in young children. Nearly 40 percent outgrew their mustard allergy by age seven.

I am puzzled why mustard allergy is so rarely reported in the United States, the world's largest consumer of mustard. I cannot recall ever seeing a case of mustard allergy. One reason for the paucity of case reports in the United States to foods like mustard is that there is no uniform reporting system for food allergy reactions similar to the programs in many European countries. I plan to look more closely for mustard reactions in cases of unexplained allergic reactions, as many victims of a mustard reaction experience anaphylaxis.

Mustard allergy may be difficult to diagnose, as mustard contains skin irritants, such as isothiocynates and capsaicin, that might produce false positive skin tests. Thus, a CAP RAST blood test or an oral challenge to mustard may the best way to confirm the diagnosis of mustard allergy.

■ Nutmeg Allergy

The nutmeg tree is native to the Moluccas, or the so-called Spice Islands, in the West Indies. It produces two spices—mace and nutmeg. This large tropical evergreen grows to an average of forty to sixty feet in height and produces about 2,000 nutmegs per year. The fruit is often collected with a long pole with a basket that resembles a lacrosse stick. Arabs were the exclusive importers of the nutmeg spice to Europe until 1512, when Vasco de Gama sailed to the Moluccas and claimed these islands for

Portugal. To preserve their nutmeg monopoly, the Portuguese restricted nutmeg tree plantings. Despite these restrictions, the French smuggled nutmeg seeds to the African island of Mauritius. In 1796, the British took over the Moluccas and spread nutmeg trees throughout the Caribbean.

Nutmeg tree planting was so successful in Grenada that it calls itself the Nutmeg Island. Grenada designed its flag in the green, yellow and red colors of nutmeg and depicts a nutmeg in one corner of the flag. Nutmeg is touted as possessing magical powers. A sixteenth-century monk advised young men to carry vials of nutmeg oil and anoint their genitals for virility. Tucking a nutmeg into the left armpit before attending a social event was believed to attract admirers. Nutmegs were used to protect against a wide variety of dangers and evils. People carried nutmegs everywhere and wore silver, ivory or wood ornaments with a compartment that housed nutmegs.

The nutmeg seed is encased in a yellow, edible fruit, the approximate size and shape of a small peach. Nutmeg is sold whole or ground. Whole nutmeg may be coated with lime to protect against insects and fungus. In small dosages nutmeg allegedly reduces flatulence and improves appetite. Whole seeds are preferable to ground nutmeg, as their flavor quickly deteriorates. Nutmeg is a favorite addition to Italian sausages, Scottish hag-

> *Nutmeg tree planting was so successful in Grenada that it calls itself the Nutmeg Island. Grenada designed its flag in the green, yellow and red colors of nutmeg and depicts a nutmeg in one corner of the flag.*

gis and Middle Eastern lamb dishes. Nutmeg is also used to flavor eggnog, fondue and béchamel (white sauce). Nutmeg oil is an additive in a wide range of commercial foods and medicines, especially colas. The more aromatic mace is a frequent ingredient of sausages and other prepared meats. Nutmeg oils are used as condiments and to scent soaps and perfumes. An ointment of nutmeg butter is used as a treatment for topical irritations and rheumatism.

■ Nutmeg Reactions

True nutmeg allergy appears to be rare. Nutmeg may trigger contact dermatitis in sensitized individuals. One group of 103 patients with suspected contact allergy to spices was tested. The highest numbers of reactions were found to nutmeg. The authors postulated that the high incidence of nutmeg allergy reflects the increasing use of nutmeg (and other spices) in cosmetics in Western society. Nutmeg abuse is well reported in the medical literature.

The symptoms of nutmeg overdose that are due to consumption of its poisonous oil include hallucinations, palpitations, and a feeling of impending doom. One thirteen-year-old female who smoked marijuana and ingested a large amount of nutmeg developed bizarre behavior and visual and auditory hallucinations. A fatal case of nutmeg poisoning was reported in a fifty-five-year-old woman who allegedly died from a nutmeg overdose.

■ Perilla Seed and Perilla Seed Oil

This fascinating seed and seed oil that comes from the mint family is a plant that grows throughout Asia, especially in Korea and the hills and mountains of China and Japan. There are both green-leafed and purple-leafed varieties which are generally recognized as separate species by botanists. The leaves resemble stinging nettle leaves, being slightly rounder in shape. It is increasingly commonly called by its Japanese name, shiso. The Japanese call the green type aojiso or oba ("big leaf") or aoba or aoshiso ("green leaf") and often eat it with sashimi (sliced raw fish) or cut into thin strips in salads, spaghetti, and meat and fish dishes. It is also used as a flavorful herb in a variety of dishes, even as a pizza topping. (Initially it was used in place of basil). The purple type is called akajiso ("red leaf") and is used to make umeboshi (pickled ume), or combined with ume paste in sushi to make umeshiso maki. Its young leaves and flower buds are used for pickling in Japan and Taiwan.

The oil from perilla seeds is high in Omega-3 fatty acids, specifically alpha-linolenic acid, as well as several phenolic compounds. With a minimum content of 50 percent Omega-3 fatty acids, perilla seed oil can serve as a vegetarian's alternative to fish oil. Perilla seed oil has been used for centuries by Asian practitioners to treat cough, colds, and the flu. It has also been used in paints, varnishes, linoleum, printing ink, lacquers, and protective waterproof coatings on cloth.

Several studies tout this seed as a potent inhibitor of the chemical mediators of allergic inflammation. Alleged benefits include reduction of allergic symptoms and asthma, relief of pain and inflammation, stimulation of immune function, and reduction in blood clotting. In one small study involving fourteen asthmatics, seven subjects consumed perilla seed oil while the other seven were given corn oil. Those taking the perilla seed oil experienced a significant reduction in allergy mediators while the corn oil participants had an increase. In addition, the perilla seed oil group showed a significant improvement in lung function within two to four weeks. As perilla seed oil is quite inexpensive, it may be a more economical item for those who want to increase their daily intake of Omega-3 oils. Perilla food products are available in the United States in many Korean ethnic markets.

There were no documented cases of perilla allergy until June 2006, when researchers from Seoul, Korea, reported the first two cases of anaphylaxis from the perilla seed. Their patients were two young men (with asthma and allergic rhinitis) who developed typical signs of anaphylaxis immediately after eating food that contained perilla seeds. Their allergy was confirmed by skin tests, CAP RAST blood tests, and a positive oral challenge that triggered a scary anaphylactic reaction (severe facial and throat swelling, hives, and dizziness) that required epinephrine administration in both cases.

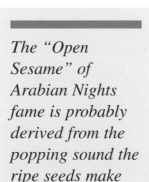

Poppy Seed Allergy

Cultivated and wild varieties of poppy seeds grow primarily in the northern hemisphere. Their oil can be pressed from the seeds. Poppy seeds are used as a bread spice and as an ingredient in salads and sauces. Skin, intestinal, and respiratory symptoms to poppy seed have been reported, but they are quite rare.

Pumpkin Seed Allergy

Pumpkin seeds are roasted and eaten as snacks. The pumpkin pulp is often pureed and eaten as a vegetable or as a pie filling. The pumpkin family includes cucumber, squash, and zucchini and is related to muskmelon and watermelon. There are only a few documented cases of pumpkin seed allergy.

Sesame Seed History

Sesame is one of the first recorded plants to be treasured for its seeds. Early Assyrians believed their gods drank sesame wine as a prelude to creating the world. A drawing on an Egyptian tomb depicts a baker adding sesame seeds to dough nearly 4,000 years ago. Around the same time, the Chinese were burning sesame oil to make soot for ink. A Chinese ointment, *shinkoh*, derived from sesame seeds, has been used for centuries to treat burns. Ancient Greek soldiers carried sesame seeds as energy boosting rations, and the Romans made a hummus from sesame and cumin. Sesame has been considered a symbol of good luck and signifies immortality to the Brahmins.

Sesame oil is highly stable—rarely turning rancid in hot climates. In southern India, it is used to anoint the body and hair. The "Open Sesame" of Arabian Nights fame is probably derived from the popping sound the ripe seeds make when they burst from their pods. The sesame plant grows up to three feet in height and has pink or bluish white flowers. Sesame seeds come in three different colors and are used as a crushed seed or a paste in Western fast foods like hamburger buns, bread sticks, pretzels, bagels, and crackers. The seed contains 50 to 60 percent oil. It is very rich in protein,

The "Open Sesame" of Arabian Nights fame is probably derived from the popping sound the ripe seeds make when they burst from their pods.

and its polyunsaturated fat is used in margarines and cooking oils. Non-culinary uses include soaps, cosmetics, lubricants, and medicines. Due to its stability and non-irritating effects, sesame oil is commonly used in pharmaceutical and cosmetic products like lipsticks and body oils.

■ Sesame Seed and Sesame Oil Allergy

Sesame seed allergy is a growing food allergy of global proportions outside of North America. Some call it, "the peanut allergy of the Middle East." The popularity of sesame seed snacks like Halva and Tahina in Israel may explain why sesame seed allergy now ranks just behind egg allergy and cow's milk allergy in Israeli children. Sesame seed allergy is three to four times more common than peanut allergy in Israeli children.

One Israeli clinic described thirty-two infants and children with sesame-seed allergy. The average age of onset was very young—11.7 months. Most children also had other allergies. Thirty percent experienced an anaphylactic reaction to sesame seed and only three outgrew it. Another Israeli group that followed seventy-four children with sesame seed allergy reported that one in five outgrew it. Sesame seeds are an essential part of the Lebanese diet, and Lebanese children have nearly four times more sesame allergy than peanut allergy.

The rise in cases of sesame seed allergy is not confined to the Middle East. Sesame seed allergy now ranks fourth behind peanut, egg, and milk allergy in Australian children. A survey of members of the Anaphylaxis Campaign-United Kingdom examined the features of sesame seed allergy among 400 members who reported avoiding sesame seeds. One hundred and fifty people reported 288 reactions to sesame seeds. Eight-nine percent reported other atopic diseases, and, notably, 84 percent were also allergic to peanuts or tree nuts. One in six (17 percent) suffered potentially life-threatening symptoms, with two-thirds of these severe reactions occurring on their first known exposure. The age of a first reaction ranged from six months to sixty-five years. The majority of reactions (91 percent) involved foods or dishes where sesame seed was a deliberate ingredient rather than an accidental contaminant.

Is sesame seed allergy less common in the United States than in the United Kingdom, or is it underreported? I suspect the latter. Despite widespread use in India and China, there are few reports of sesame allergy—possibly due to different methods of preparation or a later introduction into a child's diet.

Sesame seeds are unique. Unlike other nuts and seeds, their oil is very sensitizing, as it is not highly refined like peanut, soybean, cottonseed, or sunflower oil. Sesame oil may be more sensitizing than the seed itself and has triggered anaphylactic reactions at very low doses. Sesame oil can trigger both an immediate (IgE-type) reaction and a delayed contact dermatitis. Sesame paste, made by grinding up the seeds, is also highly allergenic. One report described a six-year-old child with eczema who had an anaphylactic reaction to a sesame paste bread sandwich. There are several reports of sesame seed cross-reactivity with hazelnut, kiwi, poppy seed, cashew, walnut, and peanut. Thus, sesame

> *Sesame seeds are an essential part of the Lebanese diet, and Lebanese children have nearly four times more sesame allergy than peanut allergy.*

seed-allergic individuals should avoid peanuts and tree nuts. Sesame seed allergy may be lifelong. One sneaky source of hidden sesame seed allergen is the bread bins in bakeries and supermarkets where plain bagels and rolls can be cross-contaminated with other baked products covered with sesame seeds. Sesame seed has been added to the list of major food allergens in Europe and Canada, but, unfortunately, not in the United States.

Sugar Beet Seeds

This seed belongs to a botanical family that includes allergenic weeds like Russian thistle and lamb's quarter. Swiss chard, a variation of the sugar beet seed, has been implicated in allergic rhinitis and bronchial asthma. The oil from sugar beet seeds is highly refined and is not usually allergenic.

Spice Allergy

As spices are derived from natural plants, they confer an authentic taste to a variety of foods. Due to the presence of pharmacologically active substances, the diagnosis of spice allergy versus an intolerance reaction may be difficult. Allergic reactions have been reported to spices, such as coriander, caraway, fennel, paprika, and saffron. Curry is not a single spice, but a combination of several spices that includes coriander, cumin, turmeric, fenugreek seeds, mustard, cinnamon, ginger, black pepper, cloves, nutmeg, cardamom, cayenne, and chili powder. Reports of curry reactions are rare. One fifteen-year-old

Curry is not a single spice, but a combination of several spices that includes coriander, cumin, turmeric, fenugreek seeds, mustard, cinnamon, ginger, black pepper, cloves, nutmeg, cardamom, cayenne, and chili powder.

Korean boy had a reaction to curry powder that was confirmed by positive skin and CAP RAST tests and an oral challenge.

Many spice allergens are similar to pollen and vegetable allergens. Individuals who are allergic to mugwort or birch pollen and celery are more likely to be sensitive to aniseed, fennel, coriander, and cumin—all from the same botanical family as celery. Several spices that may induce a contact or irritant dermatitis-like reaction include:

- Cinnamon—a common cause of contact dermatitis in bakers and candy makers
- Cayenne pepper—used in ginger ale and some liquors
- Nutmeg—a fatty oil found in soaps and perfumes
- Oil of cloves—in toothpaste, soaps, perfumes, mouthwashes, and dental preparations; may cross-react with Balsam of Peru clove
- Vanilla—made from the vanilla plant pod can trigger dermatitis, hives, and asthma in exposed workers

New and Unusual Spices

The booming specialty food industry has made exotic condiments and spices readily available for the smaller restaurants and the home chef. New spices and condiments are now the fastest growing specialty food category. In 2004, 825 new products were introduced to the marketplace. Several new specialty spices include pimenton—a paprika produced by smoking chili peppers over oak logs and grinding them into a powder. Pumpkin seed oil is made from green pumpkin seeds. Verjus is a juice made from unripened grapes. Several new vinegars are made from grape must—the skin and pulp of wine grapes. Dehydrating citrus rinds and grinding them in a blender with salt produces citrus salts. Other potentially allergenic spices include zatar, a Middle Eastern aromatic spice mixture containing toasted white sesame seeds, ground sumac, thyme, and salt.

■ Turmeric Allergy

Turmeric, a common ingredient of curry powder, is an ancient spice used as food dye and color additive. It is frequently employed in rituals of the Hindu religion and used to dye holy robes. The stems from this East Indian, ginger-like herbal plant are boiled, dried for over a week, and ground into a bright yellow fine powder. In many languages turmeric is called the "yellow root." In India, it is used to tint sweet dishes and remove fishy odors from seafood dishes. The active ingredient, curcumin, has antioxidant and anti-inflammatory properties. Turmeric ointment is sold as an antibacterial ointment in Malaysia. Turmeric water is an Asian cosmetic that imparts a golden glow to the skin. One documented case of turmeric allergy depicted a forty-four-year-old woman who reacted to a horseradish sauce and herbal potato dish that contained turmeric. ●

Other potentially allergenic spices include zatar, a Middle Eastern aromatic spice mixture containing toasted white sesame seeds, ground sumac, thyme and salt

Chapter 12

Seafood Allergy

As fish were the first vertebrates on earth, the world's lakes, rivers, and oceans have provided man with a delicious and nutritious food source since prehistoric times. From early civilization, seafood was a vital food source that was easily gathered by spearing or placing basket-like traps (nets) in rivers, lakes and oceans.[1]

The strength of the ancient Greek and Roman civilizations was in no small part due to the abundance of seafood in the Mediterranean Sea. Prior to modern refrigeration methods, only coastal communities derived the benefits from regular ingestion of seafood. The increased availability of fresh seafood, enhanced by the popularity of commercial and sport fishing, and matched with the rising appreciation of the health benefits of seafood, has led to a dramatic increase in worldwide seafood consumption.

Seafood, the best source of iodine next to salt, is an excellent source of selenium, fluoride, iron, zinc, and magnesium. Both freshwater fish and saltwater seafood, especially fatty finfish like tuna and salmon, are rich in essential Omega-3 fatty acids. Having insufficient Omega-3 fatty acids in your diet amounts to a dietary deficiency that has been linked to a wide range of health problems, including asthma, cardiovascular disease, diabetes, cancer, osteoporosis, and disorders of the nervous system. Available evidence indicates that eating small amounts of fish—

about two pounds a week—is enough to optimize health.

In the 1970s, Danish scientists observed that fish-eating Intuits from Greenland had one-tenth to one-third the heart attack rate of Danish citizens. The Intuits had lower bad cholesterol and low-density lipoprotein (LDL) levels, and higher good cholesterol and high-density-lipoprotein (HDL) levels than the Danish citizens.

Similar findings were observed on Kohama Island in Japan where residents have one of the lowest, if not the lowest, rate of heart disease in the world. Studies in France and the Netherlands found that people who eat seafood at least once a week have less dementia and Alzheimer's disease. The protective effect of fish appears to be related to cooking methods. Eating broiled or baked fish provides more protection than eating fried fish or fish burgers. Pan frying and deep frying seafood at high temperatures apparently destroy the Omega-3 fatty acids. Not everyone has fully accepted the health benefits of

> *Having insufficient Omega-3 fatty acids in your diet amounts to a dietary deficiency that has been linked to a wide range of health problems, including asthma, cardiovascular disease, diabetes, cancer, osteoporosis, and disorders of the nervous system.*

---

[1] Seafood refers to any sea animal that is served as food or is suitable for eating. This includes finfish, shellfish (like mollusks and crustaceans), and freshwater fish.

seafood consumption. Some finfish (like swordfish) contain mercury, a potential neurotoxin. While many of the mercury studies are inconclusive at best, it may be wise to limit consumption of finfish that contain high levels of mercury.

■ Non-Allergic Seafood Reactions

Unlike reactions to other foods, seafood reactions are quite varied and complex. In addition to the typical allergic reaction, seafood can trigger many non-allergic reactions. Shellfish lovers like myself who were raised in New England were taught to only eat raw shellfish like oysters and clams in any month of the year that contains an R in the name. In other words, avoid eating these tasty bivalve mollusks in the warmer months of the year, such as May, June, July, and August, where spoilage is likely to occur. Another hint: if you purchase raw shellfish such as clams or oysters and the shells are open, briskly tap them on a countertop. When they do not close, discard them. Fortunately, modern refrigeration and transport methods have reduced the risk of seafood spoilage in the warmer months of the year.

While fruit and vegetable food-borne illnesses are increasing, spoiled seafood is the still leading cause of food poisoning in the United States.

Common non-allergic reactions from seafood toxins and poisons include scombroid poisoning, the red tide toxin, and viral and bacterial contamination in spoiled seafood. While the food supply in the United States is the safest in the world, about 76 million people get sick, more than 300,000 are hospitalized, and 5,000 die each year from a food-borne illness. While fruit and vegetable food-borne illnesses are increasing, spoiled seafood is the still leading cause of food poisoning in the United States.

■ Scombroid Poisoning

Fish from the scombroid family, such as tuna, mackerel, and bonito, are commonly implicated in spoiled fish reactions, leading to the term, "scombroid fish poisoning." These warm-water fish that are non-toxic when caught have a dark oily meat that contains a chemical called histidine. When improperly processed or poorly refrigerated, these fish spoil and bacteria converts histidine into histamine. While such spoiled fish look and smell normal, cooking does not destroy the histamine.

Thus, ingestion of such spoiled fish is actually a form of histamine poisoning, and the reaction mirrors that of an acute allergic reaction. Scombroid poisoning should be suspected in anyone who develops flushing, hives, sweating, dizziness, nausea, or headache right after ingestion of the implicated fish. A burning peppery taste in the mouth and throat immediately during or after eating the fish and similar symptoms in other diners is an excellent clue for scombroid poisoning. The duration of symptoms ranges from several hours to twenty-four hours. One should suspect scombroid poisoning when such symptoms occur in someone who regularly eats finfish without experiencing any reaction.

The incidence of scombroid poisoning is undoubtedly underestimated because of its frequently mild nature, lack of mandatory reporting, and misdiagnosis as a seafood allergy. Many physicians, especially emergency room doctors who are not familiar with scombroid poisoning, tell their patients they have experienced an allergic reaction to the offending seafood. The diagnosis of scombroid poisoning is best accomplished through a process of elimination. When the patient's skin and allergy blood tests are negative to seafood, one must suspect scombroid poisoning.

If leftover fish is available, a simple histamine analysis of the suspect fish may detect high levels of histamine in the spoiled fish. Scombroid poisoning occurs in clusters—typically several cases will be reported from the same food source or restaurant. While scombroid poisoning appears to be a rare event (only nineteen cases were reported in the United States in 1999), I suspect it may be more common than believed as it is not a reportable disease. Some non-scombroid fish like mahi-mahi, bluefish, and sardines also cause this reaction.

One report described five physicians who developed typical symptoms of scombroid poisoning while attending a medical conference in New Hampshire, yet no fish in the scombroid family had been consumed. The outbreak was eventually traced to spoiled blue fish. Another outbreak in 232 persons was linked to canned tuna. The treatment of scombroid poisoning includes taking an antihistamine such as Benadryl or emergency room care in severe cases.

■ *Ciguatera* Fish Poisoning[2]

Ciguatera is a Spanish term that originated in the Caribbean basin to describe the poisoning caused by ingesting a marine snail that the early Spanish settlers named cigua. The term is now used to describe poisoning with a toxin from by a dinoflagellate (algae) that is found in larger fish that become infected when they eat smaller reef fish that have fed on algae organisms.

2 Centers for Disease Control and Prevention. *Health Information for International Travel, 2005-2006.*

Ciguatera poisoning is the world's most common form of seafood poisoning. About 50,000 to 100,000 people who live in or visit tropical and subtropical climates develop ciguatera poisoning every year. Affected areas include the Caribbean Islands, Florida, French Polynesia, American Samoa, Micronesia, Hawaii, and Australia. Fish that have been reported to cause ciguatera poisoning include amberjack, barracuda, grouper, kahala, parrotfish, sea bass, snapper, surgeonfish, and ulua.

Common symptoms of ciguatera poisoning include nausea, vomiting, diarrhea, cramps, excessive sweating, headache, and muscle aches. Sensations of burning, pins and needles, weakness, itching, and dizziness also occur. Some people experience temperature reversals (hot surfaces feel cold and cold surfaces feel hot), unusual tastes, nightmares, or hallucinations.

Since no country routinely tests for ciguatoxin in locally caught fish, travelers need to be aware of where the problem occurs and which locally caught fish have been associated with the toxin.

Rare deaths due to hypotension and cardiovascular collapse have been described. Symptoms often occur within three hours—but can occur up to a day or more—after eating the contaminated fish. Neurological symptoms may begin several days later and continue for months. People who have had a previous ciguatera poisoning develop more severe symptoms with repeated exposures.

The diagnosis is based on the clinical signs and symptoms and a history of eating fish infested with the ciguatoxin. Laboratory tests have been developed to test for ciguatoxin in fish. Since no country routinely tests for ciguatoxin in locally caught fish, travelers need to be aware of where the problem occurs and which locally caught fish have been associated with the toxin. Knowledgeable native fishermen are aware that fish caught on some reefs are more likely to be toxic and avoid fishing these areas. Ciguatoxins do not affect the taste or smell of the fish, and the toxin is not destroyed by cooking. Larger fish (over six pounds) are more likely to have ciguatoxin. Thus, avoiding consumption of very large reef fish is protective, as well as not eating parts of the fish where the toxin is concentrated, such as the liver, intestines, head, and fish eggs. Treatment of ciguatera poisoning is generally supportive and tailored to the symptoms. Irregular heartbeats, low blood pressure, and acute neurological syndromes will require emergency room care.

◼ Puffer Fish: Both Ugly and Deadly

Several fish that belong to the Tetraodontidae fish family include sunfish, porcupine fish, and the fugu or puffer fish. A puffer fish scares away its enemies by gulping down water and inflating itself to appear much larger. In my bottom-fishing days, whenever we caught a puffer fish we moved on to another spot as these ugly guys usually scare other fish away. The porcupine fish, a close relative of the puffer fish, has many prickly spines sticking out

The porcupine fish, a close relative of the puffer fish, has many prickly spines sticking out of its body that also scare its enemies away. When eaten by another fish, it inflates itself in the fish's mouth and both fish die.

of its body that also scare its enemies away. When eaten by another fish, it inflates itself in the fish's mouth and both fish die. Puffer fish are considered to be a delicacy in Japan where a single restaurant serving can cost several hundred dollars. These fish must be carefully cleaned as their skin, liver, gonads, and intestines contain a potent and deadly neurotoxin called tetrodotoxin or TXX. Consumption of as little as ten grams of TXX may be fatal. Only trained and licensed Japanese chefs are allowed to prepare puffer fish, taking particular care with the gonads, skin, liver, and intestines.

The Japanese have a rather unique way of training and certifying these chefs. They must pass a strict written exam and demonstrate the proper technique by preparing a puffer or fugu fish. Before serving it to their customers, they then must eat it. *Bon Appétit!*

Despite careful preparation, some diners experience numbness of the tongue and lips, which often disappears. In other cases, such mild symptoms are followed by headache, nausea, vomiting, and paralysis of the face and extremities. Severe cases may experience respiratory distress, convulsions, irregular heartbeat, and speech impairment; and death can occur within hours. Many victims exist in a zombie-like state of suspended animation for days while remaining completely lucid. Most victims recover within a few days or weeks with supportive treatment, but permanent disability has been described. It is estimated that there are as many as 200 cases of such poisonings a year worldwide, and half of these victims die. Even though this form of poisoning is quite rare in the United States, all puffer or fugu fish have been implicated in a fatal reaction.

■ The Red Tide

This form of seafood poisoning is confined to the East Coast of the United States, Alaska, California, and Washington state. Also known as paralytic shellfish poisoning, the red tide is caused by ingesting toxins present in bivalve shellfish like clams and oysters. The red tide toxin comes from a marine algae that multiplies when excess freshwater falls in saltwater costal marshes and changes the color of seawater to red or brown—hence the name, red tide.

The toxin-infested algae multiply and are, in turn, ingested by bivalve clams, mussels, and oysters that are then consumed by humans. The red tide toxin is one of the most potent neurotoxins known to man. Local health departments where red tide is a problem must constantly monitor shellfish beds for the presence of this toxin. Early symptoms of red tide poisoning include numbness, tingling, and burning of the lips and tongue within thirty minutes of ingestion. Such symptoms then spread to the face, neck, hands, and feet, and weakness and paralysis may ensue in two to twelve hours and may last for as long as seventy-two hours. Severe cases may require assisted breathing in an intensive care unit. Muscular weakness may persist for weeks. When untreated, up to 75 percent of red tide victims can die.

One recent case from Florida points out the dangers of the red tide toxin. A six-year-old child ate some steamed clams gathered and cooked by his family at a Florida beach during a red tide alert. He developed tingling in his hands and face followed by a severe headache, convulsions, and respiratory arrest that required intubation (placing a breathing tube into the lungs) for two days. Three other family members suffered similar but milder symptoms. The bottom line—avoid eating locally harvested bivalve shellfish during red tide alerts.

■ Neurogenic Shellfish Poisoning

This is another form of shellfish poisoning that causes intestinal and neurological symptoms. It is a milder form of red tide poisoning but lacks a paralytic component. It is usually self-limited and resolves within a few hours. The algae that triggers this reaction is ingested by filter-feeding bivalve mollusks along the southern Atlantic coast and the Gulf

> *The bottom line—avoid eating locally harvested bivalve shellfish during red tide alerts.*

of México. Unlike other shellfish poisonings, this toxin can be aerosolized by wave action along beaches and sand dunes and cause eye irritation, sneezing, nasal congestion, and wheezing that can be confused with an allergic reaction or asthma.

One study of Florida beachgoers found a significant increase in respiratory symptoms after exposure to red tides. Anecdotal reports indicate that persons with asthma are more sensitive to the aerosolized toxin. Fifty-nine persons with physician-diagnosed asthma were evaluated one hour before and one hour after going to a Florida beach on days with and without red tide exposure. Asthmatics who were using daily asthma medications were more likely to report respiratory symptoms and experience a decrease in their lung function after red tide exposure. This is the first study to objectively show adverse health effects from aerosolized Florida red tide toxins in people with asthma.

■ Domoic Acid and Amnesic Shellfish Poisoning

I have had the fortunate experience of living near the ocean for most of my lifetime. I worked and fished on many boats in high school and college, and at one time I held a highly prized commercial lobster license. Thus, throughout my medical training, I read as much as I could about seafood-driven diseases. In my recent research on seafood-driven diseases, I was completely dumbfounded upon learning about domoic acid and amnesic shellfish poisoning.

> *Fortunately, there have been no documented human cases of domoic acid or amnesic shellfish poisoning in the United States or Canada since widespread testing for this shellfish toxin began in 1988.*

Domoic acid is a relatively new toxin that has surfaced along the West Coast of the United States and Canada. Domoic acid is produced by toxic planktons or microscopic-sized algae that are ingested by clams or mussels. The contaminated shellfish are then eaten by birds, fish, sea mammals, or humans. The first outbreak of domoic acid poisoning occurred in 1987 in Prince Edward Island, Canada, where infested mussels were consumed. In that outbreak, three people died, and more than 100 developed a variety of toxin-induced symptoms. The most unusual and most serious symptom was a loss of short-term memory, hence the designation amnesiac shellfish poisoning. Unfortunately for many victims, the amnesia was permanent.

In 1991, high levels of domoic acid were detected in razor clams off the Washington and Oregon coasts. Razor clams can accumulate domoic acid in their edible tissue, and the poison lingers long after the infestation in the water is gone. In 2001, dead and dying seabirds were observed along the beaches of Monterey Bay in California. Many of the sick birds displayed unusual symptoms, suggesting a neurological toxin. Analysis of the content of the dead birds' stomachs revealed high levels of domoic acid. In February 2002, more than 500 sick California sea lions washed ashore in southern California. Marine scientists traced the condition to the domoic acid toxin. Sea lions do not eat the microscopic algae, but fish do. The sea lions eat the fish that have ingested the algae. How can such a toxin be so deadly?

The toxin becomes more concentrated as it travels through the food chain in a process called bioaccumulation. When sea lions eat fish that contain domoic acid, the toxin damages their hippocampus, a part of the brain involved in learning and memory. Sick sea lions showed a variety of symptoms, including vomiting, seizures, depression, and coma.

Many of the sea lions that died on the beaches of California were pregnant females. Domoic acid may have killed as many as twenty-one large whales that were found floating off the New England coast in July 2003. Fortunately, there have been no documented human cases of domoic acid or amnesic shellfish poisoning in the United States or Canada since widespread testing for this shellfish toxin began in 1988.

Diarrheal Shellfish Poisoning

This is the mildest and most benign form of shellfish poisoning. Symptoms begin thirty minutes to six hours after ingestion of shellfish and may last for up to thirty-six hours. Symptoms that are usually confined to the intestinal tract may be due to the consumption of bivalves contaminated by biotoxins from marine algae that flourish in the summer months. No fatalities have been reported, and full recovery occurs.

I spent one summer working at an emergency room on Cape Cod, a seacoast community in Massachusetts. Nearly every evening, one or two patients would come to the emergency room with profuse vomiting and diarrhea. Most of these patients had severe dehydration and required intravenous fluids. Most victims who had ingested shellfish (usually steamed clams) were vacationers from other inland parts of the United States, like the Midwest. They had little or no prior exposure to steamed shellfish. It was rare to see this reaction in Cape Cod natives who consumed shellfish on a regular basis, suggesting that regular shellfish consumption protected natives from a diarrheal shellfish reaction.

Less Common Forms of Seafood Poisoning

Other rare forms of seafood poisonings include clupeotoxism, a highly fatal reaction caused by a clupeidae, a herring-like fish. This poisoning occurs in the Pacific and Indian oceans in the warmer summer months. Elasmobranch poisoning is caused by ingestion of contaminated meat or liver from several species of sharks, including the Greenland sleeper shark. This disease is characterized by gastrointestinal and neurological symptoms. Red Welk poisoning is due to toxins present in gastropods in Japanese and northern European waters.

Bacterial and Viral Infections

Seafood contaminated by bacteria and viruses is responsible for diseases such as botulism, staphylococcal food poisoning, and salmonella. Shellfish harvested in sewage-contaminated waters may contain many organisms, including the hepatitis A virus. Raw and lightly steamed seafood like sushi are potential sources of bacterial and viral infections.

Vibrio is a bacterium from the same family as those bacteria that cause cholera. It normally lives in warm seawater and is part of a group of *Vibrios* that are called "halophilic" because they require salt. *Vibrio* can cause disease in those who eat contaminated seafood, especially oysters, or in individuals who have an open wound that is exposed to seawater. In healthy people, ingestion of *Vibrio* can cause vomiting, diarrhea, and abdominal pain. In immunocompromised persons, particularly those with chronic liver disease, *Vibrio* can infect the bloodstream, causing septic shock, a severe and life-threatening illness characterized by fever, chills, blistering skin lesions, and decreased blood pressure. Most *Vibrio* infections occur in the Gulf Coast states. One tip for preventing *Vibrio* infections, particularly among immuno-compromised patients, including those with underlying liver disease—do not eat raw shellfish.[3]

> *One tip for preventing vibrio infections, particularly among immuno-compromised patients, including those with underlying liver disease—do not eat raw shellfish.*

---

[3] Centers for Disease Control and Prevention. Summary of Human *Vibrio* Isolates Reportetd to CDC, 2004.

Seafood Intolerance

The last group of non-allergic seafood reactions can be classified as seafood intolerance reactions. Such reactions may occur when ingested seafood contains large amounts of chemicals such as histamine and tyramine often present in canned fish and fresh fish, such as tuna, mackerel, and herring. Such chemicals cause an intolerance type reaction.

Seafood Allergy

Seafood allergy has an important place in the history of medicine. One of the most famous experiments in the history of allergy and immunology, performed in the early twentieth century, is called the Prausnitz-Kustner or P-K reaction for short. Heinze Kustner was a German gynecologist and obstetrician who experienced itching, skin swelling, coughing, sneezing, and vomiting after eating cooked fish. His colleague Carl Wilhelm Prausnitz, a German hygienist and bacteriologist, believed the blood of allergic individuals contained a substance he called reagin, which, when combined with an allergen, produced untoward symptoms. Prausnitz brilliantly reasoned that if he transferred Kustner's serum into his own body, he would also become allergic to fish. After injecting fish extract into his arm at the same site where he had injected Kustner's serum, he developed allergic symptoms. Sixty years later, Prausnitz's protein reagin was isolated as the IgE antibody.

Until 2004 there were no accurate studies depicting the incidence of seafood allergy. The older literature stated that only one in every 100 individuals was allergic to seafood. Countries where inhabitants eat a lot of seafood like Finland and Spain reported the highest incidence of seafood allergy. A Finnish study found 3 percent of Finnish children were fish-allergic. In 355 Spanish children with food allergy, 30 percent had a fish allergy, and 7 percent were allergic to shellfish. Finfish allergy was more common in children, whereas shellfish allergy was more prevalent in adults.

The observation that allergy specialists and allergy centers in the United States were seeing more cases of seafood allergy prompted investigators from the Mount Sinai School of Medicine and FAAN to conduct a nationwide study to determine the prevalence of seafood allergy. A telephone survey of nearly 11,000 American households found that those with seafood allergy were not being spared from the ongoing food allergy epidemic. It now appears that nearly 7 million Americans have a seafood allergy. Thus, there may be more than twice as many people with seafood allergy compared to peanut- and tree nut-allergy. This survey found that boys and adult women have more seafood allergy than young girls and adult males. The highest rate of seafood allergy was found in black Americans. In contrast to peanut- or tree nut-allergy that begins in younger children, seafood allergy usually started in adulthood. Seafood allergy may be permanent, as only 4 percent of respondents reported outgrowing their seafood allergy.

The Seafood Allergy Registry

In response to the issues raised by this survey, the Seafood Allergy Registry was established through a collaborative effort of FAAN, the Jaffe Food Allergy Institute, and the University of Georgia Marine

> *There may be more than twice as many people with seafood allergy compared to peanut- and tree nut-allergy.*

Extension Service. The surveys were filled out by people with seafood allergy or by parents of children with a seafood allergy. Analysis of the first 1,000 registrants found 55 percent reported an allergy to finfish and 85 percent reported a shellfish allergy.[4] The most common finfish offenders were salmon, cod, and tuna, whereas the most problematic shellfish were shrimp, crab, lobster, and clam. The majority of registrants, both children and adults, avoided all types of seafood. Children with seafood allergy (90 percent) were more likely to have a doctor-confirmed diagnosis, including allergy skin tests, whereas only 50 percent of adults had received specialty care or undergone skin testing. Fifty percent of the reactions were classified as moderate to severe, and one in five reactions were treated with an auto-injectable epinephrine device. Fewer than 10 percent of children had a reaction in a school setting, implying that it is easier to avoid seafood than peanuts or tree nuts at school. The most common location for a seafood reaction was a restaurant—about 50 percent.

A closer look at 125 registrants who had a reaction in a restaurant uncovered that only one in five registrants disclosed their seafood allergy to restaurant personnel. Even more disturbing was the fact that one of three registrants (mostly adults) ordered seafood even though they knew or suspected they might have a seafood allergy. The bottom line of this important survey: seafood allergy is a widespread problem and a serious public health concern in the United States. Adults with seafood allergy may be under-diagnosed and under-treated, and may be big risk-takers when ordering seafood. Proper communication is essential when dining out. Considering carrying a "chef card" to describe your food allergy and always carry your auto-injector epinephrine device.[5]

■ Occupational Seafood Allergy

Unlike other food allergies, exposure to seafood in the workplace is a risk factor. Up to 30 percent of workers in seafood restaurants, seafood processing plants, and commercial fishermen may develop occupational asthma, contact dermatitis, or eczema from constant exposure to seafood products in their workplace. Methods of sensitization include direct skin contact with raw seafood and inhaling vapors during cooking and processing. A survey of occupational skin problems was carried out among 883 workers in seafood processing industries in northern Norway. The prevalence of dry, itchy, or chapped skin, eczema, and chronic sores was two times higher among production workers in the fish processing plants compared to office workers in the same plants. Major risk factors were contact with raw fish and fish juice.

The best data on occupational seafood allergy comes from the king crab industry in the northwestern United States where workers often develop asthma or contact dermatitis from direct exposure to raw crabs. Other reports have described asthma in snow crab, codfish, and oyster plant workers. I have personally treated several employees from Gorton's Seafood, located in Gloucester, Massachusetts. Most workers who develop asthmatic to seafood have to be transferred out of the production lines where raw seafood is processed. One new form of recreational or occupational

---

[4] Scott H. Sicherer, M.D., "The Seafood Allergy Registry: Providing New Insights," *Food Allergy News,* June-July 2006.

[5] To create a chef card or participate in the Seafood Allergy Registry, go to the FAAN Web Site at www.foodallergy.org.

Table 12.1. Seafood Species		
Bony Finfish	**Crustaceans**	**Mollusks**
Cod	Lobster	Abalone
Hake	Shrimp	Snails
Sardine	Crab	Limpet
Mackerel	Crayfish	Squid
Tuna	Rock lobster	Clams
Sharks		Mussels
Salmon		Oyster
Rays		Scallop

allergy to shrimp has been described. Gammarus is a freshwater shrimp often used to feed turtles. A thirteen-year-old boy and a thirty-eight-year-old man who worked in a pet food factory developed asthma symptoms after exposure to dried gammarus. An eleven-year-old girl with allergic rhinitis and mild asthma developed hives from feeding her turtles. All three patients had positive skin tests or CAP RAST blood tests to gammarus.

A Biology Lesson

Before proceeding on with the discussion of seafood allergy, let us review some basic biology. There are three major classes of seafood—finfish, crustaceans, and mollusks (see table 12.1). The most common seafood is the bony finfish, such as cod, haddock, salmon, and tuna which have a backbone or vertebrae. The term shellfish is often used to describe any seafood with a shell-like body, such as a lobster or a clam. However, there are two very different species of shellfish—crustaceans and mollusks. Crustaceans, such as lobsters, shrimp, and crabs, are the scavengers of the ocean, which live on the ocean floor. The mollusk group, which lives beneath the ocean floor, includes bivalve clams, squid, snails, mussels, oysters, and scallops. The reason for this biology lesson is that an allergy to one group of seafood does not mean you are allergic to all three seafood groups. Most health-care providers are unaware of this classification. When they encounter a patient with an allergic reaction to seafood, they instruct them to avoid all forms of seafood. I have seen scores of patients who, after experiencing an allergic reaction to just one seafood species, are advised to avoid all forms of fish or seafood. This is most unfortunate. For example, codfish-allergic individuals may still be able to go to one of the world's greatest meals, an old-fashioned New England Clambake, and enjoy boiled lobster, clam chowder, and steamed clams. Allergists can usually determine which seafood a person can or cannot safely eat by taking a medical history, applying skin tests, ordering CAP RAST blood tests, and, when indicated, conducting an oral challenge to a particular seafood.

Seafood Allergens

Several proteins have been identified as potent seafood allergens. The major allergen in finfish like the Atlantic cod is parvalbumin. This is a highly active protein that resists heating and causes symptoms after inhalation, skin contact, and ingestion. Cod is the most frequently reported cause of finfish allergy. Reactions to other finfish, such as haddock, herring, sprat, halibut, plaice, mackerel, trout, and salmon, are well recognized, as parvalbumin is present in all finfish. It has also been found in frogs and other fish species, such as ocean pout, eelpout, and eel. Most fish proteins are heat stable. Two exceptions may be tuna and salmon, as some fish-allergic patients may tolerate canned tuna or salmon. Dark finfish meat has been reported to be less allergenic than white meat. Parvalbumin is probably not the only allergenic fish protein. One case report describes a patient who reacted to marlin and tuna but was able to eat other finfish.

The major allergen in crustaceans is an interesting protein called tropomyosin. This protein is widely distributed in nature and has been well-studied in shrimp. I used to be puzzled when I would encounter a dust mite-allergic patient who had a positive skin test to shrimp, crab, or lobster, yet had no history of an allergic reaction to these crustaceans. Mother Nature has provided the crustacean family with the same tropomyosin protein as the house dust mite. When these patients had no history of a reaction to a shellfish like shrimp, I would tell them not to worry and there was no need to avoid shellfish. However, several recent reports describe crossover reactions to crustaceans in dust mite-allergic patients. In one case, a fourteen-year-old house dust mite-allergic male with mild asthma experienced respiratory failure and nearly died while running one hour after he had ingested snails. He had positive skin and CAP RAST tests to house dust mites, snails, and crab. True allergic reactions to bivalve mollusks are less common than allergy to finfish or crustaceans. Most of the reactions I have seen to mollusks such as clams, oysters, or scallops, are food intolerance-like reactions. Some mollusks such as abalone, oyster, and squid may be more capable of inducing an allergic reaction.

Most of the reactions I have seen to mollusks such as clams, oysters, or scallops, are food intolerance-like reactions. Some mollusks such as abalone, oyster, and squid may be more capable of inducing an allergic reaction.

The Bottom Line

What is the risk of cross-reactivity among the three major groups of seafood? Can a cod-allergic patient eat lobster or clams or vice versa? While some patients may be allergic to all three groups of seafood, in my experience most patients are only allergic to one of the three major seafood species.

If you are allergic to finfish, you should avoid all finfish with a backbone as there is a 50 percent chance your will react to any type of fish in this group. In general, if you are sensitive to a crustacean, like lobster, you have a 75 percent chance of reacting to shrimp or crab. However, many patients with a crustacean allergy can eat other mollusks like oysters or clams. One word of caution! Due to the wide variability in allergic crossover reactions between seafood, especially to finfish, no one who has had an allergic reaction to seafood should consider experimental ingestion of other seafood species until he or she has undergone an allergy evaluation by an allergy specialist. Such an evaluation should include a detailed medical history, appropriate skin and CAP RAST blood tests, and, when indicated, an oral seafood challenge.

Seafood Allergy Symptoms

Symptoms of seafood allergy are no different from those induced by other food allergens, except that exposure to minute amounts of allergen in cooking vapors or handling of seafood, especially in the raw state, may induce a reaction. Severe reactions can be triggered by the smell of fish in a sensitive person. Anaphylactic shock has been reported after eating foods cooked in reused cooking oil or when utensils and containers have been previously used to cook fish. While the leading cause of fatal food reactions are peanuts and tree nuts, many fatalities to seafood have been described. Unfortunately, such cases are not always published in the medical literature. The following stories gathered from newspapers throughout the world point out the dangers of seafood allergy.

Anaphylactic shock has been reported after eating foods cooked in reused cooking oil or when utensils and containers have been previously used to cook fish.

- A groom with fish allergy died after hotel party. A bridegroom, twenty-six-years old with an acute allergy to fish, who was on his honeymoon in Thailand, died within an hour of eating at a hotel cocktail party. The European manager assured him that nothing in the small eats had seafood in it. But after eating three small fish-laden spring rolls, he complained of feeling ill and collapsed. He died half an hour later in a hospital. No first aid kit and no doctor were available at the five-star hotel in Phuket.

- A forty-three-year-old man with a history of severe allergy to seafood went out with a friend to dine at a restaurant. There, he met others who offered him a slice of pizza, which had seafood topping. Within minutes of taking a couple of bites of the pizza, he complained of a tingling sensation in his tongue and swelling, itchy eyes, and difficulty breathing. He informed his companions of his allergy and rushed to the washroom, where he vomited and collapsed. He had neglected to bring with him the emergency kit that he had been prescribed. Adrenaline (epinephrine) was given at a nearby hospital, but the man died after twenty minutes of emergency resuscitation attempts.

- A twenty-nine-year-old tourist visited a restaurant with her spouse and ordered and consumed a meal of chicken. Just as the couple were about to leave the restaurant, a waiter went past their table carrying a hot, steaming, sizzling platter of shrimp "fajitas." It is part of the ambience that is intentionally fostered in such restaurants to transport steaming seafood on a hot platter past the guests: the aroma of the food and the sizzling noise produced often fills the entire dining room within seconds. On this occasion, the tourist inhaled the vapor, became short of breath and wheezy, and had to use the asthma inhaler that she normally carried with her in her handbag. Her condition did not improve, and soon afterwards she suddenly collapsed on the floor, lost consciousness, and vomited profusely. All resuscitative measures, including those by the ambulance team called to the restaurant, proved futile. Further treatment by the emergency room physicians on arrival in the hospital was similarly unsuccessful. Her past medical history revealed that the victim was asthmatic and allergic to seafood. The victim's asthma had been well controlled and she did not suffer any symptoms prior to visiting the restaurant.

An Unusual Case

Prior reports suggest that most seafood reactions occur in older children and adults. The 2002 FAAN seafood allergy survey reported only one patient under age five with a seafood or shellfish reaction. I recently evaluated a twenty-month-old, egg-allergic child with eczema who, at age fourteen months, had an acute allergic reaction during exposure to the vapor of steamed lobsters that were being cooked in the small confines of a boat galley. This child had never ingested lobsters or crustaceans before. His parents, who reside in Gloucester, a well-known fishing town in Massachusetts, routinely steamed shrimp and lobsters throughout his mother's pregnancy and while she was breast-feeding.

He had large skin test reactions and positive CAP RAST blood tests to shrimp, crab, and lobster. I suspect that either repeated inhalation of steamed crustacean vapors within his home or oral contact with his parents probably sensitized this infant to lobster. American Academy of Pediatric and United Kingdom infant-feeding guidelines recommend avoiding seafood in high-

risk children until age three. Perhaps these guidelines should be extended to recommend avoidance of vapors from cooked seafood or oral contact with caretakers who have recently eaten seafood in at-risk infants and young children.

A Red Tattoo and a Swordfish Supper

Japanese investigators recently described the plight of a forty-year-old Japanese man with a whole-body rash. His chest, shoulders, and upper arms were covered with tattoos. Two days before the rash began, he had eaten raw swordfish and alfonsino.[6] It was felt that he had a systemic contact dermatitis caused by sensitization to mercury in tattoo pigment that was aggravated by consumption of mercury-contaminated swordfish and alfonsino.

Mercury contamination of fish is a global problem. Shark, swordfish, king mackerel, alfonsino, and tilefish are known to contain high levels of mercury. According to Japan's Fishery Agency, swordfish contains approximately one part per million of mercury, while alfonsino contains approximately zero to forty-eight parts per million of mercury. Allergic reactions to metal salts used in tattooing are surprisingly frequent. Mercury, chromium, cobalt, and cadmium have been reported as contact sensitizers in tattoos. Among these, the red tattoo pigments (cinnabar and vermilion) are known to include mercury and produce a delayed skin reaction.

Systemic contact dermatitis induced by mercury has been reported in those with red tattoos after exposure to inhalation of mercury vapor, broken thermometers, mercury-containing creams, topical anti-parasitics, antiseptics, vaccines, gammaglobulin

---

[6] Alfonsino is related to the red snapper and is widely dispersed in New Zealand waters.

preparations, contact lens solutions, anti-toxins, and amalgam dental fillings. The authors concluded that physicians should be aware of the potential for systemic dermatitis in individuals with red tattoos, particularly after exposure to mercury-contaminated food. Since mercury can cause such severe eruptions, they recommend that tattooists abandon the use of mercury in tattoo pigments, and individuals with allergic reactions to red tattoos should avoid eating mercury-contaminated finfish.

■ Anisakis Allergy

Not all worms prevent allergic diseases. A new form of seafood allergy called anisakis is caused by a small white worm, or parasite, that infests the stomachs of whales, seals, and dolphins. Often called herring or cod worm disease, anisakis is often mistaken for a seafood allergy. How does it infect humans? Follow the food chain—the eggs of the parasite are released from the intestines of the infested mammals and are ingested by small crustaceans. These crustaceans, in turn, are then eaten by larger finfish. Humans, the accidental host, acquire the parasite by eating raw or undercooked finfish such as cod, herring, sardine, and mackerel. Up to 80 percent of blue whiting fish from European fishing grounds may be infested with the anisakis parasite.

Typical symptoms of an anisakis reaction include hives, swelling, and abdominal pain. This is a true allergic reaction, as patients exhibit positive skin and CAP

How do you avoid anisakis? It's relatively easy— only eat well-cooked or previously frozen finfish, as freezing or heating kills the parasite.

RAST blood tests to the parasite. Chronic forms of this disease may cause intestinal abscesses that may mimic all types of intestinal diseases. The disease is more common in Japan and Spain due to widespread consumption of raw seafood in these countries. One report suggests that anisakis may be an unrecognized cause of chronic hives. Exposure to this fish parasite can also trigger asthma and contact dermatitis in workers exposed to contaminated fish or fish meal. In one study of 578 fish processing workers, 8 percent were sensitized to anisakis.

In one study in Spain, 15 percent of blood donors had allergic IgE antibodies to anisakis. Spanish investigators recently detailed twenty-three cases of anisakis allergy. Most victims were older adults with a history of allergy. Allergy specialists and emergency room doctors should suspect anisakis allergy in unexplained cases of hives or anaphylaxis, especially if there is a history of undercooked or raw fish ingestion. Unlike other seafood reactions, anisakis allergy may be delayed for up to twenty-four hours after eating the parasitized fish. When patients with a solid history for finfish allergy come up negative on their skin and CAP RAST tests, look for anisakis allergy. It may be the reason for a high rate of missed diagnoses in allergic or anaphylactic reactions. How do you avoid anisakis? It's relatively easy—only eat well-cooked or previously frozen finfish, as freezing or heating kills the parasite.

■ Treatment of Seafood Allergy

The lessons from these seafood reactions are quite clear. There is no effective preventive treatment for seafood allergy other than patient education and complete avoidance. Unlike various fruits and vegetables where cooking may reduce or eliminate allergic potential, heated or cooked seafood can become more allergenic. This is a very important point for restaurant workers and cooks where spatula carryover from a pan or grill or steaming vapors from cooked seafood in a dining room may trigger a severe or fatal food reaction in an unsuspecting patron. Seafood-allergic individuals should be cautious when eating away from home. It may be best to avoid fish and seafood restaurants altogether because of the high risk of cross-contamination from counters, spatulas, cooking oils, fryers, or cooking grills in restaurant kitchens.

■ Hidden Sources of Seafood

Food labels need to be read carefully as any processed food may contain hidden fish or shellfish. Common hidden sources of seafood include anchovies, Caesar salads, Caponata, Sicilian relish, and Worcestershire and marina sauces. Caviar is actually the egg of certain fish species. The "crab seafood" salad you purchase in your local market is often made from surimi, an Alaskan pollock that is closely related to the cod family. Surimi is also used in imitation crab legs, hot dogs, pizza toppings, bologna, and ham. Seafood skin from monkfish and shrimp is often used as filler in food products and medications. Fish skin is used to remove particulate matter from coffee, wine, and beer in a process known as "fining." (see table 12.2).

■ Should Fish Allergic Patients Consume Fish Oil Products?

Omega-3 fatty acids may be important in reducing the risk of heart disease, rheumatoid arthritis, and cancer. They may also play a role in improving mood and memory. While cold-water fish are the highest source of Omega-3 fatty acids, there are other foods and oils that contain these fat-

Table 12.2. Hidden Sources of Seafood

Anchovies
Caesar salads
Capone and Sicilian relish
Worcestershire and marina sauces
Caviar
Surimi, an Alaskan pollock
Imitation crab legs
Hot dog
Pizza toppings
Bologna and ham
Fish skin used in fining

ty acids in smaller amounts, such as walnuts, flaxseeds, and flaxseed oil. I could not find any reports on fish oil reactions in fish-allergic patients. The only reference I could find was the Mayo Clinic Web site that stated, "People with an allergy or hypersensitivity to fish should avoid fish oil or Omega-3 fatty acid products derived from fish." I recently saw a finfish-allergic patient who reacted to a fish oil product. He had a mild systemic reaction and a positive skin test to fish oil. In correspondence with the company that made this product, I learned they make two types of fish oil.

One type is processed from sardines and anchovies, and the other brand is extracted from the liver of Norwegian codfish. This patient reacted to the sardine-anchovie-derived fish oil that you would expect to contain fish muscle protein. However, I wonder if pure cod liver oil extracts contain fish protein that is usually found in the muscle of the fish. As there are no studies on this intriguing question, I currently recommend that fish-allergic patients avoid fish oil products.

Does Shellfish Allergy Mean That You Are Allergic to Iodide?

Many individuals can experience a reaction to the X-ray dyes used by radiologists to outline various bodily organs, such as the kidneys and heart. Most older X-ray dyes contain iodide. For many decades it was taught that if you had an X-ray dye reaction, you were allergic to iodide and should not eat seafood with a high iodide content, like lobster; or, conversely, if you had a seafood allergy, you were likely to have a reaction to an X-ray dye or a topical antiseptic like Betadine. In one Florida survey of seventy-five patients with a history of a shellfish allergy, 92 percent of those surveyed believed iodide in the seafood was the triggering allergen, and two-thirds of the patients were wary of undergoing contrast studies using X-ray dyes. In my opinion, true iodide allergy does not exist. We all consume significant amounts of iodide every day in salt, meat, vegetables, dairy products and finfish.

The bottom line—there is no need for individuals who have had a reaction to an X-ray dye to avoid seafood, nor should seafood-allergic patients worry about being at risk for a reaction to an X-ray dye.

> *In one Florida survey of seventy-five patients with a history of a shellfish allergy, 92 percent of those surveyed believed iodide in the seafood was the triggering allergen, and two-thirds of the patients were wary of undergoing contrast studies using X-ray dyes.*

Is Glucosamine-Chondroitin a Problem in Seafood Allergy?

Glucosamine-chondroitin is a popular complementary medicine used to treat joint pain and osteoarthritis. Glucosamine is derived from shrimp shells, and chondroitin comes from shark cartilage. While patients allergic to seafood are usually allergic to the protein in the muscle of the seafood, not the shell, tests are not routinely performed on these products to exclude protein contamination. My literature search found a few anecdotal reports on asthma related to glucosamine-chondroitin. I did not find any reports of anaphylaxis. Unfortunately, there is no registry that routinely collects adverse effects to over-the-counter products, or dietary or herbal supplements. Thus, there is no proof that glucosamine-chondroitin products are safe for seafood-allergic patients.

Glucosamine-chondroitin products registered in Australia and New Zealand carry labels warning against their use in people allergic to shellfish or crustaceans. In one study, seventeen shrimp-allergic patients tolerated a glucosamine-chondroitin challenge. In another small pilot study, six shellfish-allergic individuals were skin tested and challenged with 500 mg of glucosamine without any adverse effects. The authors wisely point out that approximately 600 patients would have to be studied to ensure the safety of glucosamine. Thus, additional studies are needed before I give a green light to seafood-allergic patients who want to take glucosamine-chondroitin products.

Is Carrageenan a Risk in Seafood Allergy?

Carrageenan was originally obtained from seaweed or Irish moss and marine algae. Carrageenan is commonly used as an emulsifying, suspending, and clarifying agent in foods, dairy products, dressings, sauces, beverages, pharmaceuticals, cosmetics, and polishes. Carrageenan is the magic ingredient used to de-ice frozen airplanes sitting on tarmacs during winter storms.

One patient undergoing a diagnostic barium procedure had an anaphylactic reaction to the barium enema solution. At first, the latex in the enema device was suspected, but the patient did not test positive to latex. Instead, she tested positive for the carrageenan that is used as an emulsifying agent in the barium suspension. As carrageenan is not related to fish or shellfish, it does not need to be avoided in seafood-allergic individuals.

Beneath the Sea

Dr. Robert Hickey, a New Hampshire allergist, reported an interesting case of allergy to sushi, a Japanese food that consists of vinegared rice combined with various toppings and fillings, most often seafood. In March 2006, his forty-one-year-old patient experienced an acute allergic reaction within minutes of eating sushi in Hawaii requiring emergency care. The patient ate crackling shrimp, a

Additional studies are needed before I give a green light to seafood-allergic patients who want to take glucosamine-chondroitin products.

California roll with snow crab and sea urchin roe (uni), cooked eel (unagi) with fish sauce, rice, and saki mayo.

In his paper "What Lurks Beneath the Sea?" presented at the New England Society of Allergy meeting in October 2006, Hickey reported that his patient's skin and CAP RAST tests were negative to common seafood species and fresh eel. But a skin test to fresh sea urchin roe obtained from a local restaurant was strongly positive. The patient recalled slight tongue tingling and numbness while eating sushi in 2003.

The patient reported that in the late 1990s, he was employed off the coast of Maine as a commercial scuba diver to harvest sea urchins for export to Japan. While on board ship, he would frequently crack open fresh sea urchins and sample the roe for quality. Hickey astutely hypothesized that his patient became sensitized to sea urchin roe while working as a diver. Delayed hypersensitivity reactions to sea urchin stings have been reported. However, no food allergy or anaphylactic reactions have been previously attributed to sea urchin roe. This case points out the need to fully investigate suspected food and beverages and, when indicated, perform skin tests with fresh foods. ●

13

Fruit and Vegetable Allergy[1]

Many allergy specialists, including myself, now consider fruit and vegetable allergy to be the most common food allergy in older children and adults. Just like the peanut- and tree nut-epidemic, the rise in the incidence in fruit and vegetable allergy is astounding. Based on a European telephone survey of 40,000 adults, researchers estimated that 17 million Europeans had a food allergy. The most commonly cited allergy was fruit allergy (29 percent), followed by milk allergy (26 percent), and vegetable allergy (16 percent). Mount Sinai Hospital allergists in New York City described ninety-five children with fruit and vegetable allergy.

The average age of onset was five years. Most symptoms were confined to the lips, mouth, and tongue. Only four experienced a systemic reaction, and two of these reactions occurred in carrot-allergic children. The most common triggers were apples, carrots, and peaches in children who were allergic to birch pollen, melons, and bananas in ragweed-sensitive individuals. Italian allergists have reported a higher rate of systemic reactions in patients with a fruit or vegetable allergy. Unlike the peanut- and tree nut-epidemic, there are few, if any, clues for the striking increase in fruit and vegetable allergy.

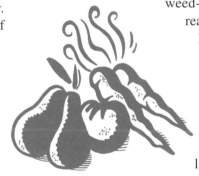

Unlike the peanut- and tree nut-epidemic, there are few, if any, clues for the striking increase in fruit and vegetable allergy.

■ The Oral Allergy Syndrome

The presence of a food allergy in patients with a pollen or latex allergy has been given several names, including the oral allergy syndrome, the pollen-food allergy syndrome, and the latex-fruit allergy syndrome. Many patients with a pollen or latex allergy complain of an itchy lip, mouth, or tongue after eating raw fruits and vegetables, such as apples, pears, peaches, celery, carrots, melons, and various tree nuts. For example, people with birch pollen allergy may have difficulty with apples, pears, and peaches; and ragweed-allergic individuals may react to melons or bananas. Mugwort-allergic patients can react to apples, carrots, celery, coriander, fennel, or melons. Grass-sensitive individuals may react to tomatoes, oranges, or melons. Many latex-allergic patients do not tolerate bananas, avocado, kiwi fruit, or chestnuts.

The cross-reactivity between these pollens, foods, and latex is due to the fact that the many food proteins closely resemble pollen and latex proteins. Several fruits and vegetables contain the

[1] Several sections in this and subsequent chapters were adapted from the informative Web site: AllergyAdvisor.com, edited by Dr. Harris Steinman, harris@zingsolutions.com.

Table 13.1. Cross-Reacting Fruits and Vegetables

Pollen	Fruit Allergy	Vegetable Allergy
Birch	Apples	Carrots
	Pears	Celery
	Peaches	Fennel
	Pears	Parsley
	Plums	Parsnip
	Apricots	
	Cherries	
	Nectarines	
	Prunes	
	Kiwi	
Grass	Melons	Potato
	Oranges	Tomato
Ragweed	Melons	Dandelions
	Bananas	Zucchini
		Cucumber
Mugwort	Apples	Celery
	Melons	Fennel
		Carrots
		Parsley
		Coriander
		Sunflower
		Pepper

protein profilin, a major component of birch pollen. Other foods share chitinase, an enzyme that protects the latex tree against insects. Offending pollens and foods vary depending on local pollen exposure and dietary habits. The highest incidence of the oral allergy syndrome occurs in northern Europe where birch pollen predominates in the spring. British allergists believe the rise in oral allergy syndrome cases in the United Kingdom may be due to the exclusive planting of male birch trees throughout Britain. While the attractive male birch trees are not as messy as their female counterparts (they do not drop their fruit on streets and sidewalks), they are more prolific pollen producers than the female trees.

Oral allergy symptoms include an itchy mouth, throat, or tongue. Handling or peeling raw fruits and vegetables may cause itchy skin, sneezing, runny nose, and watery eyes. More severe symptoms include hives, hoarseness, shortness of breath, vomiting,

The highest incidence of the oral allergy syndrome occurs in Northern Europe where birch pollen predominates in the spring.

cramps, and diarrhea. The oral allergy syndrome may be an important warning sign of a more serious reaction, as life-threatening reactions to fruits and vegetables have been reported.

Most victims can eat the offending fruit or vegetable if it is cooked, canned, microwaved, or baked. Some people can eat the fruit flesh if the skin is peeled away, as the more allergic part of the fruit may be just beneath the skin. Birch pollen-allergic patients who are allergic to raw apples can drink apple juice or eat applesauce, apple jelly, apple pie, and dried apples.

Skin tests to fruits and vegetables are often negative unless a fresh food is used in the skin test.

Exceptions to this rule include celery plants and tree nuts, where heating does not denature the offending protein. Some types of fruits cause more allergic reactions than others. Reactions to fruits and vegetables can occur anytime of the year but may be worse during the specific pollen season. Some newly described foods that trigger the oral allergy syndrome include asparagus, bell peppers, cherries, jackfruit, lettuce, and tomatoes. Skin tests to fruits and vegetables are often negative unless a fresh food is used in the skin test.

■ Oral Allergy Syndrome–Treatment

The obvious treatment is avoidance. You may not need to avoid all cross-reacting fruits or vegetables. Nuts, such as walnuts and hazelnuts, that trigger oral symptoms should be totally avoided because of a high risk of a severe tree nut reaction. Raw fruits that are usually tolerated in these patients include strawberries, blue-

berries, raspberries, citrus fruits, grapes, currants, gooseberries, guava, mangos, figs, pineapple, papaya, avocado, persimmon, and pomegranates. Vegetables that rarely trigger symptoms include cabbage, cauliflower, broccoli, watercress, radish, Swiss chard, and green onions.

Studies in birch pollen-allergic patients who have undergone allergy injections, or immunotherapy, have reported an unexpected but valuable spin-off. In one survey, nearly 80 percent of oral allergy symptoms were resolved with allergy injections. I recently conducted an informal survey of more than sixty patients in our practice with tree pollen allergy and oral allergy symptoms who underwent allergy injections to tree pollen. Approximately 50 percent felt their food symptoms were diminished after receiving pollen injections. This is not strong enough evidence to recommend allergy injections solely to eliminate

Table 13.2.
Fruits and Vegetables Usually Safe in the Oral Allergy Syndrome

Fruits	Vegetables
Strawberries	Cabbage
Blueberries	Cauliflower
Raspberries	Broccoli
Citrus fruits	Watercress
Grapes	Radish
Currants	Swiss chard
Gooseberries	Green onions
Guava and figs	
Papaya	
Avocado	
Persimmon	
Pomegranates	

oral allergy symptoms. While reactions to fruits and vegetables can be commonly linked to the oral allergy syndrome, many of these foods are capable of inducing reactions in non-pollen-allergic individuals. The following section reviews some common (and not-so-common) fruits and vegetables that can trigger an allergic reaction.

■ Apples—Myths and Legends

The apple comes from a small tree with a broad, dense, and twiggy crown. Apple flowers bloom in spring, and the fruit matures in the autumn. The wild ancestor of *Malus domestica* has no common name in English but is known as "alma"—named after Alma-Ata in Kazakhstan, the city where the apple tree is thought to have originated. This tree grows wild in the mountains of Central Asia, Kazakhstan, and China. The word apple comes from the Old English word *aeppel*, which was used to refer to any round object. On the other hand, the scientific name *malus*, comes from the Latin word for apple.

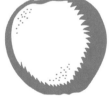

There are more than 7,500 known cultivars of apples in temperate and subtropical climates. Apples do not flower in tropical climates because they require chilling temperatures to properly grow. The Greeks grew several varieties of apples in late 300 BC, and the ancient Romans loved apples. Researchers have found the charred remains of apples at a Stone Age village in Switzerland. European settlers brought apple seeds and trees with them to the New World. Records from the Massachusetts Bay Company indicate that apples were

In 1796, Canadian John McIntosh discovered a variety of apple known as the McIntosh apple that is now enjoyed worldwide.

grown in New England as early as 1630. In 1796, Canadian John McIntosh discovered a variety of apple known as the McIntosh apple that is now enjoyed worldwide.

No other food is more steeped in legend and mythology than the apple. An integral part of legendary tales and religious traditions, apples are portrayed as a mystical and forbidden fruit. When the dark beauty Hecuba, the wife of King Priam of Troy, was pregnant, she had a terrifying dream. She dreamed she gave birth to a firebrand and awoke screaming that the city of Troy was burning to the ground. Alarmed by this, her husband consulted his son, the seer Aisacros, who told his father that the unborn baby would one day cause the destruction of Troy. Accordingly, King Priam ordered that the child should be put to death. So, after the boy Paris was born, he was given to Agelaus, the chief herdsman, to be killed. Agelaus left the child on Mount Ida to die from exposure. Upon returning five days later, Agelaus found the boy was still alive and took him home where he secretly brought him up. As a young man, Paris became famous for his extreme beauty, wit, and prowess.

At about this time, the wedding of Peleus and Thetis, the hero and the sea goddess, was being celebrated on Mount Pelion. All the gods and goddesses were invited with the noted exception of Eris, the Goddess of Strife who was a hideous and disagreeable person. Angered at being left out of the nuptials, Eris strode into the middle of the wedding feast and threw a golden apple into the assembled company. It landed

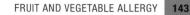

between the three most powerful god-desses, Hera, Athena, and Aphrodite. Pick-ing it up, Zeus found it was inscribed "For the Fairest." Zeus wisely decided not to judge between Hera, Athena, and Aphrodite and ordered the designated judge to be the most handsome mortal in the world. This turned out to be Paris, who was serving as a shepherd at the time. Paris agreed, and so a time was set for the three goddesses to appear to him on Mount Ida.

When the day came, Paris sat himself on a boulder and waited with a beating heart for the arrival of the three great goddesses. All at once, a great light appeared which covered the entire mountain. So the three finalists—Aphrodite, Hera, and Athena—sought him out in the meadow where he was tending his flocks. Not content to leave the out-come to the judge's discernment, the three Goddesses proceeded to offer bribes to Paris.

Helen, the subject of one of the most dramatic love stories in history, was the main reason for the ten-year war between the Greeks and the Trojans

Hera, the great queen, approached him and flaunted her beauty in front of him. Radiant with glory, she made him a promise. If he awarded her the golden apple, she would grant him wealth and power. He would rule over the greatest kingdom on earth. Paris felt the excitement of this, his ambition rose up, and he yearned for her gift.

After that, the grey-eyed Athena approached him, drawing near and bending down so that he might look into the magi-cal depths of her eyes. She promised him victory in all battles, together with glory and wisdom—the three most precious gifts a man could have. This time Paris felt his mind leap with excitement and with desire for the riches of knowledge and the glory of prowess.

Then it was Aphrodite's turn, the God-dess of love. The Romans called her Venus (hence the famous armless statue known as the Venus de Milo). Aphrodite lived on Mount Olympus with the other supreme deities and was married to the homely craftsman-god Hephaestus. Hanging back a little, she tilted her head so that her hair fell forward, concealing a blush on her face. Then she loosened the girdle of her robe and beneath it Paris caught sight of her perfectly formed breasts, white as alabaster. "Paris," she said, and her voice seemed to sing inside his head. "Give me the apple and in return I will give you the gift of love. You will possess the most beautiful woman in the land, a woman equal to me in perfection of form. With her you will experience the greatest delights of lovemaking. Choose me, Paris, and she will be yours." Paris, overpowered by the intoxication of her words and her beauty, handed her the apple without even pausing to reflect on his decision, guided only by the strength of his desire.

So it was that Paris awarded the Apple of Discord to Aphrodite, and Hera and Athena became his implacable enemies. True to her promise, Aphrodite gave him Helen, the most beautiful woman living on earth at that time. In order to capture her, Paris had to sail to Sparta and kidnap her from her powerful husband, Menelaus. After her abduction, Helen's husband and his brother King Agamemnon raised a Greek armada (1,000 ships) to sail to Troy and retrieve Helen—thus began Helen's legend as the face that launched a thousand ships. Helen, the subject of one of the most dramatic love stories in history, was the main reason for the ten-year war between the Greeks and the Trojans in which many legendary heroes, including Prince Hector, Achilles, and Paris, lost their lives at the Fall of Troy.

There are many other apple myths and legends. In Greek mythology, Atalanta refused to marry anyone unless a suitor could defeat her in a running race. One clever suitor, Milanion, accomplished this goal by dropping three golden apples that were gifts of the Goddess of Love during the race. Atalanta stopped to pick them up, lost the race, and became his wife.

An ancient Greek who wanted to propose to a woman would only have to toss her an apple. If she caught it, she accepted his proposal. In medieval times, Germanic men who ate an apple that was steeped in the perspiration of the woman he loved would succeed in his pursuit of her. In Britain, apples were closely identified with the Island of Avalon, whose name is derived from the Welsh word for apple. Avalon, where the mortally wounded King Arthur was taken to be healed, is a mythical place where there is constant sunlight, warm breezes, and lush vegetation; and the inhabitants neither age nor know pain or injury.

Although the forbidden fruit in the Garden of Eden is not identified, Christian tradition holds that it was an apple that Eve seduced Adam to share with her. The larynx in the human throat has been called "Adam's apple" due to the belief that it was caused by the forbidden fruit sticking in Adam's throat. Another reason for the adoption of the apple as Christian symbol is that in Latin, the words for "apple" and for "evil" are identical—*malum*. It is often used to symbolize the fall into sin, or sin itself. When Christ is portrayed holding an apple, he represents the Second Adam who brings life. In Adam's hand, the apple symbolizes sin. In the Old Testament, the apple signifies the fall of man. In the New Testament, it is an emblem of the redemption from that fall as represented in paintings of the Madonna and the infant Jesus.

In a Swiss story, William Tell, an archer, is arrested and then promised freedom for his people if he can shoot an apple off his son's head with a crossbow. Irish folklore claims that if an apple is peeled into one continuous ribbon and thrown behind a woman's shoulder, it will land in the shape of her future husband's initials. Danish folklore says that apples wither around adulterers. Apples are said to increase a woman's chances of conception as well as remove birthmarks when rubbed on the skin.

In the United States, Denmark, and Sweden, a polished apple is a traditional gift for a teacher. This tradition stemmed from the fact that poorly paid teachers were compensated with baskets of apples by their students. Once wages were increased, a basket of apples was toned down to a single fruit. Americans have a favorite story about an apple farmer named John Chapman. Known as Johnny Appleseed, he became famous in the 1800s when he distributed apple seeds and trees to settlers in Ohio, Indiana, and Illinois. Legend claims that Chapman traveled barefoot wearing old torn clothes and a tin pot for a hat.

> *In the United States, Denmark and Sweden, a polished apple is a traditional gift for a teacher. This tradition stemmed from the fact that poorly paid teachers were compensated with baskets of apples by their students. Once wages were increased, a basket of apples was toned down to a single fruit.*

◼ Nutritional Facts

Apples have long been considered a healthy food, as indicated by the proverb, "An apple a day keeps the doctor away." Apples may reduce the risk of colon, prostate, and lung cancer. They may also help with heart disease and weight loss and lower cholesterol levels. Apples are a good source of vitamins A and C. A ripe raw apple is easily digested and reduces stomach acidity. The apple is also an excellent dentifrice—the mechanical action of eating the fruit serving to clean both the teeth and the gums.

Most reactions occur after ingestion of fresh apples as apple proteins are denatured by canning, pulping, or heating.

◼ Clinical Reactions to Apples

Apple allergy is most frequently associated with birch pollen allergy in northern Europe and North America. Between 40 and 90 percent of patients allergic to birch pollen are also allergic to apples.

In my experience, the apple is the most common cause of the oral allergy syndrome. Symptoms may occur after low-dose exposure to apple, as demonstrated in a report of a twenty-four-year-old woman who experienced swelling of her lips and itching in her mouth after a kiss from her boyfriend who had just eaten a green apple.

In a study of 172 Finnish university students with food allergy, apple was a frequent (29 percent) cause of symptoms. The apple allergy often cross-reacts with pears, peaches and hazelnuts. In a Japanese study of 101 patients with the oral allergy syndrome and pollen allergy, the most common allergen was birch tree pollen.

In 61 percent of birch-allergic patients, a concomitant allergy to a fruit or vegetable was reported. Apple was the most prevalent allergen (97 percent), followed by peach (67 percent), cherry (58 percent), pear (40 percent), plum (40 percent), and melon (33 percent). There are differences in the allergenic potencies of different apple varieties and ripening stages of the fruits. Peels are more allergenic than pulps. Most reactions occur after ingestion of fresh apples as apple proteins are denatured by canning, pulping, or heating.

Due to the heat-labile nature of the apple allergens, you need to skin test with a fresh apple. All members of the apple family contain the toxin hydrogen cyanide in their seeds and possibly in their leaves, but almost never in the fruit. Hydrogen cyanide is the substance that gives almonds their characteristic taste. Apple seeds do not normally contain high quantities of hydrogen cyanide, but, even so, their seeds should not be consumed in large quantities. In small quantities, hydrogen cyanide stimulates respiration and improves digestion. In excess, it can cause respiratory failure and death.

◼ Artichoke Allergy

Artichokes are a good source of folic acid, vitamin C, and potassium. This low-calorie member of the sunflower, or Composite food family, can trigger reactions in ragweed-sensitive individuals. One case of artichoke anaphylaxis occurred after unintentional ingestion of artichoke. Skin tests were positive to artichoke, chicory, and endive (also plants from the Compositae family). This report suggests that this common Mediterranean vegetable may be an unrecognized cause of food allergy, especially in individuals with pollen and multiple food allergies.

■ Asparagus Allergy

Asparagus belongs to the lily family, which includes ferns and vegetables such as onions, leeks, garlic, and chives. This well-known delicacy was cultivated more than 2,000 years ago by Greeks and Romans. Asparagus is native to the marshes of southwest Europe and grows wild in southwest England, southern Russia, Poland, and Greece. Asparagus is a high-fiber, low-calorie source of folic acid and potassium. The smell in one's urine after eating asparagus is caused by excretion of methyl mercaptan. This propensity that occurs in 43 percent of people is due to inheriting a dominant gene. Asparagus, a well-known diuretic and laxative, has been touted as a folk remedy for eye ailments, toothaches, cramps, convulsions, and sciatica.

One series of twenty-seven cases from Spain described allergic symptoms after inhaling, eating, or handling asparagus. Eye irritation, nasal congestion, tightness of the throat, and coughing during cooking have been reported. Several cases of asparagus-induced hives and contact dermatitis have been reported. Gout sufferers should avoid asparagus as it contains purines that may increase the production of uric acid.

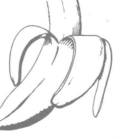

Trivia. The banana plant is not a tree. It is actually the world's largest herb!

■ Banana Allergy

Banana is a fruit of the tropical family Musaceae that grows from ten to twenty-six feet high and belongs to the same family as lilies, orchids, ginger, cardamom, and Jamaican arrowroot. The banana tree contains anywhere from fifty to 150 bananas, with individual fruits grouped in bunches known as "hands" that contain ten to twenty-five bananas each. Arabian slave traders are credited with giving the banana its popular name. The bananas that originally grew in Africa and Southeast Asia were not the eight-to-twelve-inch giants sold in supermarkets today. They were small, about as long as a man's finger. Hence, the name, *banan*, which is Arabic, for finger. The Spaniards found banana trees were similar to their plane tree and gave them a Spanish name, *platano*.

Bananas, one of the world's most popular fruits, has an interesting history. Originally grown in Malaysia, bananas were exported to India, where they were discovered in 327 BC by Alexander the Great who is credited with bringing the banana back to the Western world. Eventually, the banana reached Madagascar, an island off the southeastern coast of Africa. In 1402, Portuguese sailors discovered the luscious fruit in their travels to the African continent and brought it the Canary Islands.

Banana trees were then exported to the Caribbean island of Santo Domingo in 1516 by Tomas de Berlanga, a Portuguese Franciscan monk. It wasn't long before bananas became popular throughout the Caribbean and Central America. However, it took almost 350 years after bananas were introduced into the Caribbean before Americans tasted their first banana. Wrapped in tin foil, bananas were first sold for ten cents each at a celebration held in

Pennsylvania in 1876 to commemorate the hundredth anniversary of the Declaration of Independence. Today, most bananas are grown in tropical and subtropical countries, such as Costa Rica, Mexico, Ecuador, and Brazil.

The edible part of the banana fruit is rich in protein and contains a range of enzymes and pharmacologically active substances like serotonin. The banana is one of the best sources of potassium. Since the average banana contains a whopping 467 milligrams of potassium and only one milligram of sodium, one banana a day may help prevent high blood pressure and heart disease. Men who eat potassium-rich foods and foods high in magnesium and cereal fiber have fewer strokes and less heart disease. My late father ate a banana every morning of his life. Were it not for a lethal hip fracture at age 93, I think he would have made it to the century mark.

Bananas have long been recognized for their antacid effects that may prevent stomach ulcers. In one study, a mixture of banana and milk significantly suppressed gastric acid secretion. Bananas are a rich source of fructooligosaccharide, a compound called a prebiotic because it nourishes probiotic (friendly) bacteria in the

Men who eat potassium-rich foods and foods high in magnesium and cereal fiber have fewer strokes and less heart disease. My late father ate a banana every morning of his life. Were it not for a lethal hip fracture at age 93, I think he would have made it to the century mark.

colon. These beneficial bacteria produce vitamins and digestive enzymes that improve our ability to absorb nutrients that protect us against unfriendly microorganisms. Additional touted health benefits from bananas include a lower risk of age-related macular degeneration, osteoporosis, and kidney cancer.

■ Clinical Reactions to Bananas

Numerous reports depict allergic reactions to bananas. Common symptoms include hives, swelling, and oral allergy symptoms. Allergenicity may increase with ripeness. A fifteen-year-old girl developed anaphylactic shock, asthma, swelling, and hives after eating a banana. She had eaten a banana two weeks earlier without adverse effects. Anaphylaxis was reported in a thirty-two-year-old woman who developed severe oral symptoms, hives, and difficulty breathing. Banana reactions can occur at any age. A five-month-old boy suffered three episodes of generalized hives twenty minutes after the ingestion of a fruit puree containing apple, banana, and orange.

Skin testing showed positive results to banana and chestnut. His mother admitted she ate lots of bananas during pregnancy and while breast-feeding. Due to the presence of cross-reacting allergens in the banana fruit and the latex rubber tree (*Hevea brasiliensis),* allergic reactions to banana are quite common in people with latex allergy. In a study of banana CAP RAST levels in latex-allergic individuals, 55 percent were positive to banana. Bananas also share common allergens with other fruits, such as avocado, chestnuts, kiwi, and melons. Banana may precipitate migraine headaches due to the presence of vasoactive substances, such as serotonin and tyramine.

■ Blackcurrant Allergy

Blackcurrants are small edible berries that grow on a temperate shrub that is a member of Rosaceae family. One report from Spain described a fifty-year-old woman with an allergy to peach, nectarine, and apricot who reacted to fresh blackcurrants and blackcurrant jam.

■ Blueberry Allergy

Blueberries are a small, tasty berry that grows in the colder climates of Canada, New England, Great Britain, and New Zealand. North America accounts for nearly 90 percent of the world's blueberry production. The blueberry, is one of the most recent fruit crops to be brought under cultivation. Other similar berries include cranberry, lingonberry, bilberry and huckleberry. Blueberries have been used in European folk medicine since the 16th century. Early American settlers incorporated blueberries into their diets, eating them fresh off the bush and adding them to soups, stews, and many other foods.

Nutritional research has found that blueberries contain a number of compounds that have beneficial properties, such as prevention of urinary tract infections, antioxidant (anti-cancer) activity, reducing heart disease, strengthening collagen, regulating blood sugar, reducing replication of the HIV virus, and treating diarrhea. One survey looking at the antioxidant capacity of fruits and vegetables placed blueberries near the top of the list. Blueberries are a rare trigger of food allergy. Thus, blueberries—like raspberries, cranberries, lingonberries, bilberries and huckleberries—are usually a safe, albeit expensive, healthy alternative for fruit-allergic individuals who suffer from oral allergy syndrome. Blueberries may also improve eyesight. One study found that Israeli fighter pilots given regular doses of blueberries had better night vision. After my research on blueberries, I have added them to my breakfast meal with the hope that they will improve my putting stroke in golf.

■ Broccoli Allergy

This vegetable, an excellent source of vitamin C, beta-carotene, and folic acid, is also touted as an anti-cancer food. Broccoli provides a safe alternative for the vegetable-allergic individual, as it is a rare trigger of food allergy.

■ Brussel Sprout Allergy

Reportedly cultivated in the 16th-century in Belgium, Brussel sprouts belong to the cabbage family. They resemble tiny cabbage heads and grow in western and middle Europe, Japan, and North America. Brussel sprouts are high in vitamins A and C and also contain iron. No allergens from this plant have yet been characterized. Cross-reactivity between broccoli, cauliflower, and cabbage is possible. As Brussels sprouts rarely trigger food allergy, they provide a compatible food for many patients with vegetable allergies.

> *Blueberries may also improve eyesight. One study found that Israeli fighter pilots given regular doses of blueberries had better night vision. After my research on blueberries, I have added them to my breakfast meal with the hope that they will improve my putting stroke in golf.*

■ Cabbage Allergy

Cabbage is a vegetable with few reported allergic reactions. The close botanical relationship between cabbage, broccoli, Brussel sprouts, and cauliflower suggests that these vegetables contain very similar proteins. Another safe, albeit somewhat unpalatable alternative for vegetable-allergic individuals.

■ Carrot Allergy

The carrot, a member of the parsley family, is used in a wide range of foods, including salads, soups, and stews. Carrots are rich in sugar and have been renowned for 2,000 years for their health-giving properties and more recently for their high vitamin A content. The most frequent cross-reactions with carrot allergy have been reported in birch pollen-allergic patients. Individuals with carrot allergy may react to other members of the parsley family, such as celery, fennel, anise, caraway, dill, lovage, and parsley.

> *Excessive consumption of carrots and other yellow-green vegetables by infants and young children is the most common cause of carotenemia that produces a yellow tinge to the skin.*

In one European study, carrot allergy was reported to affect up to 25 percent of food-allergic subjects. In a Swiss study, carrot was the third most common food allergy, affecting 13 percent of food-allergic patients. It was more common than hen's egg and fish allergy. The most frequently reported symptoms are mild oral allergy symptoms, but severe reactions have been described. Anaphylaxis may occur to minute quantities of carrot, as depicted by an individual who developed anaphylactic shock due to the inadvertent ingestion of carrot hidden in an ice cream.

Overindulging in carrots may lead to an overdose of vitamin A that triggers cerebral edema (brain swelling), as described in a patient who consumed large quantities of raw carrots to lose weight. Carotenemia, also known as xanthoderma, is another adverse effect of ingesting large quantities of carrots, usually in the form of carrot juice. Affected individuals develop a yellowish-orange skin color. Excessive consumption of carrots and other yellow-green vegetables by infants and young children is the most common cause of carotenemia that produces a yellow tinge to the skin.

■ Castor Bean Allergy

The castor bean pollen from this oil-producing plant can be highly sensitizing for people living near castor bean trees. Most reports on castor bean allergy involve asthma. Unprocessed castor bean seeds are highly toxic, and severe sickness and deaths have been reported in people who have chewed the whole castor bean seed.

■ Cauliflower Allergy

It is believed that both cauliflower and broccoli were cultivated from wild cabbage by eastern Mediterranean gardeners about 400 hundred years ago. Cauliflower is a cool-season annual plant that is eaten raw cooked or added to soups and side dishes—often smothered with a cheese sauce. Cauliflower contains vitamin C, a fair amount of iron, and high levels of antioxidant and anticancer compounds. Some research has suggested that compounds in cauliflower and other members of the cabbage family may prevent macular degeneration, the leading cause of blindness in the elderly.

There are very few cases of cauliflower allergy in the literature. Investigators from Madrid, Spain, described a seventy-year-old man who suffered mouth itching, facial and hand swelling, and severe wheezing a few minutes after eating a vegetable dish (paella) containing cauliflower, green beans, and red and green pepper. His cauliflower allergy was confirmed by skin and CAP RAST tests. Another report depicted an allergic twenty-one-year-old woman who had anaphylaxis to cabbage and who had positive skin tests to cauliflower, broccoli, and mustard. A report from China described a sixteen-year-old boy with cauliflower-triggered, exercise-induced anaphylaxis. Infantile colic has been described when breast-feeding mothers ingest significant amounts of cauliflower and other members of the cabbage family.

■ Celery Allergy

Celery is another ancient plant from the parsley family. There is a widespread myth that the word celery, known as "the fast vegetable," is derived from the Latin word, *celer*, meaning fast or swift. This is entirely false. The word celery comes from the Greek word, *selinon*, meaning *parsley*. A reference to *selinon* is found in Homer's *Odyssey*. Originally grown in Italian and European gardens in the sixteenth century, celery had a stringent taste and was used only for medicinal purposes. In the late seventeenth century, European gardeners found that growing the plants in late summer and fall and storing them over the winter eliminated the strong taste. Celery still grows wild in ditches and salt marshes along western and northern European coastlines.

Celery is a very popular vegetable, used primarily in salads, casseroles and soups. When combined with salt, the resulting celery salt is often used as an alternate to ordinary salt in various recipes and cocktails. It greatly enhances the flavor of a Bloody Mary drink and Chicago-style hot dogs. The celery seed is also used as a spice.

In North America, commercial production of celery is dominated by a variety called pascal celery. Celery has a negative calorie effect. The stringy celery plant is difficult to digest. The effort to digest it burns more calories than it contains. The net loss in calories, while not significant, can assist dieting by filling the stomach and quenching hunger. Folk-medicine practitioners have promoted the celery plant to treat rheumatoid arthritis, gout, high blood pressure, urinary tract problems, and nervous exhaustion.

Infantile colic has been described when breast-feeding mothers ingest significant amounts of cauliflower and other members of the cabbage family.

Celery is a frequent cause of pollen-related food allergy, particularly in birch pollen-allergic Europeans. In Switzerland and France, 30 to 40 percent of patients with food allergy are allergic to celery; and, in one study, 30 percent of severe anaphylactic reactions to food were attributed to celery. Symptoms of celery allergy range from mild oral allergy symptoms to life-threatening reactions. I believe celery and parsley family allergy is very common in North America where we do not have reliable reporting mechanisms to collect cases of fruit and vegetable allergy.

■ Celeriac Allergy

This vegetable, derived from the root of the celery plant, was developed from the same wild species as today's varieties of celery. Italian and Swiss botanists first described celeriac in 1600 AD. While celeriac never became popular in England or the United States, it is a popular vegetable throughout Europe. Rarely eaten raw, it is well suited for soups and stews. Celeriac allergy may be more common and severe than celery allergy. Unlike many other fruits and vegetables, cooked celery and celeriac may remain very allergenic even after extended cooking. Food labeling rules now require pre-packed foods sold in the United Kingdom and the European Union to clearly label celery-containing products. Unfortunately, the new United States labeling law does not cover fruits and vegetables.

> *The original citrus fruit, the citron, is better known to most consumers in its preserved rather than in its natural form.*

Cherry Allergy

Two documented cases from Spain depicted cherry reactions in a twenty-eight-year-old woman with asthma and almond allergy and a twenty-five-year-old woman with asthma and oral allergy symptoms to kiwi fruit.

Citrus Fruits

It's generally believed that the ancestors of citrus fruits were grown 8,000 years ago in India and in the Fertile Crescent between the Tigris and Euphrates rivers in what is now Iraq. The original citrus fruit, the citron, is better known to most consumers in its preserved rather than in its natural form. Citron seeds have been found in Mesopotamian excavations dat-

ing back to 4000 BC. The armies of Alexander the Great are thought to have carried the citron to the Mediterranean region. Ancient Mesopotamians treasured citrons for their beauty and aroma. Egyptians used citrons as an embalming fluid, and Romans used them as mothballs. Jews brought them to Israel after they escaped from their captivity in Babylon some 2,500 years ago. Citrons were touted as aphrodisiacs, cures for fever and colic, and as protection against poisons.

The fragrant citron is one of the four species used in the synagogue service on the Feast of Tabernacles. In ancient times, the citron was a popular Jewish symbol on coins, graves, synagogues, and circumcision knives. A Jewish coin struck in 136 BC bears a representation of the citron on one side. After the Jewish rebellion against Rome in 66 AD, Jews dispersed throughout the Roman Empire and planted citron plants across the Mediterranean. Ancient Jewish gardeners were also responsible for the cultivation of other citrus fruits. The Romans commissioned these gardeners to develop oranges and lemons, which they did using the citron as a grafting stock. What the Talmud calls the "sweet citron" was probably an early orange. After the fall of Rome, citrus fruits disappeared from Europe only to be reintroduced by the Arabs in the 10th century.

During the great seafaring voyages of Columbus, citrus fruits were found to prevent scurvy. Columbus took citrus seeds to the New World where they were spread throughout the Caribbean. Ponce de Leon took them to Florida in 1513 and required his sailors to plant 100 seedlings wherever they landed. This undoubtedly laid the foundation of today's modern-day Florida citrus industry. The citrus family contains dozens of different fruits, including oranges, lemons, grapefruits, limes, and tangerines.

Citrus fruits are notable for their fragrance and juices. They contain a high proportion of citric acid, giving them their characteristic astringent odor and flavor. They are good sources of vitamin C and flavonoids. An orange hybrid bearing an orange and red rind with red flesh is called blood orange. The Temple orange, named after the man who created it, is a flavorful orange-tangerine hybrid. Bitter oranges, also known as Seville oranges, named after the Spanish city of the same name, are seldom seen in markets and are used chiefly for marmalade and liquors. Because of its hot, damp climate, Florida grows thin-skinned juicy oranges. In contrast, California's drier climate produces thick-skinned, sweet "eating" oranges like the Valencia and navel oranges.

The pomelo is a citrus fruit. Pale green to yellow in color when ripe, it is larger than a grapefruit and has a sweet flesh and thick spongy rind. The pomelo is also called a shaddock after English sea Captain Shaddock who introduced the pomelo seed to the West Indies in the seventeenth century. Pomelo is native to southeastern Asia and is grown commercially in California and Israel. A pomelo is the biggest of all citrus fruits. They can grow to one foot in diameter and weigh up to twenty-five pounds. Pomelos can usually be found in grocery stores in the United States from the late fall until early spring and are sometimes sold as a Christmas fruit.

The grapefruit, a hybrid between a pomelo and an orange, was given its name because it grows in grape-like bunches. Spanish nobleman Don Philippe introduced grapefruit to Florida around 1840. It is sometimes said, "A grapefruit is a lemon that had a chance and took advantage of it."

■ Citrus Fruit Allergy

There are many reports of citrus allergy in the literature. Some older studies put orange allergy in the top ten. In a study of 1,419 patients aged one year to eighteen years, 3 percent of Spanish children were reported to be allergic to citrus fruit. In my experience, orange or citrus allergy is quite unusual. The skin test to oranges may be falsely positive as I often see positive skin tests in patients who have no problems eating oranges or other citrus products.

Oranges are considered to be common allergenic fruits in China and may induce severe food allergy in sensitive individuals. Chinese investigators report that the major allergenic components of orange reside in orange seeds, not the juice. Systemic reactions developed in five Chinese patients after intradermal skin testing with orange seed extract. The authors concluded that orange seeds contain potent allergens that may induce reactions after careless chewing of orange seeds.

The symptoms of orange or citrus allergy include nausea, itching, abdominal pain, vomiting, diarrhea, wheezing, hives, low blood pressure, and anaphylaxis. Several cases of orange-dependent, exercise-induced anaphylaxis have been described. Delayed reactions from orange and lemon peel can produce hand dermatitis in food handlers. One bartender with hand dermatitis had positive skin tests to the skin of lemon, lime, and orange, but not to their

> *Spanish nobleman Don Philippe introduced grapefruit to Florida around 1840. It is sometimes said, "A grapefruit is a lemon that had a chance and took advantage of it."*

respective juices. Eleven percent of 490 patients with classic migraine reported citrus fruits triggered their headaches. The majority of these patients were also sensitive to chocolate and cheese.

■ Corn—History and Nutrition

Corn (also known as maize) is the world's most abundant grain crop. It was first grown over 5,600 years ago by the Mayan and Aztec tribes in Mexico. By 1400 BC, corn cultivation spread throughout North and South America and was an important part of the American Indian diet. The crop eventually reached what is now southern New England approximately 1,000 years ago. After Columbus received corn as a gift from the Indians he encountered in the Caribbean, he carried it back to Spain. Within a short time, corn was grown worldwide.

> *Patients with corn (or maize) allergy must be wary of a wide variety of foods, including corn sweeteners, cornstarch, some baked goods, candy, canned fruits, cereals, cookies, jams and jellies, lunch meats, syrups, baking powder, powdered sugar, sweeteners, maple syrup, wheat, and potato rice starches.*

The first Pilgrims who arrived in Plymouth, Massachusetts, probably would have starved to death had they not been given corn by the Indians. The Indians taught the Pilgrims how to grow corn and prepare corn bread, soup, pudding, and fried corn cakes. When English and German settlers arrived in the New World, they distinguished corn from other grains by calling it "Indian corn." The corn crop now dominates American agriculture. Corn is planted on roughly 70 million to 80 million acres annually in the United States, with an annual production of about 9 billion bushels that is valued at $30 billion. Popcorn comes from a special variety of corn with smaller kernels that, when heated, turns into a fluffy mass of starch and fiber. Corn is a good source of potassium, folate, and thiamine.

■ Corn Allergy

While there are many cases of corn-induced asthma and rhinitis in the literature, it was quite difficult to find cases of corn-induced food allergy. The best corn study comes from researchers in New Orleans who recruited fifty-nine patients, age five to sixty-five, with a history of adverse reactions to corn or corn products and a positive skin test to corn. Only five of the seventeen patients who completed an oral corn challenge had a positive challenge. This study concluded that although corn allergy may be rare, when it occurs it can be severe. Another survey looked at sixteen subjects with positive skin and CAP RAST tests to corn flour. An oral challenge to corn was positive in only six patients.

Professor Janice M. Joneja, a world-renowned dietician, author, and food allergy expert from Vanouver, Canada, believes that adverse reactions to corn and corn derivatives are frequently undiagnosed, and the incidence of corn allergy is greatly underestimated as skin and blood tests to corn are generally negative. She believes corn allergy is an example of a food allergy that can only be successfully and accurately identified by dietary elimination or an oral challenge. Corn may not be unique in this respect as a number of food allergens may often be overlooked when the standard allergy tests are negative. Patients with corn (or maize) allergy must be wary of a wide variety of foods, including corn sweeteners, cornstarch, some baked goods, candy, canned fruits, cereals, cookies, jams and jellies, lunch meats, syrups, baking powder, powdered sugar, sweeteners, maple syrup, wheat, and potato rice starches.

■ Cucumber Allergy

A hairy vine from the Mediterranean produces cucumbers, a small oval fruit that separates from the footstalk when ripe. Its roots and fruit have been used as a cathartic, analgesic, and anti-inflammatory agent since antiquity. The cucumber plant is also used in some parts of the Mediterranean to treat sinusitis.

Cross-reactive allergens may be responsible for the clustering of food allergies seen in patients allergic to celery, cucumber, carrot, and watermelon. While allergic reactions to cucumber are rare, one case report suggests cucumber allergy may be more common than believed. A thirty-four-year-old woman with long-standing pollen allergy and oral allergy symptoms after ingestion of fennel, cucumber, and melons was administered allergy injections to grass, mugwort, and ragweed pollen. After forty-three months of allergy injection therapy, she was able to tolerate fresh fennel, cucumber, and melon in open oral challenge tests.

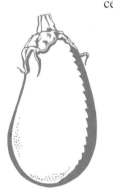

Commonly thought of as a vegetable, eggplant is actually a fruit—specifically a berry.

■ Eggplant Allergy

Eggplant, a member of the nightshade family, is related to potatoes, tomatoes, and peppers. Commonly thought of as a vegetable, eggplant is actually a fruit—specifically a berry. The eggplant is also known as aubergine, brinjal, melanzana, garden egg, and patlican. Often called "the poor man's meat," eggplant is of considerable economic importance in many tropical and subtropical parts of the world. The ancestors of eggplant were first cultivated in China in the fifth century BC. Eggplant was introduced to Africa and then Italy, the country with which it has long been associated. Eggplant cultivation subsequently spread throughout Europe and the Middle East and was brought to the Western Hemisphere by European explorers.

Although it has a long and rich history, the bitter-tasting early varieties did not always hold the revered place that it does today. The first eggplants that English-speaking people encountered were white egg-shaped fruits, hence the vegetable's name. Eggplant was initially suspected of causing madness, leprosy, cancer, and bad breath, prompting its use only as a decorative plant. Once better tasting varieties were developed in the eighteenth century, eggplant took an esteemed place in the cuisines of many European countries, especially Italy. At one time, Asian women used a black dye made from eggplant to stain their teeth gunmetal gray. The dye probably came from the dark purple eggplant that we see on supermarket shelves today.

The most common eggplant sold the United States is the large cylindrical variety. Many would agree that eggplant, with its elegant pear shape and glossy purple skin, is one of the most attractive of all vegetables. It is available year-round, with its peak season in August and September. Unfortunately, eggplant is not high in any single vitamin or mineral. However, it is very filling, supplies few calories and virtually no fat. Its meaty texture makes it a perfect vegetarian dish. Eggplant can be prepared in stews, roasted, grilled, sautéed, stir-fried, breaded, baked, pickled, or stuffed. Eggplant should not be eaten raw due to the potentially dangerous amounts of solanine and histamine in raw eggplant.

> *Greek myths state that fennel was closely associated with Dionysus, the Greek god of food and wine, and the fennel stalk passed down knowledge from the gods to men.*

Allergic reactions to eggplant in subjects with pollen allergy have been reported, especially in Europe and India. In a survey of 500 food-allergic individuals in India, sixty-six people were reported to have an eggplant allergy based on their history and skin tests. The authors suggest that the high incidence of eggplant reactions was due to the presence of histamine and serotonin in the eggplant.

Anaphylaxis to eggplant was reported in a latex-allergic, twenty-seven-year-old female doctor who experienced generalized itching and rash, shortness of breath, dizziness, vomiting, nausea, abdominal pain, and diarrhea after eating boiled eggplant. Occupational allergy to the eggplant plant has also been reported in commercial and home gardeners.

■ Fennel Allergy

Fennel belongs to the Umbellifereae family, which also includes parsley, carrots, dill, and coriander. The ancient Greeks knew fennel by the name "marathon" in honor of the Battle of Marathon that was fought in a field of fennel. Fennel was also awarded to Pheidippides, the runner who delivered the news of the Persian invasion of Sparta. Greek myths state that fennel was closely associated with Dionysus, the Greek god of food and wine, and the fennel stalk passed down knowledge from the gods to men.

Fennel has been grown in areas surrounding the Mediterranean Sea and the Near East since ancient times. Today, the United States, France, India, and Russia are among the leading producers of fennel. Fennel is composed of a stalk with a white or pale green bulb and topped with feathery green leaves that produce fennel seeds. The bulb, stalks, leaves, and seeds are all edible. Fennel is very popular in Mediterranean (especially Italian) cuisine. Fennel's aromatic taste is unique, reminiscent of licorice and anise. In fact, it is often mistakenly referred to as anise in the marketplace. Florence fennel is known as *finocchio*. It is best to consume fennel soon after purchase as it ages quickly.

The most fascinating phytonutrient compound in fennel may be anethole. This is the primary component of its volatile oil, and it has been shown to reduce inflammation and prevent cancer in laboratory animals. The fennel bulb is an excellent source of vitamin C, fiber, folate, and potassium. Herbal uses of fennel include a gargle solution, eyewash, and cough medicine. Fennel oil may be used as a flavoring in toothpastes, soaps, perfumes, and air fresheners. Fennel, an uncommon food allergen, may trigger oral allergy symptoms and exercise-induced food reactions.

■ Ficus Fruit Syndrome

An allergic reaction to figs and other tropical fruits is called the Ficus-Fruit Syndrome. Fig proteins may cross-react with latex, kiwi fruit, banana, pineapple, avocado, and papaya. The paucity of clinical reports of this syndrome is probably due to infrequent consumption of raw figs. Indoor ornamental fig plants like the weeping fig may trigger rhinitis and asthma when a latex-like protein in this plant adheres to dust particles and becomes airborne. Little is known about the prevalence of fig allergy or its association with fruit and latex allergy.

■ Genip Allergy

The genip, a bright green dimpled fruit related to the litchi and akee, has been introduced to parts of the Caribbean. It grows in grape-like bunches on large shade trees. The genip tree is very adaptable to poor soils and flourishes along roadsides. The fruit is about the size of a cherry but looks more like a small lime. For that reason, it is sometimes known as Spanish lime or *limoncillo* (little lime). However, it is neither a lime nor does in grow in Spain. The tough green skin protects a gummy, jelly-like pink pulp that houses two flattened seeds that look like a single large seed. The pulp has a refreshing grape-like flavor with a touch of acidity. Despite its pale color, genip juice stains horribly.

Genips are a good source of iron as well as fiber, calcium, vitamin A, phosphorus ,and niacin. While typically eaten fresh, they are also made into jams, jellies, pies, and fruit drinks. One of my partners recently evaluated a young Puerto Rican man who had an anaphylactic reaction to genip that was confirmed by a large positive skin test. Genip allergy may be quite rare, as he cannot find a similar case in the medical literature.

■ Grape Allergy

Grape allergy is considered to be relatively rare. Most reports come from Greece where grapes are widely consumed as a fresh fruit. Eleven Greek patients, six men and five women aged sixteen to forty-four years, experienced a total of thirty-five grape-induced anaphylaxis episodes. The most common triggers were wine, red grapes, stuffed vine leaves, and raisins. A larger study from Greece detailed sixty-one grape-allergic adults with an average age of twenty-eight years. While most patients had oral allergy symptoms, many reported anaphylaxis. These patients were frequently allergic to other foods, especially apples and peanuts. These reports suggest that grape allergy may be more common than generally thought.

> *Grapple is a new fruit drink where apple is added to a grape flavoring and water. A report of eye and throat swelling in a twenty-nine-year-old woman after ingesting Grapple was tied to the Fuji apple, not the grape flavoring used in this product.*

Grape allergy has been detected in workers handling grapes, suggesting that sensitization is more likely to occur through skin than gastrointestinal tract exposure. Grapple is a new fruit drink where apple is added to a grape flavoring and water. A report of eye and throat swelling in a twenty-nine-year-old woman after ingesting Grapple was tied to the Fuji apple, not the grape flavoring used in this product.

■ Heart of Palm

Heart of palm is a vegetable harvested from the inner core and growing bud of certain palm trees. It is costly because harvesting kills the tree. Heart of palm is often eaten in a salad sometimes called "millionaire's salad." When harvesting the young palm, the tree is cut down and the bark is removed leaving layers of white fibers around a center core. The center core is considered more of a delicacy because of its lower fiber content. A study in *Allergy* (June 2006) described a twenty-five-year-old man who developed an anaphylactic reaction fifteen minutes after eating fresh, wild heart of palm. Symptoms included generalized redness, swelling, trouble swallowing, and dizziness. He had previously eaten heart of palm as well as tinned heart of palm from South America without any adverse effects.

■ Honeysuckle Allergy

I found only one documented case of honeysuckle allergy that described an eight-year-old girl who reacted to a few drops of honey obtained from a honeysuckle bush.

■ Kiwi Allergy

Over the past few years, allergists have seen a dramatic increase in the incidence of allergy to exotic fruits, such as kiwi. Also known as the Chinese gooseberry, this fruit was initially grown in China in 600-900 AD. It was imported to New Zealand in 1930 and renamed the kiwi in recognition of the flightless kiwi bird, the emblem of New Zealand.

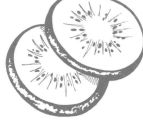

The rise in allergic reactions to kiwi and other exotic fruits, such as mango and papaya, especially in young children, is possibly related to their increased popularity and consumption.

Kiwi fruit has a long shelf life (about six months), is low in calories and rich in vitamin C.

Prior to case reports of life-threatening kiwi reactions by Dr. Henry Freye in 1991, there were only two reported cases of kiwi allergy in the literature. The results of a survey conducted by the American Academy of Allergy, Asthma, and Immunology uncovered thirty more cases of kiwi allergy, where patients ranged from three to eighty-one years of age. One interesting case described a four-month-old Italian infant who had two bouts of anaphylaxis traced to the mother's ingestion of kiwi fruit while breast-feeding. In a United Kingdom study of 245 kiwi-allergic patents, most had oral allergy symptoms but nearly one in five had a systemic reaction that required emergency care. Kiwi allergy is also on the upswing in both France and Germany.

Kiwi reactions that trigger asthma and contact dermatitis may be more severe than the typical fruit and vegetable reactions. In my experience, kiwi is a potent allergen as several of my kiwi-allergic patients had large skin test reactions to the raw fruit. There are two varieties of the kiwi fruit—the green and gold. Some researchers have proposed that the new gold variety may be less allergenic. This may not be true. Four of five patients with allergy to the green kiwi reacted when skin tested and orally challenged to the gold species.[2] The rise in allergic reactions to kiwi and

---

[2] Gold kiwi may also be marketed as Zespri and not labeled as kiwi.

other exotic fruits such as mango and papaya especially in young children, is possibly related to their increased popularity and consumption.

■ Lettuce Allergy

Lettuce is a vegetable from the Compositae family, which includes endives, artichokes, and allergenic plants such as ragweed and mugwort. Undoubtedly the world's most widely used salad vegetable, lettuce is thought to have originated in the Mediterranean region in the form of prickly lettuce. It is recorded as having been served in Persia in 400 BC. This inexpensive, low-calorie vegetable is a good source of beta carotene, vitamin C, calcium, and potassium. The sap of the lettuce plant has been used in folk medicine for its anti-spasmodic, digestive, diuretic, hypnotic, narcotic, and sedative properties.

Lettuce is most commonly served as leaves in salads and sandwiches, but it also appears in soups and stews. Lettuce allergy is very rare despite the fact that it is typically consumed raw. One chicory-allergic patient reacted to botanically related endive and lettuce. The largest series of case reports comes from Spain where fourteen patients with lettuce allergy were described. Lettuce-dependent, exercise-induced anaphylaxis has also been reported.

■ Lingonberry Allergy

Similar to cranberries, the lingonberry is touted for use in urinary tract infections. One documented case described a twenty-five-year-old woman who had two separate reactions to lingonberry jam.

■ Linseed Allergy

This plant is employed as a laxative in oils, herbal preparations, and multigrain breads. Spanish allergists described a thirty-nine-year-old woman who had a severe reaction after ingesting a spoonful of linseed grains. Unfortunately, linseed oil may not always be listed on herbal product labels.

■ Mango Allergy

Mango, an evergreen tree fruit, comes from a family that includes cashews, pistachios, and poison ivy. Mangoes have been cultivated for over 6,000 years in Southeast Asia and Indo-Malaysia. Commonly known as "the king of fruits," mangos are now also grown in California, Florida, and Mexico. Mangos are delicious peeled and eaten plain. Mango is used in vegetable and lentil dishes and as a meat tenderizer. It is a good source of beta carotene and vitamin C.

An association between latex allergy and mango has been reported. A forty-five-year-old, latex-allergic nurse developed oral allergy syndrome symptoms, eye swelling, cough, and shortness of breath following ingestion of mango. A thirty-two-year-old fruit picker developed eye swelling, facial redness, hives, and shortness of breath twenty minutes after eating a fresh mango. Several patients with mango and pistachio nut allergy have been described. Among them was a twenty-eight-year-old woman who developed a burning sensation in her mouth; swelling of the lips, face and tongue; nausea; and abdominal cramps immediately after eating a peeled mango.

Contact dermatitis of the face and lips has been described. A twenty-two-year-old female mango-eating student presented with a two-day history of a red itchy rash of the face, neck, and arms and eye swelling after peeling and eating mangoes. Patch tests to mango skin and mango flesh were positive. Complete avoidance of mango led to resolution of the eruption. The frequency of mango allergy may be underestimated because of the low consumption of mango in the Northern Hemisphere.

Manioc or Yuca Allergy

When Portuguese explorers landed in Brazil in the 1500s, they encountered the peaceful Tupi Indians. Having exhausted their own food supplies, they turned to these aborigine natives for food. One food provided by the Indians was the manioc tuber, or cassava root, the main staple of the Tupi Indian's diet. Manioc, also called Yuca, is a carbohydrate-rich food that is easy to grow but difficult to process as it is poisonous when eaten raw.

The fresh roots are cooked much like potatoes. Once peeled, they are boiled, baked, or fried. Pulverized manioc can be mixed with ground fish to produce a concoction called paçoka, or paçoca. Additional names for manioc are mandioca or yucca. A popular snack of fried, sweet manioc strips is Brazil's answer to French fries. Manioc, widely used in the West Indies and Africa, is slowly entering the American and European food market. A Brazilian friend of mine recently cooked some manioc fries for me to sample. They are quite delicious, with a somewhat sweeter taste than typical American French fries.

A Brazilian friend of mine recently cooked some manioc fries for me to sample. They are quite delicious with a somewhat sweeter taste than typical American French fries.

Fortunately for Brazilians, manioc allergy is rare. One case report describes a fifty-one-year-old asthmatic woman from Mozambique who experienced several episodes of anaphylaxis immediately after eating foods that cross-reacted with latex, including chestnut, kiwi, passion fruit, papaya, mango, peach, fig, melon, tomato, and spinach. She also reacted to boiled manioc and raw manioc flour. Her skin tests were positive to latex and to several foods, including raw and cooked manioc.

Melon Allergy

Melons belong to the gourd family Cucurbitaceae, which includes watermelons, cucumbers, and zucchini. Melons, probably natives of Asia, are cultivated worldwide in warmer regions and greenhouses. Melons are eaten raw as a dessert fruit in slices or cubes or blended with cold desserts like sorbet. Their high water content makes them poor candidates for cooking and preserving. The most common melons are watermelon, honeydew, cantaloupe, and muskmelon.

Workers who wax and clean off the small soft hairs on melons prior to shipping can develop a contact dermatitis. Melon reactions are most frequently seen in individuals with ragweed hay fever. There is a potential cross-reactivity with latex and other members of the gourd family such as zucchini and cucumber. The most common manifestations of melon allergy are oral allergy symptoms. However, hives, swelling, intestinal symptoms, and anaphylaxis have been reported. A Madrid study suggests that melon-allergic patients may be more likely to have asthma than other fruit-allergic individuals. Even though melon allergy is a common problem, especially in ragweed-allergic individuals, there are very few studies on melon allergy.

Mushroom Allergy

While there are many reports of toxic reactions to poisonous mushrooms, there are very few cases of true mushroom allergy in the literature. The difficulties of mushroom allergen research are substantial because one usually has to rely on naturally grown mushrooms. Two documented cases of oral allergy symptoms have been described. Another report depicted three patients with mushroom allergy who were also allergic to molds.

Olive Allergy

Despite widespread consumption of olives in the Mediterranean, I found only one well-documented case of olive allergy in the literature. This report depicted a nineteen-year-old woman who had several episodes of facial, neck, and hand swelling and intense itching of her palms after eating olives. She tolerated olive oil and did not have any hay fever symptoms during the olive pollen season. Olive pollen is a common trigger of hay fever and asthma throughout the Mediterranean.

Papaya Allergy

Reactions to fruits grown on the papaya tree are also increasing. The papaya tree, which originated in West India, Mexico, and Central America, is widely cultivated in tropical and subtropical areas. There are two types of papaya fruit, Hawaiian and Mexican. The Hawaiian species are commonly found in American supermarkets. A properly ripened papaya is a juicy, sweet fruit that tastes like a cantaloupe. The fruit can be used to make drinks, salads, marmalade, and candy.

Papain, an enzyme obtained from full-grown, unripe papaya fruit, has been used in medications, douche powders, and meat tenderiz-

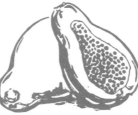

Papaya pollen is a common cause of asthma and hay fever in India. Like kiwi and mango allergy, the incidence of papaya allergy will undoubtedly increase with more global consumption of this tasty fruit.

ers. In the 1980s, chymopapain injections were a popular treatment for herniated discs. The enthusiasm for this treatment waned after papain injections caused a significant number of anaphylactic reactions and deaths. Papaya commonly cross-reacts with latex and fruit allergens, such as avocado, banana, passion fruit, figs, melons, mangos, kiwi, pineapple, peach, and tomato. While papaya allergy is thought to be mainly due to cross-reactivity to latex, it can occur on its own. Reported papaya reactions include hives and anaphylaxis. Thirty of forty-two Belgium patients with papaya allergy were also latex-sensitive. Papaya pollen is a common cause of asthma and hay fever in India. Like kiwi and mango allergy, the incidence of papaya allergy will undoubtedly increase with more global consumption of this tasty fruit.

Potato Allergy

Archaeological evidence reveals that Peruvian Indians grew potatoes approximately 4,500 years ago in the plateau and mountainous regions of Peru where it was too cold to grow wheat or corn. These Inca Indians also brewed, *chichi* beer from potatoes. After Spanish explorers brought potatoes to Europe, they became an important food source for the poor and underprivileged class. Many more affluent European countries paid little attention to the arrival of the potato as they already grew enough food to feed their population.

■ The Irish Potato Famine

The situation was quite different in Ireland, a poor country torn apart by constant warfare with its English rulers and infighting amongst the local Irish nobles. As a result, Ireland's farmers could not grow enough food to feed their people. Thus, Ireland's farmers eagerly adopted the potato as a major food source. By the 1800s, many parts of Ireland relied solely on the potato for food. This allowed the population of Ireland to grow very quickly. By 1840, the country's population had swelled from less than 3 million in the early 1500s to 8 million in the mid-1800s. Many Irish farmers warned that it was dangerous to depend on just one crop. They were right! Starting in 1845, the fungus *Phytophthora infestans* destroyed potato crops and triggered the Irish Potato Famine. During this famine, about 1 million people died from starvation or disease, and another 1 million left Ireland—mostly for Canada and the United States. Scores of Irish immigrants died on crowded, disease-infested ships that were called coffin ships.

Now one of the world's largest and economically important vegetable crops, potatoes rank fourth after wheat, rice, and maize as a staple crop. Potatoes are a low-calorie source of vitamin C and vitamin B6 as well as thiamine, niacin, magnesium, and potassium. Potatoes are not fattening unless fried or served with butter and rich sauces. The skin has the most fiber. and many nutrients are just under the skin. The potato is a rich source of starch that is used for sizing cotton and making industrial alcohol. Ripe potato juice is an excellent cleanser of silks, cottons, and woolens. The water in which potatoes have been boiled has been used to clean silver and shine furniture.

Potato belongs to the Solanaceae or nightshade family. Other members of this family include tomato, cherry, eggplant, melon, pear, paprika, bell pepper, cayenne, red pepper, tobacco, and chili. Despite worldwide consumption, reports of potato allergy are uncommon, possibly due to under-diagnosing or under-reporting. Potato allergy reactions range from mild skin and oral allergy symptoms to severe allergic reactions. Potato-dependent, exercise-induced anaphylaxis has been described. Reports of potato allergy in infants and young children include one five-month-old, breast-fed infant who developed an anaphylactic reaction after eating a cooked potato for the first time.

Another unusual report depicted a four-year-old child with potato-induced anaphylaxis that occurred after biting into a raw potato that was used in a painting project in a preschool setting. Most of the reactions that I have seen to potatoes are reactions to peeling raw potatoes. Cooked potato is usually well tolerated due to the presence of a heat-labile allergen.

The asthmatic reaction from French fries is not a potato allergy but is usually due to the addition of sulfite preservatives to potatoes to prevent browning. Unlike other fruits and vegetables, you do not

> *During this famine, about 1 million people died from starvation or disease, and another 1 million left Ireland—mostly for Canada and the United States. Scores of Irish immigrants died on crowded, disease-infested ships that were called coffin ships.*

need to use fresh potatoes for skin testing as the potency of commercial potato extract is reportedly equal to that of a fresh potato. Toxic reactions to potatoes can occur. Solanine, a naturally occurring toxin present in nightshade plants, may accumulate in greened, stored, or damaged potatoes and cause intestinal and neurological disturbances in humans and farm animals.

Sweet Potato

The sweet potato is yet another native American vegetable discovered by Columbus and his shipmates. The sweet potato is more popular in subtropical and tropical areas than the white Irish potato as it thrives in hot, moist climates, while the white potato requires a cooler climate. Sweet potatoes, first cultivated in Virginia in 1648, are generally preferred to Irish potatoes in the South. The versatile sweet potato blends with many herbs, spices, and flavorings.

Decades ago, orange-colored sweet potatoes were introduced in the southern United States. The African word *nyami* or yam, was applied to these orange-colored sweet potatoes. In my research, I was surprised to learn that sweet potatoes and yams are not botanically related to the white potato. The sweet potato is a member of the well-known morning glory family. In my initial literature search, I could not find a single case of an allergic reaction to a sweet potato. However, three recent case reports of sweet potato reactions from Spain suggest that sweet potatoes or yams may not be safe in white potato-allergic individuals.

Red Currant Allergy

Red currant berries are another food that rarely causes a food allergy. There is one case in which a forty-seven-year-old woman experienced a severe reaction and anaphylaxis after eating red and black currant jam. Her allergy was confirmed by positive skin and CAP RAST blood tests.

Sharon Fruit Allergy

The Sharon fruit, a fairly new persimmon fruit on the American market, comes from the Sharon region of Israel and South Africa. The Sharon fruit is seedless and doesn't have an astringent taste like most persimmons, and the entire fruit is edible. The texture, which resembles an apricot, can be eaten when it is firm like an apple or soft like a peach. Sharon fruit is a good source of vitamin A, sodium, potassium, magnesium, iron, and calcium. Eating one Sharon fruit a day allegedly reduces the risk of heart disease. Allergy to Sharon fruit and persimmon is rarely reported. An open challenge with Sharon fruit in seven birch-pollen and apple-allergic patients who had not previously eaten Sharon fruit was positive in six of seven cases. This study suggests that Sharon fruit may become more of a problem as Sharon fruit consumption increases.

Spinach Allergy

Allergy to spinach is rare despite widespread raw consumption. One report described a twenty-four-year-old male who had three reactions to spinach, but only when he drank alcohol.

Stone Fruit Allergy

Apricots, peaches, nectarines, and plums are all members of the Prunus family. They are called "stone fruits" because of their large, hard seed. Although stone fruit crops can provide delicious fruit from June through September, most stone fruits are native to warmer climates as they are very susceptible to injury from low temperatures. In addition, as they bloom early in the spring, the flowers frequently suffer damage from spring frosts. Thus, backyard culture of stone fruits is more difficult than that of apples or pears. Apricots, a rich source of beta carotene, iron, and potassium, are a rare cause of true allergic reactions. However, dried apricots may contain sulfites that can induce asthma in sulfite-sensitive asthmatics. Thus, sulfite-sensitive asthmatics should only purchase sulfite-free apricots.

■ Peach Allergy

The peach, a fruit that is found widely in the Mediterranean region, belongs to the Rosaceae family, which includes apples, cherries, pears, apricots, raspberries, strawberries, hazelnuts, and almonds. Peaches possibly originated in Persia, a belief fed by their botanical name, *Prunus persica*. However, historians are now in general agreement that the peach was cultivated in China in the tenth century BC. References to *tao* (a pretty way of saying peach) are found in fifth-century BC writings of Confucius. Its oval shape and delicate coloring are depicted on ancient works of Chinese ceramic art. Apparently, peaches didn't arrive in Persia until some time after 1500 BC.

> *Dried apricots may contain sulfites that can induce asthma in sulfite-sensitive asthmatics. Thus, sulfite-sensitive asthmatics should only purchase sulfite-free apricots.*

The Spaniards originally brought peaches to the New World, including Florida. The English colonists in Virginia found peaches growing wild, probably as a result of introduction by the Spaniards. American Indians spread the peach tree across the country when they were pushed west by the early settlers. Commercial peach production began in the United States in the early 1800s. In 1879, the father of the peach industry, S. H. Rumph, produced the Elberta peach from a seed of Chinese cling that he planted in the Peach Tree State of Georgia. Today, United States peach production of 300 different species is second only to apples. Americans grow almost half of the world's supply of peaches, with thirty-four states producing almost 3 billion pounds of the fruit annually.

No other fruit has added a word to our language that is synonymous with sweetness, fairness, or excellence. The term "peach" has come to mean anything that is fine and dandy, and particularly good in its class. Nothing tastes like a peach except a peach. It is both sweet and tart. This delicious, juicy, and versatile fruit grows on a low-spreading, freely branching tree that is as much admired for its beauty and the fragrance of its flowers as it is for its fruit.

Peach allergy is very common in Spain, Italy, and Israel. It was the most frequent food allergy in a Spanish survey of patients older than three years of age. Its prevalence was estimated to be between 10 and 40 percent in pollen-allergic patients. Other foods frequently associated with peach allergy include apples, pears, apricots, cherries, and plums. In the largest series of seventy peach-allergic patients, the average age was twenty years. Oral allergy symptoms were most common (86 percent), followed by hives (61 percent), and systemic reactions (26 percent). Two-thirds of the patients who were allergic to peaches were also allergic to peach pulp, and one in every three patients reported reacting to canned peaches.

Nectarine Allergy

The word nectarine comes from the Greek word "nectar," which was the drink of the gods in Greek mythology. They are essentially the same fruit as peaches, the primary difference being that nectarines have a smooth skin, and peaches are fuzzy. Nectarines, believed to be one of the oldest fruits, were grown in China over 2,000 years ago. Nectarines are a very versatile fruit and stand up well to cooking. They are also a great substitute for peaches, raw or cooked, since they do not have to be peeled prior to preparation.

Currently, there are over 150 varieties of nectarines that differ only slightly in size, shape, taste, texture, and color. Nectarines are expected to continue to gain in popularity as new varieties with better flavor, a more attractive appearance, and a longer shelf life are introduced. The smooth-skin characteristic that distinguishes nectarines is a minor genetic variation. A peach tree may suddenly produce a branch that bears nectarines and vice versa. While there is no large series of case reports of nectarine allergy, one might expect the same profile as seen with peach allergy.

Plum Allergy

The plum is another stone fruit. There are more than 2,000 varieties of plums cultivated throughout the world. These round, smooth-skinned fruits can be red, yellow, blue, green, or a purple-black color. Japanese plums tend to be yellow to crimson in color. In Canada and the United States, plums are cultivated and dried into prunes. Botanically, all prunes are plums. Oral allergy symptoms to plums have been described, but anaphylactic reactions are rare.

Swiss Chard Allergy

Swiss chard, a popular vegetable in Spain, is a member of the sugar beet family. One report of a reaction to Swiss chard described a reaction to cooked leaves in a twenty-year-old woman with a history of grass allergy and asthma. Another case depicted a fifty-year-old woman who had an asthma attack while cutting up and cooking Swiss chard. In my supermarket surveys, I notice that this vegetable is now commonly displayed in produce sections. Thus, I would not be surprised to see more cases of Swiss chard allergy.

Tomato Allergy

Tomatoes are a vine fruit of the nightshade family. Botanically speaking, a tomato is the ovary of a flowering plant, which makes it a fruit. However, from a culinary perspective, the tomato is typically served as part of the main course of a meal, meaning that it would be considered a vegetable. In 1887, American tariff laws that imposed a tax on vegetables but not on fruit caused the tomato's status to become a matter of legal importance. In 1893, the United States Supreme Court declared that the tomato was a vegetable, along with cucumbers, squash, beans, and peas. A vegetable—a culinary term that actually has no botanical meaning—was defined as a food that was served with dinner and not dessert.

Peach allergy is very common in Spain, Italy, and Israel. It was the most frequent food allergy in a Spanish survey of patients older than three years of age. Its prevalence was estimated to be between 10 and 40 percent in pollen-allergic patients.

The tomato probably originated in the west coast highlands of South America.[3] In the sixteenth century, the tomato plant was brought to Central America and southern Mexico. After their conquest of South America, the Spanish distributed the tomato plant throughout the Caribbean and the Philippines. The Spanish brought the tomato plant to Europe, where it flourished in the Spanish and Mediterranean climates in the 1500s.

Because the plant was similar to its nightshade cousins, the tomato was initially assumed to be poisonous and was mainly used as a decorative plant. Tomato leaves and stems are indeed poisonous, but the fruit itself is safe. Eventually, Italian peasants discovered that tomatoes could be eaten when more desirable foods were scarce. The tomato plant was not grown in England until the 1590s.

> *A vegetable—a culinary term that actually has no botanical meaning—was defined as a food that was served with dinner and not dessert.*

One of the earliest English tomato cultivators was John Gerard, a barber-surgeon. In Gerard's book *Herbal,* published in 1597, he noted that the tomato was eaten in both Spain and Italy. Nonetheless, Gerard still believed that tomatoes were poisonous, and they were considered unfit for eating for many years in Great Britain and the American colonies. The earliest reference to tomatoes in North America is from 1710, when herbalist William Salmon reported seeing them in what is today South Carolina. Cultured people like Thomas Jefferson ate

tomatoes in Paris and sent seeds home for planting in Virginia.

There are many legends about tomatoes. Some claimed they were aphrodisiacs; thus, the Puritans shunned them. Lingering doubts about the safety of tomatoes were largely put to rest in 1820. In a daring oral challenge, Colonel Robert Gibbon Johnson announced that at noon, September 26 he would eat a basket of tomatoes in front of a Salem, New Jersey, courthouse. Reportedly, a crowd of more than 2,000 gathered in front of the courthouse to watch him die. After eating these poisonous fruits, all were was shocked when he lived. By 1824, everyone was eating tomatoes as it was believed they kept one's blood pure in the heat of the summer.

Tomatoes are one of the most universally accepted vegetables and are second only to potatoes in worldwide vegetable production. A great variety of cultivars exist, from the tiny cherry tomato to prize-winning varieties the size of a grapefruit. Tomatoes are eaten raw or cooked, but the great bulk are processed into juice and canned goods. Tomatoes are used as an herbal remedy for a variety of conditions. The pulped fruit is a skin-wash for oily skin. The oil can be used in making soap. A spray made from tomato leaves is an effective but very poisonous insecticide.

The tomato is rich in vitamins A and C, calcium, and potassium. The skin is a good source of lycopene. Numerous epidemiological studies have demonstrated the beneficial health effects of tomatoes, tomato products, and phytonutrients. Many of these benefits have been attributed to the antioxidant and free-radical quenching activity of the carotenoids that occur naturally in tomatoes and tomato extract. Researchers at Oregon State University have created purple-fruited tomatoes that include anthocyanins—the same class of

---

[3] Andrew Smith, *The Tomato In America*, University of South Carolina Press, 1994.

health-promoting pigments found in red wine that function as antioxidants that are believed to prevent heart disease.

Many health supplement manufacturers claim that the studies on lycopene in tomatoes have shown lycopenes reduce the risk of a number of cancers, including prostate, colon, and breast. The American Longevity Company, which makes health supplements, and the Lycopene Health Claim Coalition, a group that includes ketchup manufacturer H.J. Heinz Co., petitioned the FDA to allow them to advertise that lycopenes reduce the risk of many forms of cancer. In November 2005, the FDA said it would allow claims to appear on packages of tomatoes and tomato sauce that only suggested a limited link between tomatoes and a lowered risk of prostate cancer. The FDA rejected proposals to advertise lycopene alone as having cancer-related benefits.

Tomatoes can trigger eczema and contact dermatitis. Tomato-induced, exercise-induced anaphylaxis has also been reported. Other allergic reactions to tomatoes include hives, swelling, oral allergy syndrome, asthma, rhinitis, and abdominal pain. Severe allergic reactions to tomatoes are unusual or rarely reported.

Wisconsin allergists reported two adults who experienced laryngeal edema, one of whom had an anaphylactic reaction to tomato. In December 2004, the *London Times* reported the tragic death of thirty-seven-year-old asthmatic mother of four who died from anaphylactic shock after opening a tin of tomato-containing spaghetti bolognese for her children's tea. She was aware of her tomato allergy but had assumed it was only to the raw fruit. When she realized that cooked tomatoes in the spaghetti had set off her allergy, she injected herself with EpiPen three times. Tragically, she collapsed with fatal shock, never regained consciousness, and died four days later when her life support was switched off. This unfortunate case points out that continued vigilance is required when dealing with any form of food allergy as most all foods are capable of triggering a near-fatal or fatal reactions.

◼ Turnip Rape and Oilseed Rape Allergy

Many vegetable crops, like turnip and oilseed rape, are grown to produce vegetable oils. The increasing popularity of such products has created new potential food allergens in children with eczema. One preliminary study of young children with eczema found many children had positive reactions to turnip and oilseed rape.

A study of 1,887 children screened for food allergy uncovered twenty-eight children with positive skin tests to turnip and oilseed rape. Twenty-five (89 percent) of these twenty-eight children had a positive oral challenge reaction to turnip rape. Thus, turnip and oilseed rape may be emerging food allergens in young children with eczema. ●

> *Many health supplement manufacturers claim that the studies on lycopene in tomatoes have shown lycopenes reduce the risk of a number of cancers, including prostate, colon, and breast.*

Chapter 14

Less Common Allergic and Adverse Food Reactions

The prior chapters discussed the most common forms of food allergy. As nearly 200 foods and beverages can cause an allergic reaction, this chapter will discuss the more uncommon triggers of food allergy and food intolerance reactions.

■ The History of Alcohol

Archaeologists believe that wines made from grapes have existed for more than 10,000 years, and other alcoholic drinks like mead and beer have been around even longer. Alcohol has many social purposes, including calming feuds, giving courage in battle, celebrating festivals, and seducing lovers. Historians speculate that prehistoric nomads made beer from grain and water before learning how to make bread. The Sumerians were the first civilization to develop a fixed-agricultural lifestyle. Ancient Sumerian engravings from 4000 BC depict bread being baked, crumbled into water to form a mash, and then made into a drink (beer) that made people feel, "exhilarated, wonderful and blissful."

We know that the ancient Egyptians were drinkers because they invented the first straws for drinking beer. Egyptians stored alcohol in their tombs to ease their journey into the after life. A 1600 BC Egyptian text contains 100 prescriptions describing the use of alcohol. There is evidence that Babylonians knew how to brew twenty different types of beer. The Babylonians also drew up one of the world's first legal texts that regulated drinking houses. Distilled grain spirits probably originated in China and India around 800 BC. Drinks such as brandy, cognac, and sake were created by distillation, yielding a more potent drink than beer. The distillation process did not make its way to Europe until the eleventh century.

The Greeks worshipped Bacchus, the god of wine. The Romans worshipped the same god under the name of Dionysus. The worship usually took the form of an orgy of intoxication, and their literature is full of warnings against intemperance. Roman writings record how Caesar toasted his troops after crossing the Rubicon. After Roman legions introduced beer to northern Europe around 55 BC, alcohol consumption spread.

By the Middle Ages, many monasteries made beer to nourish their monks and to sell to the people. The consumption of beer in the monasteries reached astounding levels—each monk was allotted five quarts of beer a day.

In the Middle Ages, the emphasis shifted from monastic and family brewing to

Ancient Sumerian engravings from 4000 BC depict bread being baked, crumbled into water to form a mash, and then made into a drink (beer) that made people feel, "exhilarated, wonderful and blissful."

centralized production sites (breweries) to provide hospitality for travelers and pilgrims. Home breweries became inns, taverns, and public houses. Beer became the heart and soul of almost every culture. The Middle Ages were a superstitious time, and brewing failures were often blamed on "witches brew" or the devil. The last known burning of a "brew witch" took place in 1591. By the end of the Middle Ages, most of the world had mastered the art of brewing and distilling grain into alcohol. Brewers were one of the first professionals to form a guild, and older brewmasters taught their young apprentices the proper brewing techniques. As the technology advanced, it became possible to distill spirits into purer and more potent alcoholic drinks. Many countries developed their own national spirits, such as Russian vodka, Scottish whisky, Mexican tequila, Greek ouzo, and Italian sambuca.

Colonial Americans, for the most part, showed little concern over drunkenness. In an effort to keep the American soldiers sober, the first serious efforts to regulate liquor consumption began in the Revolutionary War. The most prominent temperance spokesperson at that time was Benjamin Rush, a signer of the Declaration of Independence. Rush was the most celebrated American physician of that era and a close friend of John Adams and Thomas Jefferson. In that era, Rush had no peer as a social reformer. Among the many causes he championed—most of them several generations in advance of their time—were prison and judicial reform, abolition of slavery and the death penalty, education of women, conservation of natural resources, proper diet, and abstinence from tobacco and strong drink. In 1785, Rush was one of the first American leaders to challenge the popular belief that spirits were healthy when he wrote *Inquiry into the Effects of Ardent Spirits on the Human Mind and Body*.

In the early 1800s, the brewing industry prospered. There was nearly one saloon for every 150 or 200 Americans. To increase their patronage and profits, saloonkeepers introduced vices like gambling and prostitution. Many Americans believed saloons were offensive and noxious institutions. After the first prohibition law was passed in Maine in 1851, twelve states followed suit. Eighteen years later, the National Prohibition Party won its first seat in the House of Representatives. Three years later the Anti-Saloon League, a powerful political force in later years, was formed. Throughout the second half of the nineteenth century, several anti-alcohol measures were enforced in states all over the Union. By 1906, the prohibition movement was well underway. It was fueled by anti-alien and anti-Roman Catholic sentiments among the Protestant middle class.

The conflict between rural and urban lifestyles became more apparent with the growth of the cities that were perceived as hotbeds of crime, booze, and vice. Employers were concerned about the effects of alcohol on the efficiency of their workforce. These factors, combined with a temporary wartime Prohibition Act introduced in World War I to save grain for food, led to the passage of the Eighteenth Amendment to the United States Constitution that took away the license to do business from the brewers, distillers, vintners, and wholesale and retail sellers of alcoholic beverages.

Prohibition laws were easily enforced in rural communities where the population was more sympathetic. However, an enormous industry grew up around the production, transportation, and sale of contraband beer and liquor that was imported from Mexico, Canada, and the Caribbean. The bootleggers were uniquely named after the practice by nineteenth century travelers in the Midwest who concealed liquor in their boots when trading with Indians. "Medicinal" whiskey was readily available with real or forged prescriptions in drugstores. Denatured alcohol, legally used in other industries and treated with noxious chemicals to render it undrinkable, was "washed" of its poisonous additives and diluted with tap water. Illegal corn liquor stills produced toxic "rotgut." Coroners' reports in the first five months of 1923 revealed that nearly 100 people had perished from drinking contaminated whiskey.

Because of the complexity of their operations, bootleggers quickly organized into alliances and cartels. As the cartels grew and gang rivalry diminished, the power and profits were concentrated in fewer and fewer hands—giving birth to organized crime in America. At the time of his arrest in 1931, Al Capone's earnings were estimated to be $100 million a year. While alcohol consumption declined dramatically under Prohibition, it grew somewhat in the last years of Prohibition as illegal supplies of liquor increased and a new generation of Americans disregarded the law.

The bootleggers were uniquely named after the practice by nineteenth century travelers in the Midwest who concealed liquor in their boots when trading with Indians.

After Prohibition was finally repealed in December 1933—when the United States Congress ratified the Twenty-First Amendment—an elaborate syndicate of organized crime built on the multi-million dollar bootlegging industry survived. Organized crime then branched out into narcotics, gambling, prostitution, loan sharking, and extortion. The Twenty-First Amendment did allow individual states to control Prohibition, and a few states continued to ban alcohol. By 1966, all states had repealed these provisions, and today alcohol is regulated on a county level. Almost half of Mississippi's counties are dry, and forty-six of 254 counties in Texas are also dry.

■ Alcohol Reactions

Most starchy or sugary foods like grains, potatoes, and grapes can be turned into ethanol or alcohol by yeast fermentation. Unlike other foods and beverages except water, alcohol is not digested, but it is absorbed directly into the blood stream from the stomach. The well-touted benefits of moderate consumption of alcohol (one to two drinks a day) include a lower risk of stroke and heart disease and protection against dementia. Excessive consumption is addictive and increases the risk of heart disease, cirrhosis, and stomach and liver cancer. The most common adverse reactions to alcohol are facial flushing and a hangover headache, which may be due to the fact that alcohol is a histamine liberator.

Some patients experience intense facial flushing even after drinking very small amounts of alcohol. Flushing is reportedly more common in Asians. Several members of my family often develop a facial flush after a glass or two of wine. I call it their "Irish tan." This side-effect may be due to an enzyme deficiency, where high levels of acetaldehyde rapidly accumulate in the blood stream. A hangover is due to the high blood levels of congeners—the byproducts of alcohol fermentation. Brandy and red wine have the highest levels, while vodka contains the lowest levels of congeners.

Many patients with asthma relate that ingestion of beer, wine, or grain alcohol frequently triggers sneezing, nasal congestion, or wheezing. Wine, especially red wine, is a more frequent offender than beer or grain alcohol. In a survey in western Australia, one in every three asthmatics reported that alcohol worsened their asthma. Wines were the most frequent offenders with a response time of less than one hour. Wine-induced asthma was more common in women. The rarity of reactions to barley malt in beer is undoubtedly due to the fact that malt protein is denatured when heated and roasted in the brewing process.

I used to think that alcohol-induced asthma was due to the sulfite preservatives added to alcoholic beverages to prevent spoilage, but it was always a puzzle why all alcoholic beverages don't trigger asthma. Japanese investigators may have uncovered the answer to this observation. Alcohol-induced asthma has been well-documented in Japan as more than half of Japanese asthmatics wheeze after consuming alcohol. Researchers have found that many Japanese have a genetic enzyme defect that prevents the breakdown of acetaldehyde, a by-product of alcohol. It is postulated that the accumulation of high levels of acetaldehyde triggers the release of histamine from mast cells, leading to wheezing. Japanese researchers published a small study on thirteen patients that provides some hope for patients who enjoy imbibing beer or wine: pretreatment with antihistamines blocked alcohol-induced asthma.

Reactions to wine are usually adverse reactions to one of the 400 naturally occurring chemicals in wine. True allergic reactions to alcohol itself are rare but are described in a few dozen case reports. Many reactions are due to allergic proteins in the grapes, yeast, hops, barley, and wheat—not the alcohol itself. One report depicted a thirty-five-year-old man with a seven-year history of hives and swelling after ingestion of red and white grapes. His throat swelling and asthma began minutes after drinking a glass of Prosecco, a sparkling white wine from northeast Italy. He reported having tolerated red wine prior to this reaction. Skin tests to Prosecco, chardonnay, cabernet franc, chianti, and Nero d'Avola were positive, with the exception of chianti. In the following months, he experienced tongue edema after drinking a small amount of barbera red wine. An oral sulfite challenge was negative. This patient tolerated grappa, an alcoholic product that is obtained through fermentation, not distillation, of the grapes.

There are a few reports of an alcohol-induced rash and facial flushing in patients with eczema who were using the topical drug tacrolimus or Protopic. This should not be mistaken for an alcohol reaction, as facial flushing resolved in all cases once tacrolimus was discontinued. This reaction occurs in approximately 6 percent of patients using tacrolimus.

Japanese researchers published a small study on thirteen patients that provides some hope for patients who enjoy imbibing beer or wine: pretreatment with antihistamines blocked alcohol-induced asthma.

■ Animal Feed Allergy

Is animal feed a potential source of food allergens? Many animals are fed allergenic foods to improve their nutritional value. Cows are fed red herring to add Omega-3 fatty acids to their milk. Fish and soybean meal is added to the diet of chickens. It appears that farm-fed animals do not pass along such allergenic food proteins, as there are no reports of allergic reactions from drinking milk from fish-fed cows or eating chicken or eggs from chickens that are fed soybean or fish. The reason that cows do not pass on fish protein in their milk is probably due to their efficient digestive system, which includes four stomachs.

■ Artificial Sweeteners

Artificial sweeteners, which are non-glucose products, add sweetness without adding calories. The first sweetener was saccharin or Sweet'n Low.

Aspartame, made from two amino acids, phenylalanine and aspartic acid, also known as NutraSweet or Equal, is another zero-calorie artificial sweetener that is 180 times sweeter than sucrose. It does not cause allergic reactions in children or adults. Aspartame has been cited as a potential trigger of seizures and migraine headaches. As aspartame contains phenylalanine, it is unsafe for people with phenylketonuria, or PKU.

> *The nests are composed of an egg-like protein. Thus, bird's nest soup might be better called "bird's spit soup."*

■ Bird's Nest Soup Allergy [1]

The low prevalence of food allergy in Asia is somewhat puzzling. It may be due to a wide diversity in Asian cultures and feeding habits as well as a lack of clinical studies. In 1999, a survey of Singapore schoolchildren found the prevalence of food allergy was about 5 percent. Surprisingly, the most common food allergen in these children was a Chinese delicacy known as bird's nest soup. It appears that bird's nest soup allergy may be outgrown, as only one of forty-four adult patients in Singapore with anaphylaxis was allergic to bird's nest soup.

The history of bird's nest soup can be traced back about 1,500 years to the Tang Dynasty in China. It is believed the first bird's nest was brought back from Nan Yang (the southern country) by Chinese sailors. During that era, only the emperor and his court were allowed to consume the highly prized bird's nest. Eventually, common people were introduced to bird's nest soup.

The swiftlet bird that produces these nests is a cave-dwelling creature that grows to be 3 to 6 inches long—about the size of a sparrow. Swiftlets fly at a lower altitude, more slowly, and more erratically than most birds. Like bats, the swiftlets eat flying insects that they catch in mid air. Cave-dwelling swiftlets are the only birds to use sonar to maneuver through darkness. Not only can they navigate in total darkness, but they find their own individual nests amongst hundreds of others. Some colonies may contain up to a million birds. Their most common breeding grounds are caves and abandoned houses or buildings. During their breeding season, the swiftlet's salivary glands enlarge enormously, enabling the bird to produce extra saliva to bind a nest that takes nearly two months to construct to hold one or two eggs. The nests are composed of an egg-like protein. Thus, bird's nest soup might be better called "bird's spit soup."

The primary market for bird's nest soup is the international Chinese community. Bird's nest soup is considered to be an esteemed delicacy by upper-class Chinese families who treasure its health benefits. The peak season of demand comes during the Chinese New Year, when the gift-giver of bird's nest soup wishes the recipient

---

[1] Adrian Y, *Introduction to the Edible Bird's Nest Industry in Asia.*

a long and healthy life. It symbolizes the giver's affluence and status. Increasing wealth in the Asian region, along with the steep increase in the price of a bowl of bird's nest soup, has made this food, the "caviar of the East." The rising price—upwards of $10,000 for two pounds and $60 per bowl of soup—resulted in a decline in the swiftlet population. However, conservation efforts to control the harvesting of nests have begun to stabilize the swiftlet population.

■ Caffeine Reactions

Caffeine is a widely consumed chemical that is derived from a class of compounds called methylxanthines. It is the oldest stimulant used by humans. Legend has it that the prior of an Arabian monastery learned that the local shepherds who ate coffee plant berries did not sleep at night and were more efficient in caring for their sheep. The prior astutely ordered that coffee berries be collected and made into a beverage to keep members of his monastery awake during their long hours of nighttime prayer.

Caffeine is a mild bronchodilator that is closely related to theophylline, an older asthma drug discovered in the 1930s when German researchers were studying the anti-asthmatic effects of coffee and tea. While my literature search failed to find any cases of true IgE-mediated caffeine allergy, Dr. Harris Steinamn has reported three cases of allergic reactions to caffeine.[2] One patient was a twenty-one-year-old who reacted to coffee and caffeine-containg coke but not caffeine-free coke. The other two cases were

---

[2] AllergyAdvisor.com.

a sixty-nine-year old woman and a forty-five-year -old woman who developed hives after ingesting coffee and pain medications that contained caffeine. There are hundreds of Internet sites describing a variety of mental and psychological reactions to caffeine.

■ Caviar Allergy

Caviar consists of sieved and salted fish eggs. The best and most expensive caviar comes from the Beluga sturgeon in the Caspian Sea. Other forms of caviar are harvested from lumpfish, whitefish, and salmon. There are only a few reports of caviar allergy in the literature. In one case, an eighteen-month-old child with asthma and eczema reacted to Thai food and sushi topped with salmon roe. In another case, a fifty-one-year-old Russian male reacted to Beluga caviar. Both patients had positive skin and CAP RAST blood tests to caviar.

Another documented report described anaphylaxis in a fifty-five-year-old woman who was taking an ACE inhibitor, a beta blocker, and two heart and blood pressure drugs that can accelerate allergic reactions.

■ Chamomile Tea

Chamomile is a popular tea that is extracted from a plant belonging to the Compositae family. It has been reported to induce allergic reactions. This is not surprising, as ragweed pollen is also a member of the Compositae plant family.

■ Chocolate Reactions

Chocolate is made from beans harvested from the cocoa evergreen tree in South and Central America. These beans, which were once used as currency in South America, are now mainly grown in West Africa and Brazil. Cocoa beans were brought back to Europe by Columbus's fourth voyage to the Americas in 1502. Spanish cooks added vanilla and milk to these beans to create a "divine drink" that fought fatigue. Wherever they went, the European explorers from Columbus on found other mind-affecting drugs and brought them home with them. Tobacco was discovered on Columbus's first voyage. Cocaine was found in large areas of South America. Caffeine and LSD-like drugs were found scattered all over the world. During the next two centuries, the Europeans not only adopted nicotine and caffeine but spread them everywhere. They also imported opium. In a remarkably short space of time, western Europe was converted from an alcohol-only culture to a multi-drug culture.

> *I cannot recall ever seeing a patient with true IgE-mediated chocolate allergy unless the chocolate product contained hidden peanuts or tree nuts.*

The chocolate bar, not marketed until 1910, gained widespread popularity after it was issued to American soldiers in WWII as a "fighting food." Chocolate is not a great source of nutrients. Dark chocolate contains more antioxidants and less fat than white chocolate. Chocolate allergy is very rare considering its widespread use. The most common form of chocolate reactions is migraine headaches that are triggered by the chemicals phenylethylamine and theobromine in chocolate. Chocolate also contains significant amounts of caffeine that induces insomnia and triggers sweating and tremors in breast-fed infants when their moms eat a lot of chocolate. I cannot recall ever seeing a patient with true IgE-mediated chocolate allergy unless the chocolate product contained hidden peanuts or tree nuts.

■ Cuttlefish Allergy

This is an interesting fish that is actually not a fish. It belongs to the squid and octopus family. Cuttlefish have an internal shell, large eyes, eight arms, and two tentacles furnished with suckers to secure their prey. Cuttlefish bones are used by jewelers and silversmiths as molds for casting small objects. They are also used as bird bill-sharpeners and a source of calcium for caged birds. Cuttlefish are called the "chameleon of the sea" because of their remarkable ability to rapidly alter their skin color to communicate with their species or camouflage themselves from predators. Cuttlefish eyes are among the most developed in the animal kingdom. Domestic cuttlefish exhibit feline-like habits, such as resting, pouncing on moving prey and begging owners for food. But unlike cats, cuttlefish will try to eat other cuttlefish.

Cuttlefish allergy is rare. One report described a fourteen-year-old girl who experienced exercise-induced anaphylaxis after eating cuttlefish.

■ Garlic Reactions

Garlic, a small, pungent, onion-like plant from the lilac family, has been used as a flavoring and a medicine since 1550 BC. Only a few members of the lilac family are important food plants. The most notable of these are onion, garlic, chives, leeks, and rakkyo. Garlic's edible bulb, which grows beneath the ground, is made up of cloves encased in a parchment-like membrane. Today's major garlic suppliers are the United States, France, Spain, Italy, and Mexico.

Garlic bulbs are usually peeled, and eaten raw or cooked. Garlic salt is garlic powder blended with salt and a moisture-absorbing agent. Garlic allegedly reduces nasal congestion, blood pressure, and blood cholesterol. Folk medicine practitioners have used garlic as an antiviral, antibacterial, fungicidal, vasodilator, expectorant, diuretic, anti-asthmatic, anti-spasmodic, skin soothing tonic, and an immune stimulant. Garlic is also said to have anti-cancer activity. Some studies suggest that garlic is responsible for the low incidence of arteriosclerosis in Italy and Spain, where garlic consumption is high.

Common intolerance-like side effects of garlic include body odor, garlic breath, feeling hot, burning on urination, heartburn, and flatulence. Bad breath and body odor are caused by the essential oils in garlic that permeate the lungs and remain with the body long after garlic has been consumed. Many garlic-intolerant patients complain of a hangover reaction that may last for a day or two after garlic ingestion. Some of the side effects of garlic can be avoided by taking an aged-garlic extract sold in health food stores under the name of Kyolic. Some garlic-sensitive individuals may tolerate young or cooked garlic, as cooking may reduce or eliminate potency.

There are several cases of garlic allergy in the literature. One sixteen-month-old boy with a history of milk and egg allergy developed hives on the face and neck immediately after contact with fresh garlic. A twenty-three-year-old woman experienced a severe allergic reaction to young garlic. Garlic may trigger occupational asthma, rhinitis, and contact dermatitis in workers exposed to garlic in food processing plants. Contact dermatitis is also caused by the handling of garlic by grocers, housewives, and cooks.

■ Gelatin Allergy

Gelatin is a collection of proteins made from skin and bones of fish, beef, and pork. It is used as a stabilizer in foods, luncheon meats, medications, vaccines, and cosmetics. Many reactions to gelatin-containing foods, such as gummy bears, Jello, licorice, marshmallows, fruit yogurt, instant whipped cream, and pudding have been reported. One interesting case of gelatin allergy described a five-year-old child who had a severe reaction after eating a large number of Gummy Bears candy that contained gelatin. In a study of thirty fish-allergic patients, fish gelatin was shown to present no risk to fish-allergic patients. Gelatin allergy has also been reported to varicella (chickenpox) and MMR vaccines and intravenous fluids.

Some of the side effects of garlic can be avoided by taking an aged-garlic extract sold in health food stores under the name of Kyolic.

■ Histamine Intolerance

In her informative book *Dealing With Food Allergies*, Dr Janice Vickerstaff Joneja states that while most traditional allergy specialists are well-versed in true food allergy reactions, they come up short when confronted with food intolerance reactions. She is probably right. Conventional allergists are trained not to accept any theory or treatment unless it is documented by scientific studies. One form of intolerance that I have undoubtedly neglected is histamine intolerance.

Histamine, a natural substance produced by the body, is released from mast cells during stress and allergen exposure. This chemical is able to create widespread havoc because mast cells are found in almost all body organs. Histamine is also found in many foods, especially those that have undergone fermentation by bacteria where the amino acid histidine is converted to histamine. Such foods include processed meats, fish, cheeses, soy products, alcoholic beverages, and vinegars. High doses of histamine are toxic for everyone. Some individuals are susceptible to low levels of histamine, possibly because they lack an enzyme that breaks down histamine. The symptoms of histamine intolerance include hives, swelling, itching, and migraine headaches. Severe histamine poisoning may mimic anaphylaxis. The most common form of histamine poisoning occurs when bacteria attack spoiled fish (see scombroid poisoning on page 124). Several other foods that may contain histamine and induce a histamine-intolerance reaction include bananas, certain nuts, chocolate, shellfish, and strawberries. The bottom line—anyone who develops signs of a histamine reaction after eating such foods may suffer from histamine intolerance.

> *Several other foods that may contain histamine and induce a histamine-intolerance reaction include bananas, certain nuts, chocolate, shellfish and strawberries.*

■ Inulins: A New Fad Food

Before I started writing this book, I had never heard of inulins. They are plant-derived, naturally occurring oligosaccharide (several simple sugars linked together) that belongs to a class of carbohydrates known as fructans. Inulin is used by plants to store energy and is typically found in the stems (or rhizomes) of these plants. Plants that contain high concentrations of inulin

include asparagus, dandelions, wild yams, Jerusalem artichokes, and chicory. Inulins are the latest fad in probiotic and yogurt products. Since inulins are not very digestible, they are transported to the large intestine where they feed bacteria and promote fermentation. Inulin has been dubbed a "prebiotic" that fertilizes the bacteria in your intestine. Inulin, not chemically related to insulin, is often recommended for diabetics as it is not absorbed and does not affect blood sugar levels.

Known side effects of inulin include flatulence, bloating, cramps, abdominal pain, and diarrhea. Inulin can trigger the release of significant quantities of carbon dioxide and methane. Thus, inulin is notoriously gassy and not recommended for the socially sensitive. In one case, inulin triggered an anaphylactic reaction in a thirty-nine-year-old butcher who had experienced four episodes of anaphylaxis a few minutes after eating salsify, artichoke leaves, a margarine containing inulin, and a candy containing inulin. Another woman with a past history of allergy to artichoke presented with two episodes of immediate allergic reactions, one of which was a severe anaphylactic shock after eating health foods that contained inulin. However, the fact that inulin is a complex sugar, not a protein, makes it unlikely that inulin will become an important food allergen.

■ Meat Allergy

About 10 percent of cow's milk-allergic children may react to beef that contains traces of milk protein. True beef or mammalian allergy is rare in adults. Only a handful of cases of lamb or pork allergy have been confirmed by an oral challenge, making lamb or pork a good choice for the cow's milk-beef-allergic patient. Contact skin reactions to pork have been reported in butchers exposed to pork in meat processors. A 2006 report from France described thirteen cases of pork allergy, mostly due to pork kidney. An association between allergy to animal dander and mammalian meat have been described.

Serum albumin is probably the responsible cross-reacting allergen. A twenty-eight-year-old, dog-allergic cook experienced wheezing and hives when handling raw beef, especially during defrosting procedures. His skin test was positive to raw and cooked beef, raw lamb, cat, and dog. A sixty-one-year-old Australian woman presented with a history of hives following consumption of beef, pork, lamb, rabbit, and kangaroo. She was able to consume milk, chicken, eggs, ham, and fish without problems. A unique aspect of this case was a positive skin test to kangaroo meat, making it the first case report of kangaroo allergy. Marine mammals make up a large portion of the diet of Alaskans residing near the Bering and Beaufort seas. One report described three Intuit children with eczema who reacted to caribou and seal meat, which was often eaten raw. Another Alaskan boy reacted to meat from the bowhead whale and the bearded seal.

Poultry Allergy

I have seen a handful of individuals with poultry allergy over the past two decades. While most reactions were mild in nature, I followed one thirty-five-year-old asthmatic patient who has had severe reactions to poultry since childhood. Despite being very careful, he has experienced reactions to hidden sources of poultry, like chicken-fortified hot dogs. On one occasion, ingestion of a "ham sandwich" that actually contained turkey ham sent him to the emergency room. He is so sensitive to poultry that he reacts to the vapor from heated chicken soups and has to leave his home on Thanksgiving morning when the family bird is being cooked.

A few reports in the literature have described egg-feather allergic patients who react to poultry or bird meat in what is called the "bird-egg-meat syndrome." As poultry-allergic patients may react to other game birds, they should probably avoid all game birds. As there are few clinical studies on poultry allergy, its exact prevalence is unknown. The fact that poultry allergy is relatively uncommon may be due to the fact that most cases (like the one I described above) are not reported in the medical literature.

A few reports in the literature have described egg-feather allergic patients who react to poultry or bird meat in what is called the "bird-egg-meat syndrome." As poultry-allergic patients may react to other game birds, they should probably avoid all game birds.

Quorn Foods

Quorn foods are made by an English company that specializes in meat-free foods that contain mycoprotein, a fungus related to mushrooms, truffles, and morel. They provide a strong nutritional profile and an authentic meat-like texture. Quorn meals and snacks, which have been sold in Europe for nearly seventeen years, are now available in the United States.

Allergic reactions to this food are rare. Research suggests that about one in 100,000 to 200,000 people may react to Quorn. As it is made from a mold or fungus, it's possible that some mold-allergic individuals could react to Quorn.

■ Quinine Reactions

Quinine is a chemical extracted from the bark of the cinchona tree that grows on the slopes of the Andes Mountains in South America. In the 1500s, the Peruvian Indians commonly used cinchona bark to treat fevers. They soon realized that cinchona bark was also effective in preventing and treating malaria. It is believed that the tree's name came from the Countess of Chinchon, wife of the Spanish viceroy of Peru who, in 1638, fell desperately ill with malaria. After she was cured by the ancient herbal quinquina bark, the tree was then named the cinchona tree in her honor. Once the anti-malarial value of cinchona bark was widely recognized, supply could not keep up with demand. At one point in time, the cost of the bark powder matched its weight in gold—prompting uncontrolled harvesting and severe decimation of the cinchona tree.

At that time, no one actually knew that the potent ingredient from the cinchona tree was the alkaloid quinine. It was not until 1820, nearly 200 years after the bark was introduced into Europe for the treatment of malaria, that quinine was isolated from the bark of the tree. Quinine was commonly used to flavor foods, and a bitter tasting quinine tonic water was developed to prevent malaria. After the British colonists in India added gin to make the quinine tonic more palatable, the popularity of the gin and tonic cocktail spread throughout the world. Quinine therapy for malaria was eventually replaced by synthetic drugs, such as chloroquine and mefloquine. However, in recent years, quinine treatment has resurfaced as more drug-resistant strains of malaria have been reported.

There are very few cases of true allergic reactions to quinine in the literature. However, quinine can trigger skin rashes, kid-ney problems, and a blood disease called thrombocytopenic purpura, where blood platelets are destroyed leading to easy bruising or purpura. The mechanism of this reaction involves the binding of quinine to the platelet surface and then reacting with an antibody that, in turn, destroys the platelets. Not a true food allergy, so-called cocktail party purpura occurs in individuals who have become sensitized to quinine and develop purpura from ingestion of quinine-like medications and beverages that contain quinine. In the mid-1980s, I reported a case of thrombocytopenic purpura that occurred in one of my patients after he drank a popular quinine-containing aperitif called Dubonnet. The title of my paper was "Purpura on the Rocks."

■ Royal Jelly Allergy

Royal jelly is the food of queens—not human queens, but queen bees. Royal jelly, a milky-white gelatinous substance, is secreted from the glands of worker bees for the sole purpose of stimulating the growth and development of the queen bee. Without royal jelly, the queen bee would be no different from the worker bees and would live about as long (seven to eight weeks). With royal jelly, the queen bee may live five to seven years. After a few days of feeding, larvae that have the potential to develop into queens continue to be fed this nectar. Since queen bees are much bigger, live much longer, and are more fertile than all the other bees, royal jelly is believed to impart mystical qualities.

Royal jelly consists of an emulsion of proteins, sugars, and lipids. Royal jelly also contains vitamins, such as pantothenic acid, and minerals. It is reputed to have a number of benefits, including enhancing immunity; preventing arthritis, multiple sclerosis and asthma; slowing aging; and stimulating hair

Table 14.1. Potential Sources of Tyramine

Beer and ale	Figs	Dry sausages
Robust red wines	Raisins	Soy sauces
Chianti	Avocados	Sauerkraut
Vermouth	Commercial gravies	Salami
Homemade breads	Italian broad beans	Canned meats
Cheese	Green bean pods	Yogurts
Sour cream	Eggplant	Bouillon soup cubes
Bananas	Pickled herring	Chocolate
Red plum	Liver	

growth. Several allergic reactions from oral intake of royal jelly have been reported. They can range from hives or mild gastrointestinal upset to more severe reactions, including asthma and anaphylaxis. People who are allergic to bee pollen or honey should not ingest royal jelly.

Rice Allergy

Rice is the primary food source for many Asian and Latin American countries. Fortunately for man, rice allergy is uncommon. While rare in the United States and Europe, rice allergy has been reported in Eastern Asia and Japan. Most reports are from exposure to uncooked rice. Rice can trigger hay fever symptoms in areas where it's grown commercially. People who are allergic to rice may react to a number of other foods from the same botanical family, such as barley, maize, wheat, oats, and rye.

Tyramine Reactions

Tyramine, an amino acid found in many foods, is produced by the natural breakdown of the amino acid tyrosine. The word tyramine is derived from the Greek word *tyoos* for cheese that contains the highest levels of tyramine. Tyramine commonly triggers migraine headaches. Other symptoms include nausea, vomiting, and palpitations. There are very few cases of true tyramine allergy in the literature.

Tyramine occurs widely in plants and animals and is metabolized by monoamine oxidase. If this process is compromised by the use of blood pressure drugs called monoamine oxidase or MAO inhibitors, and if foods high in tyramine are ingested, a hypertensive crisis can result. This problem was first described by a neurologist who noticed that his wife, who was taking a MAO medication, had severe headaches after eating cheese. For this reason, the crisis is often called the cheese syndrome, even though other foods like aged wines, processed meats and yeast extracts can cause the same problem. Food with high levels of tyramine are generally preserved or aged. For this reason, you should be very wary of leftovers that have been in the refrigerator for more than twenty-four to forty-eight hours. The more aged foods become, the worse the reaction may be. Potential sources of tyramine are listed in table 14.1. ●

Chapter

15

Food Additive Reactions

As our cities and towns have grown and farms have been abandoned, it is more difficult to obtain fresh foods and produce at a local farm or market. Thus, most consumers rely on the local supermarket for our food supply. More than 3,000 food additives can be added to the foodstuffs and beverages we purchase in a local supermarket. A lot of food purists would have you believe that food additives are poisons. This concept has led to the proliferation of international food store chains that promote organic and natural foods. Some foods like poultry and meat are undoubtedly healthier when they are food additive-free. However, many foods and beverages on store shelves would quickly spoil before being sold without the availability of food additives. For example, without food additives, bread would have a shelf life of about two days before becoming stale.

The majority of food additives have been extensively tested before being added to foods. The U. S. Food and Drug Administration puts a stamp of approval on food additives with a GRAS or "generally recognized as safe" label. Thanks to our effi-

> *The majority of food additives have been extensively tested before being added to foods. The United States Food and Drug Administration puts a stamp of approval on food additives with a GRAS or "generally recognized as safe" label.*

cient immune system, relatively few food additives trigger allergic or adverse reactions. There are four basic groups of food additives.

1. Nutrients, such as iron, vitamins, and iodide that improve the nutritional value of food
2. Food preservatives that prolong shelf life by preventing spoilage by bacteria and fungi
3. Food emulsifiers, binders, and fillers that improve food consistency
4. Food enhancers and colorings that improve taste and the appearance of foods

■ Food Preservatives

Common preservatives include benzoic acid, sodium benzoate, parabens, nitrates and nitrites, sulfites, ascorbic acid, vitamin E, BHA, and BHT.[1] Most food preservatives are antioxidants that keep foods such as cereals and grains crisp and prevent them from becoming rancid after exposure to heat and oxygen. Case reports of true allergic reactions to food preservatives are extremely rare. BHA and BHT, two of the most powerful antioxidants, have been reported to cause hives and rashes, especially in aspirin-sensitive individuals.

Several food preservatives can trigger adverse, non-allergic reactions in susceptible individuals. One common food preservative reaction includes migraine headaches triggered by nitrates and nitrites that are commonly added to processed foods like sausages and hot dogs.

---

[1] For complete discussion on food preservatives, see Dr. Janice Joneja, *Dealing with Food Allergies* (see appendix)

■ Sulfite Sensitivity

Sulfites are true preservatives that, like salt, vinegar, and sugar have been used since ancient times. Sulfites preserve food flavor and color, inhibit bacterial growth, reduce spoilage, stop fresh vegetables from turning brown, and prolong the shelf life of many medications. How do sulfites work? They release the gas sulfur dioxide that preserves foods and medications. The main concern about sulfites is their propensity to trigger asthma.

Some sulfite-sensitive asthmatics have a partial enzyme deficiency that prevents the breakdown of sulfur dioxide. Sulfite sensitivity is due to an irritant reaction to sulfur dioxide vapors released when sulfites in foods and beverages are ingested and swallowed. This is a chemical reaction not a true allergic reaction. One of the worst asthma attacks I ever experienced occurred after I heated up some sulfur powder from a chemistry set I received as a Christmas gift.

■ Clinical Reactions to Sulfites

From 1980 to 1998, the FDA received over 1,000 reports of severe sulfite reactions, including twelve fatalities. Many of these reactions occurred in restaurants where sulfites had been added to foods in salad bars. The FDA contracted with the Federation of American Societies for Experimental Biology (FASEB) to examine the link between sulfites and reported health problems, including hives, difficulty breathing, and fatal asthma. In 1985, the FASEB concluded that sulfites were safe for most people but posed a hazard for sulfite-sensitive asthmatics. In 1986, the FDA prohibited the use of sulfites to

One of the worst asthma attacks I ever experienced occurred after I heated up some sulfur powder from a chemistry set I received as a Christmas gift.

maintain color and crispness in fruits and vegetables in restaurant salad bars and supermarkets. They required food companies to label sulfite agents when the concentration of sulfites exceeded ten parts per million—the equivalent of one drop of water in a bathtub. This FDA order was extended to other foods, like pickles and bottled lemon juice.

■ Hold Those Fries!

In 1987, the FDA proposed revoking the GRAS status of sulfite agents on fresh potatoes and French fries. This triggered a protracted court battle in which the potato industry prevailed. The experience of a sulfite-sensitive asthmatic described in a recent FDA consumer report reinforces the need to label sulfite-containing foods.

> My boyfriend and I were at a hamburger joint, and I had a burger and fries. About 10 minutes after we finished eating, my throat began to itch. I grabbed my [asthma] inhaler but I could feel my throat constricting. I couldn't breathe and started to panic. When I passed out, my boyfriend flagged down a passing police car. The officer radioed for an ambulance, and I was rushed to the hospital. I was revived with a massive dose of epinephrine to counteract the reaction caused by the sulfite solution the potatoes had been soaked in before frying. I know enough to stay away from wine, shrimp and other foods that contain sulfites, and take note whenever I don't feel right after eating something. But I never expected French fries to be sulfited. I've had allergic reactions to sulfites before, but this time I came close to dying.

In 1993, the FDA mandated that sulfites be disclosed on the labels of packaged foods. When food is sold in bulk form, like a barrel of dried fruit or raw shrimp, store managers must post a notice that lists the ingredients so consumers can determine if a product has been treated with sulfites.

■ Incidence of Sulfite Sensitivity

Doctors are constantly urged to report adverse drug reactions to the FDA. However, with sulfites and other food additives, reporting is erratic at best, so it's difficult to say just how many people are at risk. Doctors Donald Stevenson and Ron Simon estimate that 5 to 10 percent of all adult asthmatics may be sulfite sensitive. If their figures are correct, there may be 500,000 sulfite-sensitive asthmatics in the United States. Asthmatics who are dependent on cortisone drugs are more prone to sulfite reactions.

When patients tell me that they have no problems drinking beer or wine or eating fresh shrimp, I usually dismiss the possibility of sulfite sensitivity.

At first I doubted these estimates and thought sulfite-induced asthma was a rare problem. But once I started looking, I found so-called "restaurant-induced asthma" was not all that uncommon. Fortunately, the incidence of sulfite reactions in asthmatics declined dramatically after the FDA banned their use in salad bars, restaurants, and supermarkets. A clinical history is the best way to diagnos sulfite sensitivity as skin and blood tests are not very helpful. When patients tell me that they have no problems drinking beer or wine or eating fresh shrimp, I usually dismiss the possibility of sulfite sensitivity. In some cases, an oral challenge may be needed to refute or confirm the diagnosis of sulfite sensitivity.

■ Common Names and Hidden Sources of Sulfites

The only way to prevent a sulfite reaction is avoidance. Regulations require manufacturers who use sulfites to list them on their product labels. When eating out, ask the chef or server if sulfites are added to foods before or during preparation. If you want to eat potatoes, order a baked potato rather than hash browns, French fries, or any dish that involves peeling the potato. Common names and hidden sources of sulfites are listed in table 15.1.

■ Sulfites in Medications

While some eye drops, creams, and oral medications contain sulfites, most reports on sulfite drug reactions come from injectable medications, like epinephrine; cortisone drugs; local and general anesthetics; and antibiotics. Note: injectable epinephrine should never be withheld in an emergency situation in patients with sulfite sensitivity as the benefit of this life-saving drug far outweighs any theoretical risk of a sulfite reaction!

■ Does Sulfite Sensitivity Cross-React with Sulfa Drugs?

There is no evidence that sulfite-sensitive individuals will react to sulfa drugs. Likewise, there is no increased risk of a sulfite reaction in patients allergic to sulfa drugs. Confusion arises when a patient is labeled as having a sulfa allergy. Sulfa allergy refers to an allergy to a class of antibiotic drugs known as sulfonamides. With the exception of sulfasalazine, an older drug used to treat ulcerative colitis and Crohn's disease, and Celebrex, a newer NSAID, all sulfonamides are antibacterial drugs.

Table 15.1. Common Names and Hidden Sources of Sulfites

Names	Hidden Sources
Sulphur dioxide	Beer, wine, cordials
Sodium sulfite	Fruit juices, soft drinks, instant tea
Sodium bisulfite	Lemon and lime juice, vinegar, grape juice
Sodium metabisulfite	Dried or French-fried potatoes
Potassium metabisulfite	Gravies and sauces, fruit toppings, Maraschino cherries
Calcium sulfite	Pickled onions
Calcium bisulfite	Maple syrup, jams, jellies, biscuits, and bread
Potassium bisulfite	Pie or pizza dough
	Dried fruit like apricots, grapes, and raisins
	Crustaceans like shrimp
	Mincemeat, sausage meat or hamberger patties

■ A Day Without Sulfites?

As the saying goes, "A day without wine is like a day without sunshine." Were it not for sulfites, it would indeed be a very cloudy world for wine lovers. Romans were the first to recognize the value of the sulfites that they added to wine to prevent spoilage. When grapes are harvested, they have wild yeasts on their skins. While yeasts ferment the grape juice and convert it into wine, it is almost impossible, especially in warm climates, to know precisely what effect those yeasts will have on the quality of the wine. Some yeasts turn the best grapes into unspeakably bad wine, and other yeasts are so weak that they fail to convert the grape sugar into alcohol, thus leaving unwanted sugar in the wine.

Only the bravest of winemakers rely only on wild yeasts to make wines. Instead, they kill the wild yeasts with sulfites and then add laboratory-grown yeasts designed for making wine. Many wineries add sulfites immediately before bottling to prevent further fermentation in the bottle. As a rule, sulfites levels are higher in casks than in bottled wine and higher in white wine versus red wine. Some winemakers produce sulfite-free wines. Most wine lovers like myself who have sampled these sulfite-free wines would revert to imbibing beer if sulfite-fortified wines were not available.

Most countries require wineries to label wines that contain sulfites. As sulfites are added in small amounts, between twenty and 150 parts per million, only the most sulfite-sensitive individuals will react to sulfites in wine. Sulfite-induced asthma in wine drinkers may be overestimated. In one study, only four of twenty-four asthmatic patients with a history of wine-induced asthma reacted to sulfite additives in wine. In a second study, wine-sensitive asthmatics challenged with sulfite-fortified wine had no change in their lung functions, suggesting that sulfite-induced asthma from wine and beer may be overestimated.

■ Food Binders and Fillers

Food binders, or fillers, are organic compounds that improve the consistency of foodstuff. Such compounds include carrageenan, gum arabic, karaya, tragacanth, gum carob, locust bean, mannitol, and moisture enhancers, such as propylene glycol, glycerine, and sorbitiol. While isolated case reports have linked these chemicals to allergic reactions, most binders and fillers are safe. One interesting binder known as "confectioner's glaze" is derived from secretions from the female Indian "lac" bug. This shellac-like substance prevents candies, jellybeans, ice cream cones, avocadoes, and citrus fruits from drying out.

> *There is one case report of a reaction to saffron, a yellow dye from the flower of the crocus plant. Similar concerns about other food dyes have also been proven to be unfounded with the exception of carmine dye.*

■ A Big Mac Attack

In May 1978, a letter to the *New England Journal of Medicine* from doctors at McGill University described a thirty-five-year-old woman who had a severe anaphylactic reaction while eating a Big Mac. With the cooperation of McDonald's of Montreal, the woman was tested with the secret ingredients in a Big Mac, including egg, beef, wheat, garlic, mustard, lettuce, tomato, onion, and sesame seed. All tests were negative. However, testing with gum tragacanth was positive. Gum tragacanth is added to foods to give bulk. The natural gum tragacanth is a sap that comes from Middle Eastern legumes and is produced in Iran. Tragacanth swells to form a stiff gel that is used as an emulsifying agent in pills, hand lotions, and lubricating jellies. Older literature (late 1940s) reports several reactions to drugs containing tragacanth gum. Interestingly, since these reports there have been very few cases of documented reactions to tragacanth.

■ Food Dyes

The largest group of food additives is food dye, which enhance the color and appearance of foods. One dye, tartrazine (FD&C Yellow Dye No. 5), was touted as a significant asthma trigger in the 1970s. This dye, a derivative of coal tar, is commonly used to color foods like margarine yellow. Controlled studies have proven that this yellow dye is not a risk for asthmatics. There are a few case reports of reactions to annatto dye, which comes from the fruit of the annatto tree. This yellow dye is used to add color to margarine, cereals, cheese, ice cream, and many beverages. Additionally, there is one case report of a reaction to saffron, a yellow dye from the flower of the crocus plant. Similar concerns about other food dyes have also been proven to be unfounded with the exception of carmine dye.

■ Carmine Dye Allergy

One of the more interesting food dyes is carmine, a natural red dye that is derived from the dried bodies of the female cochineal insect, a parasitic beetle that lives on the prickly pear cactus plant. At sexual maturity (approximately 100 days), the female insects' bodies are filled with eggs that contain the greatest concentration of the carmine dye. Just before they lay their eggs, the insects are brushed off the cactus, collected, and dried. It takes about 70,000 beetles to make one pound of carmine.

These insects and cactus plants are native to Mexico, where Cortez discovered the Aztecs using cochineal insects to color their food, clothing, and bodies. This red dye then became an important trade item as it was ten times stronger than the dyes used in Europe at the time. The cochineal trade declined with the introduction of synthetic colors in 1856. However, in the 1990s, a preference for natural food dyes led to a resurgence of natural colors such as carmine. Carmine-derived colors include red, strawberry red, orange, and magenta. Currently, large cactus plantations in Mexico, the Canary Islands, and Peru are devoted to carmine production. Carmine-containing substances may not be listed on food labels, as neither carmine nor cochineal extract are FDA-certifiable color additives. The FDA only requires man-made colorings to be listed on labels. Carmine dye is also used in cosmetics and textiles.

■ The Popsicle Patient

In 1997, University of Michigan allergists described an interesting case of carmine allergy. Their patient was a twenty-seven-year-old female who, after ingesting a Good Humor SnoFruit Popsicle colored with carmine, experienced nausea and itching within minutes, followed by hives and low blood pressure. She exhibited a positive skin test and oral challenge to carmine and negative tests to other components of the Popsicle. Over the past few years, several cases of carmine allergy and anaphylaxis have been reported in the medical literature and at national allergy meetings. Doctors from the Naval Medical Center in San Diego, California, described three women who reacted to red-colored candies or fruits. Two reported prior contact reactions to red eye shadow. The eleven other cases in the literature were also women.

Thus, red-dyed cosmetics may be a common route of sensitization in carmine-allergic patients. Unlike other food dyes that are synthetically manufactured, this natural dye may now be the most common cause of an allergic reaction to a food dye.

Carmine is a potential sensitizer in an occupational setting. Eighteen cases of occupational asthma have been described. A forty-two-year-old male butcher presented with a five-year history of eye irritation, nasal congestion, and asthma after occupational exposure to food additive dusts. Prick tests were positive to carmine and carmine-containing additives. Common beverages that use this dye include Dannon Boy grapefruit juice and Tropicana Ruby Red grapefruit juice. The FDA is considering requiring natural dyes to be labeled on all products. This may trigger food and beverage manufacturers to stop using carmine altogether as many consumers may be reluctant to purchase or ingest foodstuffs derived from unsightly insects or beetles. Potential carmine-containing are listed in table 15.2.

Carmine-containing substances may not be listed on food labels, as neither carmine nor cochineal extract are FDA-certifiable color additives. The FDA only requires man-made colorings to be listed on labels.

■ Food Enhancers: A Bad Rap for MSG?

Monosodium glutamate (MSG), the most extensively researched food additive, has been the subject of hundreds of studies over the past thirty years. While most studies have shown MSG to be very safe, bad press has led the public to believe that

Table 15.2. Carmine-Containing Products

Candy blushes	Artificial crab and lobster products
Vitamins	Cherries in fruit cocktails
Ice creams and popsicles	Yogurts
Lipsticks	Syrups
Homeopathic medications	Liqueurs
Juice drinks	Vinegar
Eye shadow	Puddings
Fruit fillings in baked goods	Lumpfish eggs
Strawberry-colored milks	Caviar
Port wine cheese	Processed meats

MSG is a dangerous food additive. More than 1,200 years ago, Asian cooks discovered that many foods tasted better when they were prepared in a soup stock made from seaweed. In 1908, Japanese scientists discovered that the compound in seaweed that was responsible for enhancing food flavor was an amino acid called glutamate, also known as monosodium glutamate, or MSG. The Japanese have a particular name for the taste of glutamate, they call it, *unami*. There are many misconceptions about MSG. It is neither a tenderizer nor a preservative, and it is not used to make food look attractive. MSG is, purely and simply, a food enhancer. MSG does not change the flavor of a food but masks unpleasant tastes and brings out agreeable flavors by stimulating the tongue's taste buds.

Many people erroneously believe that MSG is made from chemicals; it is not.

MSG is, purely and simply, a food enhancer. MSG does not change the flavor of a food but masks unpleasant tastes and brings out agreeable flavors by stimulating the tongue's taste buds.

MSG is produced by fermentation, the same process used to make beer, vinegar, soy sauce, and yogurt. Fermentation begins when natural products, such as molasses from sugar cane or sugar beets, and food starch from tapioca or cereals, are fermented in a controlled environment with bacteria called *Corynebacterium glutamicum*. The crude glutamic acid produced in this process is filtered, purified, and converted into pure white crystals of monosodium glutamate. MSG is the sodium salt of an amino acid called glutamic acid, or glutamate. Amino acids are the building blocks of protein needed for proper metabolism and brain function. Because we make our own supply of glutamic acid, about fifty grams per day, it is called a non-essential amino acid as opposed to essential amino acids that are only available through dietary supplementation.

■ Unami—The Fifth Basic Taste

In medical school, I learned that there were four basic tastes: sweet, sour, salty and bitter. While researching this book, I was surprised to learn that a fifth basic taste, unami, had been included by researchers at the University of Miami. The unami taste from glutamate is the pleasant flavor we enjoy from eating tomatoes, cheese, meat, milk, seafood, mushrooms, peas, broccoli, and other vegetables. Infants are apparently born with only two sets of taste buds. The first detects the sweet taste of the lactose sugar in their mother's milk and the second taste senses the unami, or glutamate. Breast milk is rich in free glutamate—containing about twenty times the amount found in cow's milk. If breast milk didn't taste good, no baby would want to breast-feed.

The unami flavor is not exclusive to Asian foods. English anchovy sauce and Australian vegemite are rich sources of glutamate. Italian cuisine, enriched with tomato sauces and cheeses, provides more glutamate than most MSG-fortified Asian meals. Many criticize the addition of MSG as a short-cut method of enhancing the flavor of food. However, the addition of the right amount of MSG, as little as one-fifth of a teaspoon, enhances the flavor of foods by bringing out the natural unami taste. Overuse of MSG or use with poor quality ingredients result in a poor tasting product. Like sugar and table salt, MSG has no distinctive smell.

■ Less Salt or More MSG?

Many individuals completely eliminate salt in an attempt to lower blood pressure and reduce weight. The trade-off is reduced palatability. Here is where MSG may help. While not a salt substitute, using a small amount of MSG may allow you to slash salt intake without compromising flavor. Research has shown that low-salt diets are more acceptable to the dieter when a small amount of MSG is added. Like all bodily functions, our sense of taste and smell declines with age. This process normally begins at about age sixty and becomes more pronounced in our 70s. As a result, food choices may change and lead to inadequate food intake, especially for senior citizens placed on low-salt diets. Thus, MSG may enhance the diet of elderly people by making foods more appetizing.

Overuse of MSG or use with poor quality ingredients result in a poor tasting product. Like sugar and table salt, MSG has no distinctive smell.

■ The Chinese Restaurant Syndrome

In April 1968, Dr. Robert Ho Man Kwok, a researcher at the National Institutes of Health, wrote a letter to the *New England Journal of Medicine* in which he described his own reactions after eating at various Chinese restaurants, especially when northern Chinese cuisine was served. Kwok's symptoms, which lasted for about two hours, consisted of numbness in the back of his neck and arms, general weakness, and palpitations. The title of his letter was the "Chinese Restaurant Syndrome."

Kwok's report triggered numerous replies from many fellow physicians who described similar reactions. Eventually, this syndrome was linked to MSG. The common symptoms of MSG sensitivity are a burning or tingling sensation in the back of the neck, forearms, face, and

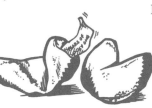

chest; chest pain; heart palpitations; headache; nausea; rapid pulse; and wheezing. Symptoms are usually dose-related and occur immediately after ingestion or up to forty-eight hours later. An MSG reaction is more likely to occur when MSG is ingested in a large quantity or in liquid form, like a clear duck or wonton soup. Alcohol, exercise, and menstruation may intensify an MSG reaction. Some authorities believe the Chinese Restaurant Syndrome is not due to MSG and lay the blame on the high salt and histamine content of various Chinese foods.

■ Clinical Studies on MSG

Overall, MSG has been given a bad rap. In the early 1980s, an association between MSG and asthma was raised when several reports described patients who developed asthma-like symptoms after ingesting Chinese food. This observation prompted researchers from the Scripps Clinic in La Jolla, California, and the Alfred Hospital in Melbourne, Australia, to study asthmatics who perceived their symptoms were triggered by MSG-containing foods. The results of these studies, which used doses of up to five grams of MSG (the equivalent of three quarts of wonton soup), conclusively found that MSG did not trigger asthma.

In 2001, one of the authors of the Melbourne study, Dr. Rosalie Woods, reviewed all the literature on the alleged link between MSG and asthma and stated, "Current evidence suggests that the notion of MSG-induced asthma is extremely rare. Adults with asthma do not need to restrict MSG intake. As it is virtually impossible to avoid MSG altogether, this should ensure that people with asthma enjoy a wide variety of foods and, hence, consume a diet that is nutritionally adequate."

Researchers at Harvard University tested 130 people who believed they were sensitive to MSG. In two separate tests nineteen reacted to five grams of MSG (an enormous dose), but not to a look-a-like, MSG-free placebo. Twelve subjects agreed to be retested. Only two of the twelve reacted to the large dose of MSG in the retest. "Our research confirmed that some people are sensitive to MSG, but it's not common and the symptoms are extremely mild," said a Harvard researcher, Dr. Raif Geha.

Headache is another disorder commonly attributed to MSG. Reports imply that MSG is a vasoactive substance, meaning that it constricts or dilates blood vessels and may trigger migraine attacks. Such claims have not been confirmed in controlled studies. A critical review in the *Annals of Behavioral Medicine* concluded that there is no evidence to support an association between MSG and migraine headaches. On the basis of these studies and my own professional experience, I do not consider MSG to be an important trigger of food allergy, asthma, or migraine headaches.

Years ago, researchers discovered that vitamin B6-deficient animals did not properly process MSG. The incidence of MSG-sensitive-B6 deficiency in humans is unknown. Some individuals with MSG-sensitivity may benefit from vitamin B6 supplementation. In one study, eight out of nine subjects stopped reacting to MSG when they took fifty milligrams of vitamin B6 a day.

■ Common Names and Hidden Sources of MSG

Glutamate is found in virtually all natural foods, including meat, poultry, fish, cheese, milk, and vegetables. The average American consumes between 0.3 and 1.0

Table 15.3. Common Names and Hidden Sources of MSG

Names	Hidden Sources
Hydrolyzed protein	All natural foods
Autolyzed yeast	Avocadoes
Calcium caseinate	Meat
Glutamate	Poultry
Gelatin	Fish
Hydrolyzed soy protein	Cheese
Monosodium glutamate	Milk
Monopotassium glutamate	Tomatoes
Sodium caseinate	Mushrooms
Textured protein	Many vegetables
Yeast extract and yeast food	Seafood, especially shrimp
Flavor enhancers, like Accent	
AJI-NO-MOTO, Japanese seasoning	

gram of glutamate per day. Don't be fooled by product labels that claim no MSG, as current labeling laws do not require it to be listed on all products. The FDA requires that MSG-containing ingredients be listed with their common names. The term MSG is reserved for the ninety-nine percent pure forms of glutamic acid and sodium. Common names and hidden sources of MSG are listed in table 15.3

■ Bon Appétit!

In the United States, Australia, and New Zealand, no food additive, including MSG, is approved for use until safety has been established by governmental agencies. The Federation of American Societies for Experimental Biology in the United States concluded that there was no difference between the naturally occurring free glutamate found in mushrooms, cheese, and tomatoes, and the MSG found in hydrolyzed proteins and soy sauce. The report concluded that MSG is safe for the general population. MSG has been on the FDA GRAS list for forty years. It sits alongside pepper, sugar, vinegar, and baking powder. Similar acceptance of the safety of MSG is reflected in food laws in Europe, Australia, and New Zealand. The bottom line is that despite what you read on the Internet or print media or hear on talk shows, MSG is relatively harmless for most individuals. ●

The bottom line is that despite what you read on the Internet or print media or hear on talk shows, MSG is relatively harmless for most individuals.

Chapter

16

Risky Restaurants

Many restaurants and food service establishments have learned about the food allergy epidemic the hard way—by settling costly lawsuits. Several cases of near-fatal or fatal food allergy reactions in eating establishments throughout the world have been brought before the courts. Due to clear-cut evidence of gross negligence, numerous food service providers have settled these cases out of court.

In 1992, the widow of a Farmington, Minnesota, man who died from an allergic reaction to peanut butter received $450,000 in a settlement with a Twin Cities restaurant.[1] The man died within ninety minutes after taking a few bites from an egg roll at a Chinese restaurant. Before he ate it, a waitress assured him that the roll was not fried in peanut oil. However, the waitress did not know that the egg roll recipe had been changed to include peanut butter, often used to keep egg rolls from falling apart. After the man developed an allergic reaction, his wife and mother summoned the manager who disclosed that peanut butter was in the egg roll.

The man drove himself to a near-by urgent care center where he went into shock. His throat swelled, he stopped breathing, and was subsequently pronounced dead. The man's wife sued the restaurant. As a part of the settlement of $450,000, it was agreed that the restaurant would change the language on its menu to alert customers and disclose allergic ingredients in food. The man had a prescription

for epinephrine, but it was unclear whether he injected himself with it.

■ The Dumb Waiter

The following case illustrates the devastating consequences for both a diner and a restaurant when poorly educated waitstaff (dumb waiters) handle questions from patrons about food allergens.

A.F. was a thirty-two-year-old female with chronic asthma and a history of peanut- and tree nut-allergy since childhood. In June 1990, after eating a Danish that contained hidden nuts, she began to wheeze. She then drove herself to a local emergency room where she was treated with epinephrine, Benadryl, and SoluMedrol (a cortisone drug). She improved rapidly and was discharged in about two hours. This proved to be a mistake. On the way home, her symptoms recurred—a classic biphasic reaction. She drove herself back to the hospital and collapsed in the parking lot, where she was found in acute respiratory arrest. She was admitted to an intensive care unit, placed on a respirator and subsequently recovered. Over the next four years, her asthma was relatively stable. In January 1992, while dining at a restaurant in a local mall, she ordered a dish with pesto sauce, which according to her waiter, "did not contain any nuts." Tragically, the pesto sauce contained hidden nuts. She immediately experienced a severe anaphylactic reaction and arrived in the local emergency room in a comatose state. She died sev-

[1] *Star Tribune* (Minneapolis MN), August 8, 1992.

eral days later. The family of the unfortunate woman sued this well-known New England chain for 10 million dollars. The case was ultimately settled out-of-court for an undisclosed amount.

■ New Laws

Thanks to the efforts of proactive food allergy organizations, such as FAAN and the Food Allergy Initiative (FAI), the federal government and many states have proposed or implemented laws to protect unsuspecting food-allergic consumers. In August 2004, President George Bush signed the Food Allergen Labeling and Consumer Protection Act (FALCPA) that became law in January 2006. FALCPA was the result of years of cooperative effort involving the food industry, FAAN, FAI, the FDA, concerned families, and the United States Congress.

The FALCPA law ensures that allergens and ingredients disclosed on labels are understandable to the average consumer and take the guesswork out of what's in a food package. Food manufacturers must identify in plain English language the presence of the eight major food allergens that are responsible for nearly 90 percent of all allergic reactions. They must also indicate the presence of food allergens in food additives, such as spices, flavorings, and colorings. Those eight allergens are milk, eggs, peanuts, tree nuts, fish, shellfish, wheat, and soy. The FALCPA law requires the FDA to conduct follow-up inspections and issue reports to ensure that food manufacturers comply with practices to reduce and eliminate cross-contact with any major food allergens that are not the intentional ingredients of the food.

FALCPA applies to all foods sold in the United States, including imported foods. The FALCPA law does not cover kosher foods, seeds, spices, or non-packaged foods, such as meats and poultry. Many food manufacturers have implemented measures to comply with the FALCPA law. Both the Kellogg and Campbell soup companies have reformulated several products by taking foods allergens like fish gelatin out of their recipes rather than listing them on their labels. The new law has caused some companies to fess up.[2] Dr. Cathy Kaprica, McDonald's director of global nutrition, recently stated that their famous French fries include a natural flavoring that is made in part from extracts of wheat and dairy products. McDonald's had previously listed the fries as being free of milk, wheat or gluten proteins.

The FALCPA bill also benefits the estimated 2 million Americans with celiac disease by defining "gluten free" and permitting the voluntary labeling of products as "gluten free" no later than 2008 when manufacturers must meet new government standards before being allowed to use the term "gluten free." The act provides needed information for school nurses, teachers, caregivers, the food service industry, and restaurants to help millions of food allergic students and restaurant patrons to avoid food allergens. The European Union is also enacting new labeling

The FALCPA law requires the FDA to conduct follow-up inspections and issue reports to ensure that food manufacturers comply with practices to reduce and eliminate cross-contact with any major food allergens that are not the intentional ingredients of the food.

---

[2] *Wall Street Journal* (New York), February 18, 2006.

laws. Unlike the FALCPA law, European laws will require celery, sesame seed, and mustard to be listed on ingredient labels.

■ New State Laws

Several states have taken matters into their own hands. In January 2005, the state of New Jersey passed a law directed to boards of health, restaurant managers, and wait-staff. This law calls for the creation of a public information campaign known as Ask Before You Eat. This law is designed to inform the public about food allergies and anaphylaxis. The law also calls for the New Jersey Department of Health and Senior Services to create a fact sheet on nut allergies that will be distributed to local health boards and restaurants. Connecticut has enacted a law to develop guidelines for schools that Connecticut school boards had to implement by July 2006. Similar legislation is pending in Massachusetts, Vermont, Tennessee, New York, and North Carolina.

Certainly, the ultimate responsibility for avoiding an offending food lies with consumers and their families. However, sloppy practices by food establishments have resulted in tragic outcomes and costly lawsuits.

The thrust of all this legislative activity is that food service providers must train their managers, chefs, kitchen, and wait-staff about the risks posed by food allergies. This responsibility applies not only to restaurants, but to bakeries, coffee and donut shops, delicatessens, commercial airlines, cruise ships, ice cream shops, hospitals, camps, college cafeterias, and food caterers—in other words anyone involved in serving food to the general public. Certainly, the ultimate responsibility for avoiding an offending food lies with consumers and their families. However, sloppy practices by food establishments have resulted in tragic outcomes and costly lawsuits.

■ New FDA Food Codes

Every four years the FDA publishes a code for more than 3,000 regulatory agencies that oversee food safety in restaurants, grocery stores, and nursing homes. FAAN has been working with the FDA as well as representatives of airline caterers, grocery stores, national restaurant chains, consumer advocates, and the National Restaurant Association to modify the Model Food Code which is a set of recommendations and regulations for states to consider adopting in whole or in part. The newest FDA directive mandates that persons in charge of food-serving establishments must demonstrate knowledge of the major food allergens as defined by the new federal FALCPA law enacted in January 2006. The bottom line: every restaurant needs to have someone well-versed on food allergy in-house on every shift.

■ Risky Restaurants

Most accidental food exposures occur outside the home in restaurants, bakeries, ice cream parlors, and school and college cafeterias. A survey of 129 registrants of the National Peanut and Tree Nut Allergy Registry maintained by FAAN highlights the risks of eating out. Most reactions outside the home were due to accidental ingestion of peanuts (67 percent) and tree nuts (24 percent). Symptoms often began within five minutes after eating the food and were severe in nearly one-third of the victims. The riskiest loca-

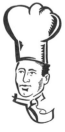

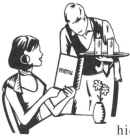

tions were Asian restaurants, ice cream shops, and bakeries. Fifty percent of the time allergenic foods were hidden in desserts, sauces, dressings, and egg rolls. One in every four reactions was due to food sharing or cross-contamination by spatula carry-over. The biggest problem was a lack of communication between the patron and the food establishment. Less than half of the victims let the food establishment know they had a food allergy. All the players in this game—including the patient or family, the food manufacturer, the food purchaser, and the food serving establishment—have a definitive role in preventing reactions outside the home.

Another FAAN survey looked at 125 registrants from their National Seafood Registry. Shellfish was the most common trigger (60 percent) in seafood and Asian restaurants. Only 21 percent of the victims let the restaurant know they had a reaction. Two-thirds of the diners re-ordered specific seafood despite the fact that they had a previous reaction to the food.

A study of fifty-nine restaurant managers, chefs, and servers uncovered a need for more education of restaurant personnel. Only one-third had some form of food allergy training. Twenty-five percent of those surveyed believed a small amount of allergen was safe, and 34 percent erroneously thought that fryer heat destroyed food allergens. Forty-six percent thought a buffet was safe if it was "kept clean." Seventy-six percent felt they were capable of providing a safe meal, and 54 percent felt they could manage a food allergy emergency but had a poor knowledge about the risks posed by food allergy.

■ Role of the Food Manufacturer, Purchaser and Provider

Food manufacturers, food purchasers, and food providers must comply with the FAL-CPA law and label all products that contain the more allergenic foods. The food purchaser must be sure that products purchased by the food service provider do not contain any hidden food allergens. Owners and managers of food service establishments must train their chefs and waitstaff on how to protect food-allergic patrons from experiencing allergic reactions. An informal poll of several of my friends in the restaurant business revealed that they had little knowledge of the risks posed by food allergy. Most were unaware that national food allergy and restaurant organizations have pooled their resources to educate and train restaurant and food service professionals about food allergies.

In an effort to educate and train restaurant and food service professionals regarding the complexities of food allergies, the Food Allergy Initiative has funded the Food Allergy Training Guide for Restaurants and Food Services. This guide, compiled by a cooperative effort of the National Restaurant Associa-

An informal poll of several of my friends in the restaurant business revealed that they had little knowledge of the risks posed by food allergy. Most were unaware that national food allergy and restaurant organizations have pooled their resources to educate and train restaurant and food service professionals about food allergies.

tion (NRA) and the Food Allergy & Anaphylaxis Network (FAAN), consists of a video and manual material (Spanish and English versions are available), which contain information for "front of the house" and "back of the house" staff. In addition to providing important allergy information, the video offers clear visual scenarios illustrating strategies for handling food-allergic customers from the moment they review the menu, place their order, and receive their food. There are several how-to demonstrations in food preparation and food service and a section on what to do in an emergency situation.

Renowned industry leaders, such as Chef Marcus Samuelsson of Aquavit and Sirio Maccioni of Le Cirque 2000 in New York City; Chet England, director of quality assurance of the Burger King Corporation; and Steven Grover, vice president of Health and Safety Regulatory Affairs of the National Restaurant Association, are interviewed in the video. They convey the importance of education and training for food allergies and offer assurance not only to food-allergic consumers but to all consumers that they will be provided a meal that is safe and to their requested specifications. To purchase the Food Allergy Training Guide for Restaurants and Food Services contact FAAN (see the appendix).

■ National Restaurant Association Guidelines

The following guidelines for food allergy awareness are adopted from guidelines published by the National Restaurant Association.

- People with food allergies must completely avoid allergenic foods. Even one bite can lead to a serious reaction or even death. That's why it's so important that restaurants work to ensure that a customer with an allergy is not served an item that he or she is allergic to. This not only protects the customer, but prevents costly lawsuits.

- Advise staff to pay close attention when a patron says he or she has a food allergy. Most allergy suffers are very knowledgeable about the foods they cannot eat. If you're not certain what food items an allergy encompasses, ask. For example, if a person asks whether an egg roll was fried in peanut oil, staff members should ask if the diner is allergic to all peanut products. In one incident at a Miami restaurant, a server assured the customer that the egg rolls were not fried in peanut oil, but failed to mention that peanut butter was used to seal the dough. The customer died from an allergic reaction. Servers should be able to describe a menu item and its ingredients upon request. Staff members should know what ingredients are in an item. In some cases, it may be helpful to show guests product labels so that they can assess the situation for themselves.

- If a server does not know whether a menu item is free of a potentially offending food substance, he or she should say so and refer the guest to a manager or a chef designated to answer such questions. Ideally, there should be a designated point person on staff during each shift who is prepared to answer questions about ingredients. However, if no one knows for certain whether an allergen is in an item, admit that and recommend ordering another item.

- Train your staff about potential allergens. Common allergens include eggs, fish, milk, peanuts, shellfish, tree nuts (including almonds, Brazil nuts, cashews, chestnuts, hazelnuts, hickory nuts, macadamia nuts, pecans, pine nuts, pistachios and walnuts), and wheat.

- Avoid cross-contaminating foods with potentially allergenic foods.
- Food for allergy sufferers should be prepared and served without any contact with allergens.
- Train kitchen staff to use a prep table that has not been exposed to the allergen and clean their cooking utensils after working with potentially allergenic foods.
- Train chefs to prepare allergen-free versions of items upon request. Be aware that many chefs use peanut butter to salvage burnt spaghetti, soups, and gravies
- Never include a possible allergenic food as a "mystery ingredient."
- A customer cognizant of her allergy to peanuts ordered chili in a Rhode Island restaurant. She never suspected that the secret ingredient used to thicken the dish was peanut butter. She died minutes later of anaphylactic shock.
- The trend toward "creative cookery" and the use of nontraditional ingredients, such as nuts in cheesecake, increases the chance that customers will ingest offending foods. To avoid these problems, try to include such ingredients in the menu item's name or description.
- Don't make casual product substitutions. For example, don't substitute peanut oil for canola oil. A regular customer with a food allergy will not think to ask whether a dish he or she has been enjoying for years has been altered.
- Read labels carefully. It's not good enough to guess what ingredients are in a product. For example, a barbecue sauce may contain nuts, but many people might not think to check the label. Just because a product was safe last month or last year doesn't mean that it's safe today. Food manufacturers often change ingredients.
- Complex foods such as sauces, dressings and garnishes may cause an allergic reaction. Serve these items on the side to allergy sufferers.
- Be aware that even a minute amount of food can set off a severe allergic reaction. For example, if a customer specifies that he or she is allergic to walnuts, it's not enough to simply scrape the walnuts off the top of a piece of cake you are serving.

■ Role of the Patient and Family

The ultimate responsibility for preventing an allergic reaction while eating away from home lies with the patient or his or her family. Many patients and families have major hang-ups about eating out. However, if appropriate steps are taken, there is no need to be a stay-at-home diner. FAAN has published an excellent manual, *Traveling with Food Allergy*, that details how to safely dine out and travel with food allergy. It lists contacts and resources for foreign travel, including foreign terms for many allergenic foods. The FAAN manual outlines the following steps to take when eating away from home.

- Be aware of hidden allergens.
- Know the symptoms of an allergic reaction.
- Know how to treat an allergic reaction.
- Always carry an antihistamine and injectable epinephrine.
- Develop a Food Allergy Action Plan (FAAP), especially for children at school, camp, or older students who go away to school.
- Carry a chef card designed by FAAN.
- Don't put yourself in harm's way. When ordering food, keep it simple! Avoid fancy dishes, fried food, sauces, and desserts.
- Let the manager or chef know about your food allergy.

- Eat American, avoid Asian, Oriental, and Indian restaurants.
- If you are severely allergic to seafood, go to a steak house.
- Watch out for peanut butter that may be used to improve flavor on steaks.
- Avoid bakeries, delis, and ice cream shops.
- Go through a buffet line first to avoid chances of a cross-contamination reaction.

■ Food Allergy Symptoms

Restaurant staff should know how to recognize the symptoms of an allergic reaction or anaphylactic reaction.[3] Such symptoms usually appear within one to fifteen minutes after consuming the food but may develop over a period of hours. While many allergic reactions to food are mild, many individuals experience severe life-threatening reactions. The most common symptoms of a food allergy reaction include:

- Itching in and around the mouth
- A tightening of the throat (airway blockage)
- Wheezing and hoarseness
- Shortness of breath
- Appearance of red welts or hives
- Swelling of the eyelids, lips, hands, or feet
- Nausea, cramping, or vomiting
- A sense of impending doom
- A drop in blood pressure
- A loss of consciousness

In the United Kingdom, over three-quarters of anaphylactic reactions to foods occur in catering premises where food labeling is unregulated, and the liberal use of peanut products is common.

■ Gambling Your Life on a Take-Away Meal

In the United Kingdom, over three-quarters of anaphylactic reactions to foods occur in catering premises where food labeling is unregulated, and the liberal use of peanut products is common. A clever study in Northern Ireland investigated the ability of take-away food establishments, when so requested, to provide a safe meal for a peanut-allergic customer. Two different food officers from twenty-six health departments in Northern Island asked for two different meals in sixty-two take-away establishments. The first officer asked for a meal likely to contain peanuts. A short time later, the second officer requested a peanut-free meal. Sample pairs from these sixty-two food outlets were then analyzed for peanut protein. Of the sixty-two meals that were sold following a request for a peanut-free meal, thirteen meals contained peanut protein.

The study concluded that one in every five times that peanut-allergic consumers visited a take-away establishment, they were gambling their lives on a take-away meal. The Irish report cited two cases of improper serving that were settled in the courts. A restaurant owner in Hull was fined 2,000 pounds for serving a peanut-allergic student a chicken korma dish containing peanuts. A twenty-eight-year-old woman who reacted to a curry dish that contained peanuts after the waiter assured her that a dish was peanut-free, received 7,500 pounds and an out-of-court settlement from a London Indian restaurant.

---

[3] Please refer to chapters five and six for a complete discussion on the diagnosis and treatment of anaphylaxis.

■ A Sad Shopping Story from North Carolina

The danger posed by take-away meals is exemplified by this sad story from North Carolina.[4]

Early one Saturday afternoon, Gina Marie Hunt, an eighth-grader from Concord, North Carolina, excitedly called her grandmother, who was also shopping nearby in the Concord Mills Mall. The story says she had found a $50 sweater on sale for $5. She then went to a food court with a friend to get some Chinese food. After eating an egg roll, Gina realized she was having an allergy attack and she called her grandmother on her cell phone and stated, "I'm throwing up, we have to go home." Gina, who also had asthma, then used her asthma inhaler that she kept in her purse. According to her mother, she was not carrying her syringe of auto-injectable epinephrine. One of the reasons she may not have had her epinephrine with her was that she was not able to carry epinephrine with her in her school that was only staffed by a school nurse two days a week. About 20 minutes later, Gina collapsed. By the time her grandmother found her, Gina was lying on her stomach on the floor of the mall. A nurse came by and performed CPR. Cabarrus County paramedics then gave Gina three epinephrine shots and took her to the Northeast Medical Center where she was pronounced dead.

Her grandmother stated, Gina was "caught up in the moment" and forgot to ask whether the food at the Chinese restaurant contained peanut products. Her mother stated, "For whatever reason, she chose to eat at a place she had never eaten before." According to her mother, there may have been a language problem when she ordered her food and she might have been served an egg roll by mistake.[5] The day before she had her fatal reaction, she was in an ice cream parlor and admonished the server for not cleaning the ice cream scoops between servings.

When Gina was two years old, allergy tests revealed that she was gravely allergic to peanuts. "When people opened up packages of peanuts, her face started to swell," her mother said as she recalled a plane trip during which Gina had an allergic reaction that prompted doctors to test her for allergies. "Her face was turning red."

After her diagnosis, Gina's food consumption was closely guarded. Her mother scrutinized food labels and interrogated restaurant employees before her daughter put anything in her mouth. Gina's mother even asked Northwest Cabarrus Middle School officials to make sure that Gina would ride in a bus with no peanut snacks or peanut butter sandwiches on field trips. But as Gina got older, there were times when her mother was not around to protect her. The other tragic part of Gina's story is that she was placed on the anti-IgE asthma drug Xolair a few years before she died. Her mother told me that her asthma greatly improved after she was started on this drug. Unfortunately, her medical insurance company discontinued her coverage for Xolair (that may also prevent severe food anaphylactic reactions) one year before her fatal reaction because of concerns about the costs of this drug.

Now, Gina's mother, local health officials and parents of peanut-allergic chil-

---

[4] *Charlotte Observer*, January 26, 2005.

[5] Personal communication, January 2006.

dren are calling on restaurants to post warning signs when they use peanuts as added ingredients in foods. Her mother's loss has driven her to take action and petition North Carolina lawmakers to protect others who might not be old enough or informed enough to protect themselves. Fred Pilkington, executive director of the Cabarrus Health Alliance, was cited as saying that restaurants aren't required to post such warnings, adding, "It's an excellent idea because teenagers don't always ask questions like that, and they don't know they're getting a peanut product." Gina's mother appropriately states her daughter's death should be a wake-up call for restaurants, and she's not resting until something is done. She has launched an online petition asking the state to require restaurants to train their employees on the dangers of food allergies and post warning signs if peanuts are used on the premises.[6] Currently, some local restaurants voluntarily post signs alerting customers if they use peanuts or peanut oil in their food. Gina's unfortunate story only reinforces the need for more education in the food service industry. As an aside, peanut products will be suspended at all Charlotte-Mecklenburg County school cafeterias by the 2006-2007 school year because of a growing number of children with this potentially deadly food allergy.

■ Take-Home Messages for Restaurant Owners and Managers

Restaurants owners and managers need to pay attention—big time! The majority of near-fatal and fatal anaphylactic reactions to foods occur away from home in food service settings, especially restaurants.

---

6 www.PetitionOnline.com

Therefore, eating establishments have both an ethical and a legal responsibility to provide a safe environment for their patrons. The basic steps that food service establishments should implement to achieve these goals are listed below.

- If peanuts and tree nuts are not an essential part of your cuisine, eliminate them from your kitchen. Consider advertising as a "nut-free restaurant;" it may increase business.
- List all important food allergens (The Big Eight) on your menu, especially when hidden in desserts, cakes, and sauces.
- Display the FAAN poster, "*Food Allergies: What You Need to Know* ."
- Teach managers, waitstaff, and chefs how to communicate with patrons with food allergies. Allow patrons, especially children, to bring their own dishes.
- Teach your kitchen staff how to avoid cross-contamination from grills, stoves, and utensils when cooking, processing, and serving the more allergenic foods. Do not bake pastries on the same cookie sheet. Use separate frying oils for various dishes, especially seafood. Clean grills and service areas between uses.
- Do not slice cheese and meats on the same equipment.
- Avoid exposing patrons to food vapors, especially steamed seafood.
- Train staff members to call for emergency aid (911) if they see a customer in distress. Post emergency numbers at all telephones. To ensure rapid response by the emergency squad, list the name, address, and telephone number of your restaurant beside each telephone.
- If GI symptoms (nausea, cramps, vomiting, and diarrhea) occur, do not allow the victim to go to the bathroom unattended.

- If a patron collapses, lay the victim down and elevate the legs—do not sit the victim up! Several reports of deaths when recumbent victims assumed the upright position have occurred due to a loss of blood flow to the heart. This so-called "empty heart syndrome" is due to shock or loss of fluid volume.
- Check the airway to be sure there is no obstruction. If cardiorespiratory arrest occurs, perform CPR, and, if your staff is so trained, employ an automatic external defibrillator device (AED).
- Many food service establishments have trained their staff in CPR and the use of AEDs. Consider training your restaurant staff on how to use auto-injectable epinephrine devices as most victims of severe food reactions do not have these devices with them at the time of their reaction. Lay persons administering injectable epinephrine in an acute emergency situation should not be concerned about liability from administering epinephrine as they are protected by Good Samaritan laws in most states.

■ New on the Menu—Allergens

The following article, "New on the Menu: Allergens" by Jenn Abelson, was published in the *Boston Globe* on May 14, 2006. It succinctly summarizes the problems faced by both the allergic consumer and food establishments.

Kayla McCarthy has given up on eating out. The eleven-year-old's nut allergies landed her in the hospital three times in the past six months after she ordered foods like pizza and ice cream that she and her family thought were safe. "I'm scared about what's going to happen," McCarthy said. "Restaurants need to do a better job with people like me, people with food allergies."

Across the country, restaurants are wrestling with how to accommodate a growing number of customers with food allergies who are demanding greater knowledge about the ingredients and preparation of food they order. Food allergy advocates say they want restaurants to take responsibility for what they serve—the way they take responsibility for when to stop serving alcohol to customers. But many restaurants say frequent menu changes and language barriers among workers make it difficult to disclose food allergens in all dishes. And they fear lawsuits if they make a mistake.

It's the latest battleground in the food allergy movement that in recent years has transformed almost every space where food is available—from supermarket aisles to school cafeterias. Seeking a middle ground, many establishments in the past year have posted warnings that they are not allergy-free environments, and some, including Massachusetts-based Ninety Nine Restaurants and Uno Chicago Grill, recently started to list ingredients in dishes that cause allergic reactions on their Web sites or in their menus.

Lawmakers nationwide are mounting pressure to put procedures in place that would train workers about food allergies and hold restaurants to specific standards. In Massachusetts, after more than two years battling state lawmakers, the Massachusetts Restaurant Association says it's willing to take what could be the industry's most aggressive steps toward accommodating people with food allergies.

These initiatives, which legislators hope will become law, include placing warnings on menus that advise customers with food allergies to inform waiters; adding a video about food allergies to the training program for state-certified food managers; and posting signs near food handlers that explain the most common food allergies and ways to avoid contaminating food, such as using new utensils and separate fryers.

A growing recognition of life-threatening food allergies has prompted schools to enforce no-sharing policies at lunch. And a new federal food-labeling law requires manufacturers to disclose whether products contain any of the top eight food allergens: milk, eggs, fish, crustacean shellfish, peanuts, tree nuts, wheat, and soy. Still, these proposed steps for Massachusetts restaurants fall short of the initial bill filed by state Senator Cynthia Creem, which called for all food handlers to receive training on the consequences of food allergies and for restaurants to list on menus food items that cause allergic reactions. During negotiations over the past two years, the bill was watered down because the Massachusetts Restaurant Association resisted such measures.

Peter Christie, president of the Massachusetts Restaurant Association, said it would be too costly to conduct widespread training and list allergens on menus given high employee turnover and frequent menu changes. It's especially difficult, the association says, for mom-and-pop venues that do not write down recipes and places that employ servers and food handlers who do not speak English. "I understand it's an emotional issue. People's lives are at stake," Christie said. "But this is a litigious society in which we live. If you misinform a customer, you're subject to a suit. We as an association don't want someone to be sued because they didn't put down an ingredient." Already McDonald's is facing several lawsuits by customers with food allergies after the fast food chain admitted this year that its French fries contain milk and wheat ingredients, which is contrary to prior statements.

At Arizona-based Coldstone Creamery, customer requests prompted the ice cream restaurant chain to provide on its Web site and in its stores information about allergens on its menu. The company also increased employee training on food allergies, according to Nola Krieg, Coldstone's associate tastemaster. At the same time, Coldstone didn't want to give customers the impression that it could ensure safe products. This spring, the chain put up signs telling customers that its products may contain traces of peanuts, tree nuts, soybeans, wheat, or eggs from manufacturing and preparation. The company used to instruct workers to serve people with food allergies by using new utensils and new ice cream to prevent cross-contamination. Now workers are told to do so only if the customer insists and to warn them that there are no guarantees that the product won't cause an allergic reaction.

Over the past two years, Blue Ginger chef-owner Ming Tsai, who is also a national spokesman for the Food Allergy and Anaphylaxis Network, has created an elaborate system at his Wellesley, Massachusetts, restaurant to accommodate people with allergies. When a customer with a food allergy asks about a dish, the server checks the restaurant's Food Bible, a binder that contains every menu item with every ingredient and highlights any food allergens. Then the server asks Tsai or the manager whether the dish can be made safely. The server prints out a meal ticket with red type indicating that this is a food allergy meal and highlights the ticket with a marker.

Tsai or the manager on duty initials the ticket, which stays next to the plate until it is served.

Tsai, whose six-year-old son David has several life-threatening food allergies, said businesses in the hospitality industry have an obligation to serve everyone. But even he's been turned away from restaurants that don't want to take the risk of serving his son. "People used to discriminate based on skin color and wheelchairs. Nowadays there is discrimination against people with food allergies," Tsai said. "But creating policies to accommodate people with food allergies isn't going to put restaurants out of business. It's going to save lives."

■ The Food Allergy Buddy Card

The National Restaurant Association announced a collaborative effort with Supermarket Guru to promote the Food Allergy Buddy Dining Card program.[7] This program underscores the restaurant industry's continuing efforts to meet the needs of its customers by promoting a

---

[7] See appendix for more details on Supermarket Guru.

proactive commitment to food allergy safety. The Food Allergy Buddy Dining Card is a public service that allows consumers to easily communicate specific food allergies to restaurant waitstaff and chefs when dining in one of the nation's 900,000 restaurants.

■ School, Camp and College Cafeterias

Lunchrooms, camp canteens, and cafeterias, especially school and college cafeterias, are hot spots for the unsuspecting food-allergic students or campers as many near-fatal and fatal reactions have occurred in these locations. Children and young adults get careless when eating away from home. They don't carry their auto-injectable epinephrine or watch what they eat. The risks of an accidental exposure in schools, summer camps, and college campuses can be reduced with close cooperation among the student, parents, camper, and school and camp personnel. Preventive and educational measures for schools, colleges, and summer camps are fully covered in chapter 18. ●

Chapter 17

Additional Tips for Food Allergy[1]

■ Don't Be Killed By A Kiss.

In her excellent book *The Allergy Bible*, Linda Gamlin warned how food-allergic patients could be "killed by a kiss." Gamlin described a young man with a fish allergy who required emergency care after kissing his girlfriend who had just eaten mackerel. Most reports of this type involve children with peanut or tree nut allergy. In June 2002, Dr. Rosemary Hallett described seventeen patients who reacted to peanuts or tree nuts after being kissed by someone who had recently eaten peanuts or tree nuts.

Reactions began rapidly after the kiss (all in less than a minute). All seventeen victims reported localized itching, swelling, or hives in the kissed area. Four subjects reported wheezing. One child immediately developed a large hive at the exact site where he was kissed on the cheek by his mother just after she had tasted some pea soup that she was cooking on a stove. Minutes later, he developed flushing, generalized hives, swelling, and severe wheezing. He required epinephrine administration in a local emergency room.

A telephone survey by a Swedish group of allergists found that approximately 10 percent of 1,139 food allergic children and adults reacted to close exposure to peanuts or by kissing someone who had just eaten peanuts. A case from the Mayo Clinic in Minnesota described a twenty-year-old waitress with a known food allergy to shrimp and lobster. After a very passionate kiss from her boyfriend who had eaten shrimp one hour before, she developed severe swelling of her lips and throat, intestinal cramps, wheezing, and low blood pressure that required emergency care. In another incident, a peanut-allergic child experienced a severe allergic reaction after his aunt who had just eaten some peanuts kissed him.

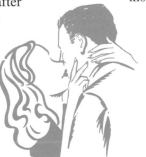

Two studies highlight the risks of transfer of a food allergen by saliva. Investigators gave two full tablespoons of peanut butter to non-allergic volunteers and found peanut allergen in their saliva up to $4^1/_2$ hours after ingestion, even after brushing their teeth. In another study in breast-feeding mothers who were fed peanuts, peanut allergen was detected in the mother's saliva six to eighteen hours after peanut ingestion. It seems logical to conclude that peanut proteins may also be present in other biological secretions long after the peanuts are ingested.

> *Thus, lips, saliva and other bodily fluids can transfer an allergenic food protein from one person to another and cause a near-fatal or fatal reaction.*

[1] This chapter contains additional tips on how the food-allergic individual, family, and caretakers can minimize the chances of accidental exposures to food allergens in everyday life.

In one poorly documented report of semen-transferred food allergen, there was no way of proving it was due to oral contact. Thus, lips, saliva and other bodily fluids can transfer an allergenic food protein from one person to another and cause a near-fatal or fatal reaction. Food-allergic individuals should inquire what their partners have recently eaten before kissing or engaging in any form of sexual activity. One recent paper concluded that peanut-allergic patients, particularly adolescents, must be counseled regarding the risks of kissing someone who has recently eaten peanuts, even if they have brushed their teeth. Practical advice may include brushing teeth and waiting a number of hours before kissing.

Dr. Scott Sicherer and his colleagues at the Jaffe Institute are conducting a study to determine the amount of peanut protein that may reside in the oral cavity over time following the ingestion of peanut protein. Another goal of this study is to determine efficient ways to clean the mouth after a meal so that saliva is unlikely to contain relevant amounts of food allergens.

■ The Bottom Line

The first symptom of a devastating food allergy reaction in asthmatic patients is often wheezing. Naturally, the victims' first impulse is to reach for their asthma rescue inhaler. However, in these devastating cases, the usual mode of death is cardiovascular collapse (shock and low blood pressure) where the asthma rescue medicine is of no value whatsoever, and life-saving epinephrine is essential for survival. I tell all my at-risk patients (especially young adult asthmatics with a peanut or tree nut allergy) that if they do not have their auto-injectable epinephrine device with them at the time of an accidental food ingestion that they might very well die.

Some colleagues think this somewhat overzealous, blunt approach may frighten patients or their families. So be it! In my opinion, a scared patient is more likely to be a compliant patient.

■ Know When NOT to Hold-Em!

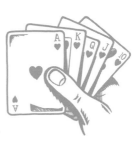

The increasing popularity of poker has led to several reports of cross-contamination by fellow card players consuming peanuts or tree nuts at the poker table and transferring peanut protein from the playing cards to the allergic person's hands or mouth. Reports of allergic reaction in a card player whose cards were contaminated by fellow players eating peanuts were recently highlighted in an article entitled "Peanut Allergy from Playing Cards—A Loosing Hand."

Dr. Ute Lepp and his colleagues described the experience of a man who needed treatment after experiencing swelling in his lips and tongue and shortness of breath while playing cards. The man was allergic to peanuts but said he had not eaten any peanuts. His card-playing companions also knew of his allergy and said they had not eaten any peanuts in front of him, and the peanuts had been stashed out of his way. However, once the patient said he had licked his thumb to help separate the cards, doctors got a clue as to how the patient was exposed. Lepp proposed that the cards contained traces of peanut protein from the fingers of the patient's opponents, which then reached the patient's mouth when he tried to separate the cards. As trace amounts of peanut protein can trigger a reaction, enough was present on the cards to cause symptoms. Thus, food-allergic card players should ask fellow players to avoid eating or handling offending foods during card games.

■ Beware the Backyard Barbecue

The family or neighborhood barbecue is another risky place for food allergy sufferers. Remind the host of your food allergy. Make sure the chef understands the risk of spatula carryover. If you are unsure what will be served, bring your own food or eat at home before going to the cookout. When there is a buffet line, ask to go through first to avoid cross-contamination reactions. Always bring your auto-injectable epinephrine device to the cookout.

■ Well Done Please

Thermal processing or cooking enhances texture and taste and kills potential pathogens. Heating a food can either increase or decrease its allergic potential. Foods that may become less allergenic when heated include most fruits and vegetables and some beef products. There are no reports of allergic reactions to homogenized or freeze-dried beef. Foods that are unaltered by heating include peanuts, tree nuts, seafood, and wheat. Pasteurization does not remove milk protein that may be hidden in hot dogs, meatballs, ham, sausages, bologna, tofu, and tuna. Celery and celeriac (a European form of celery) are not rendered less allergenic by heating. Seafood

Airborne seafood allergens have caused several fatal reactions. Salmon and tuna may be rendered less allergenic by heating and canning procedures.

proteins are very heat-stable and often become more allergenic when heated. Airborne seafood allergens have caused several fatal reactions. Salmon and tuna may be rendered less allergenic by heating and canning procedures.

■ Read Those Labels!

Throughout this book, I have listed names and hidden sources for important food allergens. The only way for someone with food allergies to reduce the risk of a potentially life-threatening allergic reaction is to completely avoid foods that contain the allergens. Food-allergic consumers are forced to decipher food labels every time they shop, a terrifying and dangerous process that is made even more difficult by confusing technical language used in ingredient statements.

One Food and Drug Administration survey looking for undeclared peanut, egg, and milk protein in food manufacturing plants found 25 percent of food ingredients were not properly labeled. A study at Mount Sinai School of Medicine in New York City demonstrated that after reading a series of labels, only 7 percent of parents of children with milk allergy correctly identified products that contained milk, and only 22 percent identified products that contained soy protein. There are many reports of adverse food reactions related to faulty labeling. Sixteen percent of 489 people surveyed at a food allergy conference reported they had allergic reactions because of misunderstood label terms, and 22 percent had a reaction to allergens not specified on food labels. Be aware that labels may vary from country to country. Canada uses the term, "may contain." In the United Kingdom the label may state: "not suitable for nut allergy sufferers." In the United States three formats are used: "may contain," "manufactured on shared equipment," or "shared facility."

The local supermarket is the best place to hone your label-reading skills. For example, be aware that albumin refers to egg; caseinate refers to milk; and textured vegetable protein refers to soybean. The term "natural flavors" could refer to peanuts, tree nuts, or any other food protein. The new FALCPA law that requires food manufacturers to identify the eight major food allergens in plain English will undoubtedly ease the burden of label reading.

■ Crossover Reactions

One of the more difficult tasks confronted by the allergy specialist is determining the relevance of cross-reacting food allergens. Many foods, pollens, and chemicals (like latex) share common proteins that may lead to positive skin and CAP RAST tests and allergic reactions. On the other hand, a positive skin or blood test does not always mean you will react to that particular food. Fortunately numerous clinical studies on potential cross-reactions between legumes, tree nuts, seeds, seafood, grains, meat products, fruits, pollens, and latex have helped to sort out the risk of cross-reactions between various food groups.

If you are allergic to cow's milk, you have a 90 percent chance of reacting to goat or sheep's milk but only a 10 percent chance of reacting to beef products. Only 5 percent of patients allergic to hen's eggs will react to chicken or poultry products. More than 50 to 75 percent of patients allergic to one finfish will react to other finfish. Crustacean-allergic patients have a 50 to 75 percent chance of reacting to other crustaceans.

Crossover reactions among crustaceans, finfish, and mollusks are uncommon. Only 5 to 10 percent of peanut-allergic patients react to other legumes (peas or beans) or soy products. But there is a one-in-three chance of reacting to another tree nut. Most wheat-allergic patients (80 percent) tolerate other grains like rye, barley, oats, rice, and corn. There is a high rate of crossover, about 90 percent, between fruits and vegetables that are members of the same food family. Warning: Do not self-experiment by ingesting potential cross-reacting foods without the advice and consent of an allergy specialist. The table compiled by Sicherer (see table 17.1) succinctly summarizes the odds of a crossover reaction between the major animal and plant food allergens.[2]

■ Danger in the Sky

The close confines of an airplane cabin are another precarious environment for passengers with food allergies. FAAN interviewed thirty-five people and families who experienced a reaction to peanuts in airplanes. Fourteen reactions were due to ingestion, seven were due to touching peanut particles, and fourteen patients described reactions after inhalation of peanut particles. Most reactions were first-time exposures in young children.

Researchers from the University of California-Davis surveyed 403 people with a food allergy. Ten percent reported an in-flight allergic reaction, including several

2 *Journal of Allergy and Clinical Immunology*, December 2001.

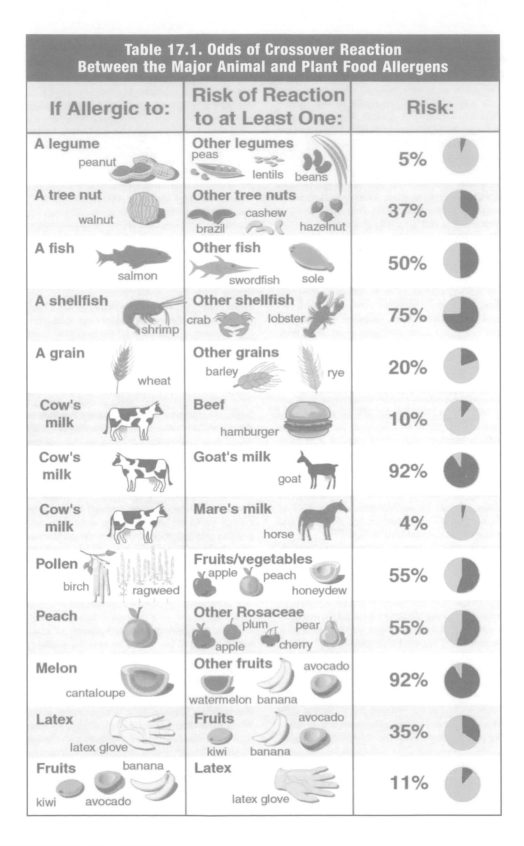

Table 17.1. Odds of Crossover Reaction Between the Major Animal and Plant Food Allergens

If Allergic to:	Risk of Reaction to at Least One:	Risk:	
A legume — peanut	Other legumes — peas, lentils, beans	5%	
A tree nut — walnut	Other tree nuts — cashew, brazil, hazelnut	37%	
A fish — salmon	Other fish — swordfish, sole	50%	
A shellfish — shrimp	Other shellfish — crab, lobster	75%	
A grain — wheat	Other grains — barley, rye	20%	
Cow's milk	Beef — hamburger	10%	
Cow's milk	Goat's milk — goat	92%	
Cow's milk	Mare's milk — horse	4%	
Pollen — birch, ragweed	Fruits/vegetables — apple, peach, honeydew	55%	
Peach	Other Rosaceae — plum, pear, apple, cherry	55%	
Melon — cantaloupe	Other fruits — avocado, watermelon, banana	92%	
Latex — latex glove	Fruits — avocado, kiwi, banana	35%	
Fruits — kiwi, avocado, banana	Latex — latex glove	11%	

anaphylactic events that required emergency landings. Most of these forty-four victims had an FAAP in place. While they were advised to carry epinephrine, many foolishly kept it in their checked luggage, not their carry-on baggage. Only 30 percent had injectable epinephrine with them in the airplane cabin at the time of their reaction. In one episode, the plane had to make an emergency landing after injectable epinephrine did not control a woman's symptoms. This patient, who had a lifelong allergy to peanut and tree nuts, reacted to pistachio nuts that were hidden in a sauce. Another patient required overnight hospitalization after a plane made its scheduled landing, and two others required emergency treatment when they landed. Seventeen patients had reactions to peanuts, three to walnuts, two to macadamia nuts, and one to cashews. The reactions from airborne exposure that accounted for most of the peanut-induced reactions were mild, mainly consisting of itchy eyes and nose. However, eight patients (including two of the people with self-described severe reactions) reported wheezing when fellow passengers were eating peanuts. Only eight passengers, including three who required emergency treatment, notified flight attendants of their reactions.

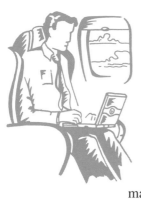

Many peanut-sensitive patients reported several mild episodes when peanut bags were opened but considered their reactions were not worthy of reporting to a flight attendant. One unfortunate passenger who experienced an in-flight nut reaction was dead on arrival when the plane landed at London's Heathrow Airport.

■ Timely Tips for Frequent Flyers

- If you are peanut-allergic, call the airline in advance. Most airlines will not serve peanuts on a flight when requested in advance. Fortunately, many airlines no longer serve peanut snacks.
- Book your flight early in the day. Morning departures are less likely to serve peanut snacks.
- To avoid check-in delays, always carry medical documentation that your auto-injectable epinephrine is a prescribed medical device, not a potential weapon.
- Carry a separate set of medications and your FAAP in your carry-on luggage.
- Wipe down serving trays and seat handles, and cover the seat with a coat.
- Look for discarded foods in the pockets in front of your seat.
- Bring your own food.
- Check out what your fellow passengers are eating. Airlines cannot guarantee a peanut-free flight as they cannot control what foods fellow passengers bring on board.
- Fly coach class. First-class passengers may be more at risk due to better air circulation and flight attendants may serve heated or roasted mixed nut dishes in flight.

■ Can You Fly Peanut-Free?

In 1998, the United States Department of Transportation (DOT) mandated that the major American airlines provide "peanut-free zones" for passengers with peanut allergy. The Air Transport Association, Congress, and the peanut industry strongly resisted this DOT directive that stemmed from the 1986 Air Carrier Access Act, a law guaranteeing disabled passengers full access to airlines. After getting complaints from peanut-allergic sufferers, the DOT reviewed a 1996 Mayo Clinic study that found peanut protein present in ventilation system filters after 5,000 hours of flight. "Particles of the allergen—in this particular case, peanuts—are small enough to actually float in the air," said Dr. David Tanner of the Atlanta Allergy & Asthma Clinic. "If they land on someone who is allergic, land in their eyes or in their nose, they can cause an actual allergic reaction."

Public awareness was heightened by several media reports on food anaphylaxis in public places and one death on an aircraft due to nut anaphylaxis. Southern peanut farmers and some lawmakers roasted the DOT over this new order.[3] A spokesman for the Southern Peanut Farmers Federation stated, "The order singles out peanuts over other foods that may cause allergic reactions. We think it's an unfair regulation because it singles out one product—our product—as opposed to all the other food allergens out there. If they do want allergy-free zones, we would like them to include all foods that are potentially allergens."

Airline officials maintained that the policy will not cause problems for peanut lovers on planes as long as they aren't booked on one of the handful of flights that includes a peanut allergy victim. "It's truly no big deal," said a Southwest Airlines spokesman. "Some people are upset by what came out of the government, but in terms of our operation, we'll just go with the flow." For Southwest, providing buffer zones was impossible because this airline uses open seating. Southwest continued what it has been doing for five years—operating peanut-free flights whenever any passenger notifies the airline of an allergy in advance.

A United Airlines spokesman stated that United was studying how best to comply with the directive. So far, United has simply banned peanuts from flights with identified allergic passengers. Continental and Alaska Airlines have stated they will remove peanuts from entire flights when such a request is made in advance. The DOT concluded there was not enough evidence to ban peanuts from flights, and the proposed ban was never implemented. At the time of this writing, domestic airlines that no longer serve peanut snacks include American, United, Northwest, Jet Blue, Delta Shuttle, US Air Spirit and ATA.[4] International carriers that do not serve peanuts include Aer Lingus, Alitalia, and British Airways. There are many reasons why a complete ban would not be effective and why patient education is a more useful proposal.

- Only body searches would guarantee a peanut-free flight.
- "Peanut Free" promotes false security that encourages complacency.
- A ban moves away from education and awareness to enforcing the ban.
- There are many other food triggers like sesame seeds, milk, eggs, fish, and wheat.

■ Cruise with Care

One of the more enjoyable aspects of taking a cruise is the wide array of fine cuisine that is available around-the-clock. Several tips for safely planning a cruise where food selections may be bewildering include:

---

[3] Stephanie Oswald and the Associated Press, "Hold the Peanuts: Government Order for Nut-Free Zones," *CNN.COM*, September 24, 1998, www.cnn.com/ TRAVEL/NEWS/9809/04/peanuts.

[4] "New Focus on Peanut Allergies," an episode of *Good Morning America*, November 30, 2005.

- Develop an FAAP before you cruise.
- Use a travel agent who transmits your concerns to the cruise line.
- Give a copy of your list of all allergenic foods to avoid and your FAAP to the cruise director.
- Be sure the ship has a medical facility capable of treating allergic reactions.
- Make sure you have additional travel insurance coverage should you have a reaction and require medical care or air evacuation.
- Provide the ship's medical facility, maitre d', and head chef with your list of food allergies and your FAAP.
- Eat your meals in the main dining room where the staff is aware of your food allergy.
- Avoid eating in cocktail areas and bars where food ingredients may not be listed or well-controlled.
- Before retiring, review the menu for the next day.
- When going ashore, carry your FAAP, medications, and a prepared box lunch.
- Bring your own cooler with alternative meals and desserts. When traveling with a food-allergic child, be sure all caretakers are aware of the child's food allergy and FAAP.

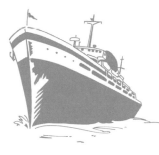

The bottom line: Don't leave home without it. Always carry several extra auto-injectable epinephrine devices, especially when traveling to undeveloped or Third World countries.

■ Don't Leave Home Without It!

A survey of seventy-five allergy specialists belonging to the World Allergy Organization by Dr. Estelle Simons found that many areas of the world have limited or no supplies of auto-injectable epinephrine kits for patients at risk of anaphylaxis. Widespread availability of auto-injectors in the United States, Europe, Canada, and Australia contrasts with a limited availability in Asia, South America, and Africa. Survey results revealed the cost for auto-injectors ranged from $30 to $110 and could vary twofold within the same country. The purchase cost in some countries was equivalent to a month's salary for many patients.

In the Asia-Pacific region, unusual triggers of anaphylaxis include buckwheat, bird's nest soup, royal jelly (ingested bee product), insect stings, bites from jellyfish, unusual bugs, and green ants. Simons' investigation raised concerns for individuals at risk of anaphylaxis who may develop an episode when traveling internationally, use their auto-injector, and subsequently be unable to obtain a prescription refill. The bottom line: Don't leave home without it. Always carry several extra auto-injectable epinephrine devices, especially when traveling to undeveloped or Third World countries.

■ Consult A Dietitian

Food allergies mandate that offending foods be eliminated from one's diet. Teaching the food-allergic patient and family to maintain good nutrition while avoiding healthy foods, such as eggs, milk, peanuts, or tree nuts, is a major challenge as many allergenic foods contain essential vitamins and nutrients. While written information on appropriate diets is widely available from books, health food stores, and publications of FAAN, the best trained professional to deal with your diet is a certified dietitian. These professionals are college graduates who have completed postgraduate training that is followed by an internship and a national certifying examination. A dietitian will review one's diet and make appropriate changes to replace nutrients present in the avoided foods. The dietitian will check caloric intake (including carbohydrates, protein, and fats) and maintain a proper balance between these three essential parts of your diet. The dietitian can answer questions regarding cooking, eating out, grocery shopping, reading labels and identifying hidden allergens, and providing recipes using non-allergic foods. Personal counseling and reading cookbooks is an essential part of developing a sound program for food allergen avoidance.

■ Timely Tips for Patients and Parents

When Grocery Shopping

- Do not buy a food if you do not understand the label.
- Call the food manufacturer with any questions about ingredients.
- Beware of imitation seafood and processed foods.
- Learn how to read kosher labels.
- Avoid selecting bakery goods from bulk bins.
- Be careful in delis where the same slicer cuts both meats and cheeses.

While at Home

- Do not bring allergenic foods into the home.
- Designate a special shelf for the food-allergic family member.
- Use stickers provided by FAAN for safe and unsafe foods.

- Order FAAN's *Food Allergy News Cookbook*.
- Avoid cross-contamination when cooking.
- Study allergy-free recipes.
- Cook special meals first.
- Cook and freeze allergy-free meals and desserts.

Train Your Babysitters

- Educate them about food allergy—have them read this book.
- Teach them how and when to administer auto-injectable epinephrine.
- Teach them how to read labels.
- Put out a tray of safe foods and snacks.
- Always leave contact and emergency phone numbers.

Travel Tips and Vacations

- Bring your auto-injectable epinephrine, allergy medications, and FAAP.
- Stay at motels or inns with kitchen facilities.
- Bring a cooler, toaster oven, or camp stove to store and cook your own foods.
- Order your salads dry, and use your own salad dressings and oils.
- Plan ahead when dining out. Contact the manager or chef in advance.
- Go to resorts with nearby medical facilities.
- Avoid remote cabins.
- Read FAAN's *Traveling with Food Allergy*.

■ Trick or Treat, Smell My Feet, Give Me Something SAFE to Eat.

Several holidays raise the threshold of an accidental reaction to a hidden food. Halloween parties and trick-or-treating pose a big risk when a wide array of candy is passed out to hungry trick-or-treaters.

Many non-allergic candies are processed on the same machines used to make milk, peanuts, and tree nuts containing candy. Parents should not allow children to eat from their bags of goodies until the parents have carefully checked their treats out. Request your neighbors and friends to hand out non-allergenic foods and candy.

Have your child carry a sign that states, "Trick or Treat, Smell My Feet, Give Me Something SAFE to Eat!" Better yet, get involved with FAAN's National Halloween Trick-or-Treat Kids' Program. In 2004, FAAN instituted a nationwide program for Halloween—the 2004 Trick or Treat for Food Allergy Halloween Coin Collection Program. FAAN members nationwide embraced the program that was established to provide a food-free activity for children who have food allergies. Young FAAN members participated by asking friends, school staff, relatives, and neighbors for coins instead of treats to support food allergy research and education. Participating children qualified for prizes, such as T-shirts and gift certificates.

■ Scoop Safely

The ice cream parlor is another minefield for individuals who are allergic to peanuts or tree nuts. Rinsing an ice cream scoop with water will not remove potent allergens after scoops have been used to serve ice creams containing peanuts or tree nuts. Several of my patients have had accidental exposures and reactions in these establishments. Be careful with toppings. It may be wise for asthmatic, peanut-allergic, or tree nut-allergic patients to avoid ice cream parlors altogether. Some ice cream parlors provide protection. Ben and Jerry's franchises post a sign that alerts allergic customers to notify their scooper of their food allergies before they are served. Also, many ice cream parlors offer a soft-serve ice cream or frozen yogurt option. Upon request, the server will usually be willing to find the soft-serve packaging so the customer can read the ingredients.

■ Hospital Food

In my medical school and residency days, the term "hospital food" was strictly an oxymoron. Today, many hospitals and medical centers offer elaborate four-star menus from foods prepared in large kitchens for consumption in patients' rooms or hospital cafeterias. Choices for food-allergic patients and employees require close communication with hospital dietitians, checking all food trays, or bringing your own food from home. For those interested in obtaining more information on food allergies and hospitals, I recommend *The Food Allergy Training Guide for Hospital and Food Service Staff* written by Shideh Mofidi, MS, RD, and edited by FAAN. This publication is a comprehensive guide for capturing food allergy information from patients and distributing the information to the kitchen staff to help them prepare allergen-safe meals for patients and hospital staff.

■ A Not-So-Best Man

JB is a twenty-four-year-old patient of mine who was attending his brother's wedding reception as the best man. He had a history of mild asthma and several prior allergic reactions to various foods, including tree nuts. Somewhat to my amazement, he had never sought emergency or specialty care for these reactions—many of which were quite severe. At the beginning of the wedding reception, he developed burning in his throat and swelling of his face, lips, and tongue minutes after ingesting hors d'oeuvres that contained hidden nuts in a pesto sauce. As an auto-injectable epinephrine device was not available, he was put in a taxi for transport to a local hospital that, fortunately, was only one block away. On the way to the hospital, he lost consciousness; and, on arrival at the emergency room, he required immediate intubation (placing a breathing tube in the throat) and life-saving intensive care for the next twenty-four hours.

Thankfully, he fully recovered from his life-threatening reaction. Allergy tests revealed he was very allergic to several species of tree nuts, including pine nuts. This near-fatal reaction points out that food-allergic patients should not deny their problem and be very cautious when attending celebrations or functions where hidden food allergens are abundant.

A good rule of thumb to follow when going to Grandmother's home for Thanksgiving Day dinner is, "Don't eat it if you can't see it!"

Thus, weddings, Bar Mitzvahs, birthday parties, and family holiday dinners are hot spots where a wide array of foods are served and eaten. Family Thanksgiving gatherings are especially hazardous, as foods, such as gravy, vegetables, mashed potatoes, and exotic pies prepared by different family members, may hide deadly allergens. A good rule of thumb to follow when going to Grandmother's home for Thanksgiving Day dinner is, "Don't eat it if you can't see it!" I highly recommend FAAN's book, *Food Allergy News Holiday Cookbook*, which provides a wide range of safe recipes and meal plans for year-round holiday celebrations.

Chapter 18

Managing Food Allergies at School, Camp, and College

The ongoing food allergy epidemic has hit parents, caretakers of children, schools, colleges, and camp personnel the hardest. Child-care centers, schools, summer camps, and colleges offer a transition from one's home to the outside world, where children and young adults learn to develop healthy friendships and social skills and improve their self-esteem and self-confidence. However, transferring from the safe confines of one's home to a school, camp, or college environment can be a traumatic and bewildering experience for the food-allergic student or camper, and his or her family.

Some schools may offer resistance to putting protocols and policies in place to keep the allergic child safe. Several years ago, I met with teachers and school administrators from a local school district to address the problem that a teacher did not want a particular child with a severe peanut allergy enrolled in her classroom. After I reminded this group that this food-allergic child met the definition of having a disability and was covered by the Americans with Disabilities Act, they promptly put programs in place that ensured the safety of this child in their school. Food allergies are covered under Section 504 of the Rehabilitation Act of 1973 that prevents discrimination based on a disability in any program receiving federal funding. In 1990, the federal government extended these rights to cover students in schools that do not receive federal funding. Thus, all private schools and child-care centers must obey these federal regulations even if they do not receive federal funding.

When a particular school does not have a food allergy program in place, parents may want to file a 504 plan. This 504 plan is a written agreement between the parents and the school that outlines steps to keep the student safe while allowing full access to all school activities. To obtain a 504 plan, parents should contact the 504 coordinator in their school district. They will need a letter from their doctor outlining the food allergy problem. The 504 coordinator will then refer you to a school nurse who can offer you an individualized 504 plan or arrange a meeting with the 504 team to establish safe guidelines for your child.[1]

> *All private schools and child-care centers must obey these federal regulations, even if they do not receive federal funding.*

■ Food Reactions at School

In 2000, a joint study from the Jaffe Food Institute in New York City and the Food Allergy and Anaphylaxis Network (FAAN) described the clinical features of allergic reactions to peanuts and tree nuts in school and day-care settings. One hun-

---

[1] "Students with Food Allergies: How the Laws Can Help" (FAAN: Fairfax, VA).

dred families who enrolled in FAAN's Peanut and Tree Nut Registry detailed 124 allergic food reactions that took place at school. The vast majority of reactions (115) were due to peanuts; only nine were triggered by tree nuts. Nearly two-thirds took place in a day-care or preschool setting. For one in every four victims, it was their first reaction; and one in every four reactions was classified as a severe reaction. A total of 32 percent had experienced one prior reaction, 37 percent had had two, and 31 percent had had three or more reactions. Sixty percent of the reactions were due to ingesting the offending food, 25 percent were caused by direct skin contact, and 15 percent were triggered by inhaling food particles.

Ninety percent of these reactions required treatment. Antihistamines were given in 84 percent of the incidents, and epinephrine was administered in 28 percent. A school nurse was available for only 23 percent of the reactions. Cooked or baked products served at birthday or holiday celebrations triggered many reactions. Other sources of accidental exposure included arts, craft, science projects involving peanut butter, and poorly supervised field trips and bus rides.

Most schools in this survey were not prepared to deal with a food allergy reaction. Only one in every three students had a food allergy action plan (FAAP) or treatment plan in place. Treatment delays were a result of delayed recognition of a reaction, attempting to call parents first, not following emergency plans, and, in one case, an inability to administer auto-injectable epinephrine. This study concluded that peanut and tree nut reactions were common in school and day-care environments, and that school personnel needed more education on how to recognize and treat food allergy reactions.

■ School Nurse Studies

Another FAAN survey confirmed what many individuals in the medical and school communities have believed for years: food allergy is a growing health and safety concern in the classroom. Nearly 44 percent of the school nurses surveyed reported an increase in students with food allergies in elementary schools over the past five years. More than one-third of the school nurses indicated that they had 10 or more students in their school with a food allergy. Nearly 90 percent stated that, compared with other health issues, food allergy in school-age children was a serious issue.

A Massachusetts Department of Education study analyzed the use of auto-injectable epinephrine in 109 school districts. During a two-year period, there were 115 administrations of epinephrine in the elementary schools. Most reactions were due to accidental ingestion of peanut or tree nuts and took place in a classroom. Students were usually treated in the school nurse's office, and 80 percent were sent to an emergency room. Many reactions (75 percent) were classified as severe. However, one in every four reactions occurred on the school playground, traveling to or from school, or on field trips. The following case illustrates the dangers of food reactions in poorly prepared schools.

BF was a nine-year-old male with asthma and nut allergy who was given some peanut candy by a classmate in school. Ninety minutes later he went to the nurse's office complaining of abdominal pain. Unfortunately, the school nurse was not aware of his peanut allergy. Within twenty minutes, he began to vomit and have difficulty breathing. Three hours after ingesting the peanut-laced candy, he died in a local emergency room.

Clearly this preventable death that took place in an ill-prepared school points out the need for more education of all caretakers of children as well as the need to administer epinephrine immediately after the symptoms begin, even if the symptoms are mild in nature. Fortunately, the efforts of FAAN, the Food Allergy Initiative (FAI), the National Association of School Nurses, and several state departments of education have led to the development of sophisticated guidelines to educate school personnel and protect food-allergic schoolchildren. Today, most of the schools I deal with have progressive programs in place to ensure the safety of all students with food allergies. As we shall discuss, each player in this game, including parents, students, school nurses, teachers, administrators, cafeteria workers, coaches, trainers, gym instructors, and even school bus drivers must be part of a team approach that ensures the safety of the food-allergic student in a school setting.

Child-Care Centers

Preschool and child-care centers are the most difficult sites for ensuring the safety of a food-allergic child. Potential problems in child-care centers include:

- A lack of a full-time school nurse
- Students grabbing food from their classmates
- Students picking discarded food off the floor
- Students licking food-contaminated toys
- Teachers using eggs, milk, and peanuts in lesson plans

In one survey of 85 Chicago day-care centers, only 55 percent of center directors and 48 percent of teachers had ever received training in the recognition and treatment of a food allergy reaction. Nearly 70 percent of the centers kept auto-injectable epinephrine devices in a locked closet. Forty-four Chicago center directors and teachers were tested before and after attending a seminar on food allergy and anaphylaxis. Before the seminar, only 24 percent knew how to properly administer epinephrine. After the seminar, 77 percent could properly inject it into the outer thigh muscle. The seminar also improved their overall knowledge of anaphylaxis. However, a follow-up study twelve months later revealed a marked decline in the ability of these child-care providers to diagnose and treat anaphylaxis. One year later, only 31 percent knew how to correctly administer epinephrine. This survey points out the need for repeated educational efforts in this area. All schools, especially preschool and elementary grades, should consider showing FAAN's child-directed videos on food allergy to the classmates of the allergic child.[2]

> *All schools, especially preschool and elementary grades, should consider showing FAAN's child-directed videos on food allergy to the classmates of the allergic child.*

Sabrina's Law

In May 2005, representatives from three Canadian political parties unanimously passed a bill that required Ontario schools to develop a policy for students with life-

---

[2] *Alexander, The Elephant Who Couldn't Eat Peanuts*, videocassette, produced by Food Allergy & Anaphylaxis Network (Fairfax, VA: 1994) and Anne Muñoz-Furlong and Mariel Christine Furlong, *How Lenny Found Out About his Food Allergy* (Fairfax, VA: Food Allergy & Anaphylaxis Network, 2001).

threatening allergies.[3] The bill, which took effect in January 2006, is called Sabrina's Law in memory of Sabrina Shannon, a thirteen-year-old student who died after eating French fries in her school cafeteria.

In 2001, Sabrina, an honor student with asthma and severe milk, soybean, and peanut allergies, helped produce a documentary on food allergy. In September 2004, she died shortly after eating French fries served with a pair of tongs suspected to have been in contact with cheese in her school cafeteria kitchen. It was just the second time she had ever eaten in her school cafeteria. She did so only after verifying with the cafeteria staff that the fries had been cooked in vegetable oil. When the reaction started, Sabrina thought she was having an asthma attack, and the administration of injectable epinephrine was unfortunately delayed. Her EpiPen auto-injector syringe apparently was in her school locker.

After Sabrina's death, her parents, Sara and Mike Shannon, crusaded to increase public awareness of their daughter's condition. Their efforts prompted Dave Levac, a former high school principal and Canadian legislator, to introduce a law forcing schools to establish an emergency plan for students prone to anaphylaxis. Sabrina's law is the first of its kind in North America. The law requires Ontario school boards to have strategies in place that reduce the risk of exposure to anaphylactic agents including:

- The school system must have a plan for disseminating information about life-threatening allergies.
- They must conduct regular training on how to deal with life-threatening allergies for school employees and others who are in regular contact with students.
- School principals must develop an individual plan for each student who has an anaphylactic allergy.
- School principals must ensure that parents, guardians, and students are asked to supply information about any life-threatening allergies.
- School principals must maintain a file for each anaphylactic student and monitor proper storage for emergency EpiPens.

Ontario school personnel may be preauthorized to administer medication or supervise a student while the student takes medication in response to an anaphylactic reaction when the school has current treatment information and the consent of the parent, guardian, or student. It is the obligation of the parent, guardian, or student to ensure that the information in the student's file is kept current and includes the medication that the student is taking. If a school employee has reason to believe that a student is experiencing an anaphylactic reaction, the employee may administer epinephrine or other prescribed medication, even if there is no preauthorization. The law states that no action for damages may be instituted in relation to an act done in good faith or any neglect or default in good faith in response to an anaphylactic reaction unless the damages are the result of an employee's gross negligence.

■ An Australian Experience

In September 2004, Alex Baptist died after an anaphylactic reaction while attending his local kindergarten.[4] It's suspected that he inadvertently came into contact with trace amounts of peanuts. When Alex was

[3] Lee Greenberg, *Ottawa Citizen* (Ontario, Canada), May 17, 2005.

[4] Helen Dalley, *Sunday This Week Reporter* (Victoria, Australia), September 18, 2005.

a toddler, he had been diagnosed as being peanut-allergic and was prescribed an EpiPen. What's frightening about Alex's story is that once they understood the potential severity of Alex's allergy, the family did what medical experts told them would keep their child safe. Alex never left home without his EpiPen, and his parents told everyone who came in contact with their son that exposure to the slightest trace of peanuts could potentially kill him. While their home state of Victoria, Australia, was woefully lax in forcing schools and preschools to adopt proper management plans and care training for anaphylaxis, the Baptists' kindergarten supported his parents' vigilance and only allowed fruit into the school. An FAAP—clearly detailing what to do if Alex had a reaction, swelled up, or stopped breathing—was prominently displayed in the kindergarten. The family says they were assured that the teachers were properly trained to use an EpiPen.

But on the day of Alex's reaction, things went horribly wrong. Nigel and Martha Baptist believe that somehow Alex was exposed to peanut butter and that the childcare staff failed to administer his life-saving epinephrine. Martha Baptist told *Sunday This Week* that Alex became distressed and had trouble breathing on the playground soon after morning tea. He collapsed and lost consciousness—showing characteristic symptoms of an acute allergic reaction. Martha Baptist says she was told that when a teacher went to administer Alex's EpiPen, the teacher accidentally jabbed it into her finger instead. "We don't believe that Alex got his adrenaline (epinephrine)," said Martha Baptist.

But what shattered Alex's parents is that they believe no second attempt was made to administer adrenaline (epinephrine) belonging to another child at the kindergarten. "It does concern us because there was another EpiPen in the cupboard and a decision was made not to give that to Alex," said Martha Baptist. Alex's grief-stricken father Nigel Baptist said: "It's just so hard for us to comprehend; you know that anyone could not give it to our Alex who was there lying, dying on the floor." Despite receiving CPR from teachers at the kindergarten, Alex had stopped breathing by the time an ambulance team arrived and could not be revived.

Michael Vassili, a lawyer acting for the Baptist family, believes that the kindergarten staff had not been adequately trained to manage the crisis: "Anyone who was properly trained would know that that child needed adrenaline, he needed the EpiPen immediately. If there was an EpiPen there, proper training would have guided the appropriate person to the EpiPen, and it would have been administered." Dr. Rob Loblay, head of the RPA Hospital Allergy Clinic in Sydney, Australia, believes the events surrounding Alex Baptist's death highlight a common concern among child caretakers and teachers faced with treating an anaphylactic reaction. "Am I legally liable if I use an EpiPen when it hasn't been prescribed or use another child's EpiPen? These are unfounded fears and so we need to sort of address that issue as well."

■ A Legislative Groundswell

The important advocacy efforts of FAAN have started a legislative groundswell at both the state and federal levels in the United States.[5] State representatives in Vermont enacted a law that requires schools to implement food-allergy management strategies, such as staff training, emer-

---

[5] For updated information on these legislative issues, or to find out how you can help enact new laws in your state, e-mail FAAN's director of legislative and regulatory research (see appendix).

gency preparedness, and meal substitutions. Similar legislation has also been introduced in New Jersey. Connecticut recently enacted a law to develop guidelines for the management of students with life-threatening food allergies. Each local and regional board was required to implement a plan based on the state guidelines by July 1, 2006. A similar law was signed in Tennessee in June 2006. One bill under consideration in Massachusetts would require all public schools to have a full-time school nurse. It won't be long before all 50 states enact some sort of legislation on this important issue.

> *One bill under consideration in Massachusetts would require all public schools to have a full-time school nurse. It won't be long before all 50 states enact some sort of legislation on this important issue.*

■ The Food Allergy and Anaphylaxis Management Act

In October 2005, Rep. Nita Lowey (D-NY), a long-time advocate for food-allergic victims, introduced the Food Allergy and Anaphylaxis Management Act of 2005 (H.R. 4063). Representative Lowey was the initial sponsor of the Food Allergen Labeling and Consumer Protection Act (FALCPA). The law calls on the federal government to create national guidelines for schools regarding the management of students at risk for anaphylaxis. As policies vary from state to state and school to school, these federal guidelines will serve as a model for school districts or individual schools.

■ Managing Life-Threatening Food Allergies in Schools

Some states and school districts have taken matters into their own hands and have published proactive guidelines for managing life-threatening food allergies in the school setting. The Massachusetts Department of Education has published an excellent monograph entitled *Managing Life Threatening Food Allergies in Schools.* A task force of medical professionals, school administrators, school nurses, teachers, and food service directors created this manual that focuses on a team approach. It addresses ways to assist schools to develop protocols for the care of students with food allergies and life-threatening allergic conditions.

In 2006, the Ann Arbor, Michigan, Public Schools Food Allergy Task Force published a comprehensive sixty-six-page monograph, *Guidelines & Practices: Managing Life-Threatening Food Allergies in Elementary School Children.* The goal of this manual is to establish a set of consistent practices within the Ann Arbor school district. The manual outlines how to develop a collaborative partnership among the school, families, and medical personnel to provide a safe and healthy learning environment that enables parents and their children with food allergies to make the transition from the safety of their homes into the expanding world of schools.

This manual precisely outlines the roles and responsibilities of specific individuals—from the school administrator to school custodian and bus drivers—in a detailed checklist format. In addition, the manual contains several templates for composing letters to classmates, families, and parents; detailing how to respond to a student with life-threatening allergies; and much more. If your school or school district wants to develop a food allergy plan for students with food allergies, I recommend using FAAN's manuals and the Massachusetts and Ann Arbor publications as models for developing such guidelines. In the following section, I will outline the roles and responsibilities of specific individuals in the management of students with food allergies.[6]

■ Role of Parents or Guardians

Prevention starts at home. The parents' first job is to develop an Individualized Health Care Plan (IHCP) that should include reports from primary health-care providers or allergy specialists that details the student's allergy and medication program. The best plan is the Food Allergy Action Plan (FAAP) developed by FAAN that describes the signs, symptoms, and appropriate treatments of allergic reactions (see appendix, page 271). The FAAP provides informed consent and contact numbers for parents, guardians, and health-care providers. Responsible parents should review the IHCP and FAAP with the school nurse and classroom teacher each year prior to the opening of school.

Parents must provide schools with a minimum of two up-to-date EpiPens or Twinject devices and be sure that these devices are stored in unlocked cabinets and are accessible to all school personnel during and after school hours. Parents should provide safe snacks for classroom parties,

and, whenever possible, accompany food-allergic children on field trips.

In addition, parents must teach students:

- How to recognize the symptoms of an allergic reaction
- How to communicate clearly as soon as possible when reactions begin
- How to read labels
- To avoid food-sharing at lunchtime
- To stress the importance of hand-washing before and after eating
- To report teasing, bullying, and threats to an adult authority
- To not share their auto-injector devices with other students
- How to say "no thank you" when offered food not from home

Responsible parents should review the IHCP and FAAP with the school nurse and classroom teacher each year prior to the opening of school.

■ Role of the Student

Steps responsible students can take to play a role in managing their food allergies:

- Assume responsibility for avoiding allergens.
- Do not trade or share foods in the classroom or cafeteria.
- Do not eat foods that do not come from home.
- Wash your hands before and after eating.
- Know the signs and symptoms of allergic reactions.
- Inform school personnel after accidental exposures.
- Make sure the school staff is aware of your food allergies.
- Develop a relationship with school nurses, principals, and classroom teach-

---

[6] Most of the material in this section is condensed from the publications of FAAN, the Massachusetts Department of Education, and the Ann Arbor, Michigan, Public School District. To obtain the Massachusetts publication, contact the Massachusetts Department of Education at 350 Main Street, Malden, MA 02148, telephone 781-338-3000, or via the Internet at www.doe.mass.edu. The Ann Arbor manual can be downloaded from the Web site of Ann Arbor, Michigan, Public Schools: www.aaps.k12.mi.us

ers related to the management of your food allergies.

- Sit just behind or to the right of drivers when riding in a school bus.
- Know where epinephrine auto-injectors are kept in the school.
- When permitted, always carry your auto-injectable epinephrine devices.
- Be sure up-to-date auto-injectors are present in your backpacks.

■ Role of School Administrators

The buck stops at the top. The school administrator (or principal) has the ultimate responsibility for providing a safe environment for food allergic students. He or she must:

- Provide training and educational seminars for all school personnel.
- Educate the school community about life-threatening allergies.
- Provide emergency communication for all school activities.
- Provide a full-time nurse in schools enrolling allergic students.
- Support a proactive relationship between students, families, and school nurses.
- Develop and implement plans for responding to potentially life-threatening food allergy reactions.
- Ensure that all substitute teachers are made aware of children in classes with food allergies prior to the start of the day.
- Provide special training for food service and custodial personnel.
- Inform caretakers if students have allergic reactions at school.
- Ensure that students are placed in classrooms where teachers are trained to administer auto-injectable epinephrine.
- Only hire substitutes and assistant teachers who have been fully trained

and have no reservations about administering emergency medications.

- Have emergency communication plans for contacting nurses when nurses are not on-site.
- Carefully complete all overnight field trip permission requests to reflect food allergy concerns.
- Eliminate unscheduled and unplanned classroom celebrations or food rewards.

■ The School Nurse— A Tom Brady

Any school enrolling a child with a significant food allergy needs a full-time school nurse. If your child's school does not have a full-time nurse, transfer to a school in your district that has complete nursing coverage. Once the parent provides the school nurse with an IHCP and an FAAP, the school nurse becomes the Tom Brady (i.e. quarterback) in this ballgame. The school nurse must not only thoroughly and regularly communicate with the parents and the student, but must teach all school personnel how to handle a food-allergic student. This requires meeting individually or in groups with the school principal, classroom teacher, food service director, cafeteria staff, coaches, trainers, gym instructors, custodians, local emergency response team, and school bus drivers. The school nurse must be organized, thorough, and persistent, as there are many key players in this game. Furthermore, some of the players may be resistant to new or different protocols that are necessary to keep these students safe.

Role of the School Nurse

The school nurse must:

- Know the student's needs, medications, and physician's orders.
- Have immediate access to local EMTs and emergency rooms.
- Be sure that up-to-date auto-injectors are readily accessible in unlocked locations even after school hours.
- Train other school personnel how to use these auto-injectors and determine which responsible students can carry their own devices.
- Maintain a list of trained school staff in the main office.
- Educate new personnel as needed and re-educate previously trained staff twice a year.
- Introduce yourself to the students and show the students how to get to nurses' office and how to communicate should symptoms occur.
- Make sure there are contingency plans in place for substitute nurses.
- Conduct fire drill-like practices to prepare the school staff to deal with anaphylactic emergency reactions.
- In large schools where telephone communication is inconsistent or if the school has a remote gym, playground or playing field, school personnel should be supplied with radios or cell phones to contact the school nurse quickly and easily.

Should Students Carry Epinephrine Auto-injectors?

Currently, many states have laws or regulations that allow students to possess (and self-administer) their prescribed epinephrine in schools, provided that certain conditions—such as consent from parents, physicians, school nurses, and local school boards—are met. Such policies help ensure that life-saving auto-injectable epinephrine will be quickly accessible during anaphylactic emergencies. The states that have passed such laws are listed on FAAN's Web site under "advocacy." If your state is not on this list, it doesn't necessarily mean that students cannot carry their epinephrine at school. It only means that there is no statewide law or regulation specifically allowing it.

Allowing students to carry certain prescribed medications is becoming more common to ensure immediate access to these life-saving devices. Keeping auto-injector devices in nurses' offices or student's lockers can have devastating results as typified by the death of Sabrina Shannon who died in her school cafeteria. In my opinion, if overly restrictive policies lead to delays in administering auto-injectable epinephrine, schools that insist on such policies could be held libel for bad outcomes.

Good Samaritan Protection

Most states have Good Faith or Good Samaritan laws to protect individuals who render emergency assistance in good faith, with no expectation of payments, and who hand patients over to appropriate medical personnel (such as EMTs or school nurses) as soon as possible. Some states have recently enacted Good Samaritan laws that specifically refer to auto-injectable epinephrine. A Connecticut law allows camps, day-care centers, and before- and after-school programs to train employees in epinephrine administration upon written requests of parents or guardians and extends Good Samaritan protection to these individuals in the event that they administer epinephrine during an emergency. A Rhode Island law extends Good Samaritan protection to school bus drivers and school bus monitors who administer auto-injectable epinephrine. A similar Wisconsin law applies to all school employees, volunteers, and bus drivers. Illinois, Michigan, Maine, and New Hampshire have recently enacted laws that help ensure that auto-injectable epinephrine is readily accessible to children attending recreational camps. The American Academy of Pediatrics' Ad Hoc Committee on Anaphylaxis in the School recommends "allowing a child with a history of anaphylaxis to carry epinephrine with him or her at all times, and self-administering it if a reaction occurs. If this is not feasible, epinephrine should be available not only in the nurse's office but in the classroom or cafeteria where it is more likely to be needed."

> *The American Academy of Pediatrics' Ad Hoc Committee on Anaphylaxis in the School recommends "allowing a child with a history of anaphylaxis to carry epinephrine with him or her at all times, and self-administering it if a reaction occurs. If this is not feasible, epinephrine should be available not only in the nurse's office but in the classroom or cafeteria where it is more likely to be needed."*

■ Role of Classroom Teacher

The classroom teacher, especially in child-care centers, preschools, and elementary grades where eating is often allowed in classrooms, is quite likely to be the first person (responder) to encounter a student having an allergic or anaphylactic reaction. Like the school nurse, the classroom teacher should be aware of the student's ICHP and keep the student's FAAP (with a photo) accessible at all times. The teacher must learn the signs and symptoms of an allergic reaction and know when and how to administer auto-injectable epinephrine. In addition, the classroom teacher must:

- Make lunch a pleasant experience for the student.
- Encourage the student to be independent.
- Sit down with the child and explain labels and need for caution.
- Prohibit food sharing and food trading.
- Ask parents not to send allergen-containing snacks to school.
- Encourage parents to provide safe foods for parties.
- Insist on hand-washing before and after eating.
- Designate peanut- and tree nut-free tables.
- Wash eating surfaces after contact with foods.
- Avoid using food in arts and craft projects.
- Use disposable plates and utensils.
- Use non-food items for prizes.
- Secure trash cans at recess.
- Educate volunteers, students, substitute teachers, and aides.
- Educate classmates to avoid endangering, isolating, stigmatizing, or harassing students with food allergies.
- Encourage parental involvement in class parties and special events. Notify parents of allergic children when such parties will be held.
- Coordinate field trips; invite parents of allergic children on trips.
- Prohibit eating on school buses and vans.
- Be sure all volunteers, students, and substitute teachers are informed of stu-

dents' allergy. Carry the student's IHCP and FAAP on trips and outings.

- Ensure there is someone with a cell phone on field trips and outings, especially on the bus.
- Work with the school principal and nurse to educate classmates, parents of classmates, colleagues, and other school staff regarding risks and proactive steps for the prevention of food allergy reactions.

The PAL Program

FAAN has launched an innovative program called "Be A Pal, Protect a Life from Food Allergies." The PAL program's mission is to educate classmates of the food-allergic student. It teaches them to avoid sharing foods, to wash their hands after eating, and how to recognize an allergic reaction in their classmates. See FAAN's Web site www.foodallergy.org/ for a free download on this worthwhile program.

Some Reassuring Studies

In my lectures to parents and caretakers of children with food allergies, their overwhelming concern is potential accidental exposure by inhalation or skin contact to allergenic foods. Researchers at the Jaffe Institute have provided some reassurance for parents and caretakers. They allowed thirty peanut-allergic children to sniff disguised peanut butter from one foot away for ten minutes, and none of the children reacted to the peanut butter. They then applied a pea-sized amount of peanut butter to thirty peanut-allergic children for one minute and found a hive-like reaction in one in every three children. None of the children experienced a systemic allergic reaction. A recent paper from Iran also provides some reassurance. Iranian investigators applied a peanut butter patch test

to 321 peanut-allergic children for fifteen minutes. While 41 percent had a positive skin test reaction, none of the children had a systemic reaction. These studies suggest that inhalation of peanut butter vapor or direct skin contact to peanut butter may not be a major risk for most peanut-allergic children.

Additional studies have analyzed methods of removing peanut protein from hands, dishes, and table surfaces. Plain soap and water were very effective at removing peanut protein, as were wet wipes and commercial cleansers like Lysol, Formula 409, and Target Cleaner. Washing or cleaning with plain water or waterless antibacterial soaps did not remove peanut protein. Another study that searched for peanut protein on twenty-two student desks, thirty-six eating areas and thirteen water fountains detected peanut protein on only one water fountain. Investigators were unable to detect peanut protein above an open container of peanut butter. Additional studies have failed to find any peanut allergen near shelled and unshelled peanuts.

The Home Economics Class

The home economics or cooking class may be an especially hazardous classroom for the peanut-allergic or tree nut-allergic student. In May 2001, a sixteen-year-old student from Amesbury, Massachusetts, died in a home economics class at school shortly after eating a rice dish that contained hidden walnuts. He had a long history of asthma and nut allergy. His parents have filed a multimillion dollar lawsuit against the town and the school district. Thus, teachers who supervise home economic classes should enforce a strict peanut- and tree nuts-ban when students with these allergies are enrolled in the courses.

Role of the Food Service Director and Cafeteria Workers

As typified by the unfortunate death of Sabrina Shannon, eating in a school cafeteria can be a hazardous situation for students with food allergies. Hidden ingredients, cross-contact between foods and utensils, and allergens left on lunch tables are causes for concern. The food service staff must attend all meetings on food allergy.

Some authorities advise posting a sheet with students' names, photos, and food allergies in classrooms and cafeterias. I am in favor of this approach as long as it does not violate privacy laws and promote discrimination and ridicule by fellow students. The United States Department of Agriculture (USDA), the federal body that oversees the national school lunch program, has a guidance document entitled *Accommodating Children with Special Dietary Needs*. In this document, the USDA recommends that children with life-threatening food allergies be given safe substitute meals based upon instructions from the childrens' physician.

> *Some authorities advise posting a sheet with students' names, photos, and food allergies in classrooms and cafeterias. I am in favor of this approach as long as it does not violate privacy laws and promote discrimination and ridicule by fellow students.*

The responsibilities and roles of food service directors include:

- Know which foods to avoid and which to substitute.
- Ask parents to provide a list of prohibited foods.
- Develop a system to check all ingredient labels of food items.
- Designate a kitchen area where allergy-free meals are prepared.
- Train cafeteria staff about cross-contamination with utensils.
- Identify the students in cafeterias lines to ensure the selected food is safe. Some schools require these students to identify themselves to food service staff. Others code lunch tickets as a way of alerting cafeteria staff to food-allergic students.
- Develop cleaning procedures for tables before and after lunch.
- Use designated sponges or cleaning cloths for the allergy-free tables.
- Use non-latex gloves in food service areas.
- Assess the need for allergy-free eating areas or tables.
- Publish advance copies of the weekly menu.
- Provide menus for parents or guardians.
- Have at least two staff trained in auto-injectable epinephrine use who are always present in the cafeteria.
- Know where the auto-injectors are located.
- Pay attention to students' complaints of any discomfort that might be the early signs of an allergic reaction.
- Know how to handle emergency situations.

Role of Coaches and Trainers

Coaches and athletic trainers have an added responsibility to protect food-allergic student athletes as they often supervise students after school hours in gymnasiums, on playing fields, at night, and on weekends when school nurses are not available.

Responsibilities of coaches and trainers include:

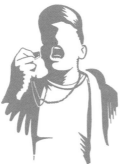

- Attending staff meetings with the school nurse
- Keeping copies of students' IHCP and FAAP
- Ensuring communication lines (cell phones) are available
- Keeping epinephrine devices in trainers' medical kit
- Knowing how to handle emergencies and administering epinephrine
- Knowing local emergency procedures

Role of Bus Drivers and the Transportation Department

- Send a representative to all staff meetings regarding food allergy.
- Provide bus drivers with the student's FAAP.
- Train school bus drivers how to manage a life-threatening reaction, including auto-injectable epinephrine administration.
- Ensure that each bus is equipped with two-way communication devices. If this is a radio, ensure that the transportation office is always manned during times the children ride the buses.
- Know the location of the closest emergency medical facility when transporting students.
- Maintain a no-eating policy on the bus.
- Bus drivers should not hand out food treats, even on special occasions.
- A student with life-threatening food allergies should sit immediately behind or to the right side of the bus driver where he or she can be easily seen by the driver.
- Students with life-threatening food allergies should be introduced to the bus driver.

- No student should be excluded from a field trip due to risk of a food allergen exposure.

Rachel's Story

The following story was written by my editor, Rachel Butler.

When my son was in kindergarten (in Hingham, Massachusetts,) the bus drivers made a huge fuss about having to have an Epipen on the bus and having to be trained on their use. (They went to the newspapers and nearly went on strike.) Finally, they had to ask for volunteers to drive certain buses and pay them more to be trained and responsible. Then one day, the head of transportation—one of the more vocal opponents—was driving my son's bus as a substitute. A bee flew in the window and stung her, she is allergic! So, she went to my son's medical kit and took a dose of his Benadryl. She called me sheepishly later that day to relate what had happened. I was never so happy to say, "Oh, no problem, I'm so glad it was there for you when you needed it!"

Timely Tips for Field Trips

A few years ago, Nathan Walters, a nine-year-old boy from a Spokane, Washington, elementary school, was on a field trip with about fifty classmates.[7] Despite knowledge of his peanut allergy, he was given a snack full of peanut products for lunch. He handed the peanut butter and jelly sandwich and mixed nuts back to his teacher but ate what appeared to be a sugar cookie that contained hidden peanuts. It was reported that he started wheezing, used his asthma inhaler, and was put on

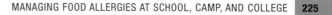

[7] James Kraemer, *The Seattle Times*, May 28, 2001. (Reprinted with permission.)

the bus to rest. When his condition worsened, one of the chaperones, a licensed practical nurse and an adult volunteer began driving him home. During this trip, his condition deteriorated and emergency care was sought but was unsuccessful in saving his life. A settlement between Nathan's parents and the Spokane School District was reached. The school district agreed to make a $25,000 donation to FAAN and a financial payment to the family. The school district also agreed to modify its field trip lunch order request form so students with special needs could be provided appropriate peanut and tree nut-free menus and lunches.

Students are not the only ones at risk on a school bus. A thirty-seven-year-old Canadian bus driver who suffered from severe allergic reactions to airborne peanut particles had problems breathing after a student eating toast coated with peanut butter boarded his bus. Students helped administer an EpiPen, and the driver was rushed to a nearby hospital and reportedly recovered. In Massachusetts, the *Cape Cod Times* recently reported that a first grader's bus driver must wipe off a child's assigned seat daily. This student has a severe peanut allergy as well as allergies to other nut products and soy.

When one considers all the horseplay and sloppy eating practices that take place on school buses, which are often undermanned or poorly supervised, it would seem prudent to ban all food products in vehicles transporting students (or bus drivers) with a peanut- or tree nut-allergy. School field trips where trained nurses are not available will require even closer supervision.

■ Role of Field Trip Supervisors
- Review the student's IHCP and FAAP.
- Brief the staff and chaperones before the event or trip.

- Ensure that a trained staff person is assigned to chaperone the student with allergies.
- Ensure that auto-injectors and instructions are taken on field trips.
- Check medication expiration dates.
- Know the signs and symptoms of allergic reactions.
- Know how to use injectable epinephrine.
- Know the location of the nearest hospital
- Carry a cell phone for emergency calls.
- Invite parents of allergic children to go on the field trip.
- Consider ways to wash hands before and after eating.
- Use hand wipes when food is consumed on the trip.
- Avoid meals with peanuts and tree nuts.
- Give the FAAP to the bus driver.
- Ensure that the bus driver has been trained to administer epinephrine.

Take all complaints of the allergic child seriously. If a student has an allergic reaction, activate emergency procedures immediately. Remember, if epinephrine is administered but not needed, the student may experience increased heart rate and nervousness but no other significant consequences. If epinephrine is needed but not administered, the student may experience a near-fatal or fatal allergic reaction.

■ Coping At College
When the food-allergic student leaves home for the first time to attend a boarding school or college, special steps need to be taken to build a solid foundation for self-management. Unfortunately, many college students adopt a careless and cavalier attitude, thinking that they are immune to severe anaphylactic reactions. Additional risks in this age group include alcohol and

fast-food consumption. Many near-fatal and fatal food reactions reported over the past few years have occurred after accidental ingestion of peanuts and tree nuts by college students who were fully aware of their food allergy. Most, if not all, of these incidents occurred in students with asthma who were not carrying injectable epinephrine at the time of their reaction. Thus, college-bound, food-allergic students who will be independent for the first time in their lives, should have a sound grasp of the fundamentals of food allergy. Student should know how to use medications and when to seek additional care for acute reactions. This is especially important if students have asthma.

Parents and the student should notify the college or university of the student's allergies in advance by providing an IHCP and a FAAP. The student's health-care provider or allergy specialist should prepare a summary of the student's medical history and a current list of medications that allows college health-care workers who are unfamiliar with the student's medical background to follow a sound treatment program. The student should be proficient in the self-management of his or her food allergy, including knowing how to avoid unsafe foods, recognize the symptoms of a reaction, and treat an allergic reaction. The student should know how and when to tell someone he or she may be having an allergic reaction and carry an auto-injectable epinephrine device at all times. Friends, roommates, and resident advisors should be made aware of the student's allergy and learn how to administer epinephrine.

College administrators and the school health facility should be aware of the federal disability laws. They must review health records submitted by the student and identify a core of team staff in health services, dining services, residence living, and security to work with the student to establish and implement a management plan. These staff members should be taught food allergy basics, including symptoms, instructions for administering medications, and emergency medical procedures. Resident assistants should be able to identify such students and know how to access emergency care. Lastly, this core team should develop a prevention plan once a reaction has occurred.

■ Be A Happy Camper

Summer camps pose another site where the risk of accidental exposure to food allergens is high as most campers are younger children who require close supervision. Parents, camp doctors, nurses, counselors, and campers must work together to minimize the risk of an accidental ingestion of offending foods.

The student should know how and when to tell someone he or she may be having an allergic reaction and carry an auto-injectable epinephrine device at all times. Friends, roommates, and resident advisors should be made aware of the student's allergy and learn how to administer epinephrine.

Parents should select a camp with a full-time nurse or, more ideally, a full-time physician. The camp should be a reasonable distance from an EMT response unit and a fully equipped emergency room. Ill-prepared volunteer ambulance crews may service remote camps. Avoid outward-bound wilderness adventures. Provide at least two epinephrine auto-injectors and check the expiration date of all medications.

Approach camp personnel just like you would school staff by providing the camp with an ICHP and a FAAP. The key contact is the camp nurse (or doctor) who should ensure that all camp personnel—including camp counselors, lifeguards, drivers, cafeteria workers, and fellow campers—are informed of the camper's food allergy. Identify a core emergency response team. Arrange to have this team meet with parents and the camper prior to the first day of camp. Assure that all who will be in contact with the camper know of the camper's allergy and know how to recognize and treat an allergic reaction.

The camp dining room or cafeteria should be closely monitored. Food service and kitchen staff must be made aware of any camper with a food allergy and discuss meal plans with parents and/or the camper. A camper with food allergies should go first in a buffet line to avoid cross-contact and eat in a designated allergy-free area. The camper should know how to identify unsafe foods and how to read labels, especially in the camp canteen. Be sure emergency medications accompany the camper and counselor on field trips. Enforce a "no eating" policy in camp vehicles. Medications must be stored in the correct temperature range as they are ineffective when left in the sunshine, inside a hot vehicle, or refrigerated.

Medications must be stored in the correct temperature range, as they are ineffective when left in the sunshine, inside a hot vehicle, or refrigerated.

■ A Down-Under School Camp Tragedy

On March 18, 2002, Rahman Hamidur, a thirteen-year-old Australian eighth grader left home with 140 other students for a five-day educational camping trip.[8] On the night of March 20, 2002, the campers gathered to play games. They were divided into groups to answer trivia questions and perform specific challenges. The object of the challenge was to be the first to finish tasks, like pushups and blowing up balloons. Hamidur found himself at the front of the group undertaking a "peanut butter challenge." Each competitor had to eat a heaped spoonful of peanut butter in the shortest time to win the heat. While Hamidur was aware that he should not eat peanut products, he was unaware of the gravity of eating peanuts and the possibility of an anaphylactic reaction.

When Hamidur collapsed moments after ingesting the peanut butter, no one was aware that they were dealing with the catastrophic symptoms of anaphylaxis. Despite valiant efforts by teachers to save his life, there was no life-saving auto-injectable epinephrine device on hand, and Hamidur died before an ambulance crew could give him proper treatment. Hamidur's initial diagnosis in 1993 was "allergic asthma, eczema and an allergy to dust mites." He suffered severe asthma attacks and was often treated at a local hospital. He was under the care of a general practitioner who had referred Hamidur to a number of specialists over the years. However, his parents did not follow through with these referrals and instead sought the assistance of a homeopathic practitioner in 1999.

---

[8] Adapted with permission from Ninemsn Australia. Helen Dalley, reporter, and Ann Bucher, producer. "When Food Can Be Fatal: Update," September 18, 2005 Sunday This Week.

At the urging of Anaphylaxis Australia, a coroner's inquest of Hamidur's death was initiated.[9] The reason for the inquiry was that Hamidur was not properly diagnosed with peanut allergy and therefore was at risk of an anaphylactic reaction. The school was ignorant of the fact that peanuts could be "life-threatening." It was not until Hamidur was thought to be having an anaphylactic reaction was the ambulance called. The school was not equipped with an EpiPen to treat such emergencies. Hamidur's death led to a lengthy inquiry. In September 2005, Magistrate Jacqueline M. Milledge recommended that staff and student training in the area of allergy awareness be implemented immediately in all public and private sector schools to ensure such preventable tragedies never happen again. These training programs should include:

- Identifying students at risk
- Allergy prevention
- Risk management
- Recognizing anaphylaxis
- Emergency treatment (particularly the use of the EpiPen)
- All staff in preschool and child-care centers undertaking allergy and anaphylaxis awareness training to ensure the safest environment for their children who may be at risk
- A system of accreditation to recognize teachers and other staff who have undertaken the training program
- All schools and child-care facilities undertaking risk assessment for all educational and recreational activities
- An audit of all schools and child-care facilities to identify children who suffer allergies
- All schools requiring parents or guardians to immediately alert them to any allergies or medical conditions that may affect their children
- Recording information in a central register accessible by all staff and continued updating
- Implementing the "Be A Mate Program" devised by Anaphylaxis Australia
- Amending the Anaphylaxis Guidelines to read: "If the form indicates the student has an allergy/s or has either been hospitalized or prescribed an EpiPen or both, a meeting should be organized with the parent"
- The current program of Registered Nurse Educators under the auspices of the Department of Health be continued and expanded to ensure all educators receive timely and expert guidance on the issues of allergies and anaphylaxis management
- That the Anaphylaxis Working Party develops a universal set of competencies for anaphylaxis training
- An awareness campaign for all medical practitioners, in both general and specialist fields, to alert them to the significant dangers of food and other allergies, and the possibility of an anaphylactic reaction. It should be impressed on these practitioners the need to have children tested for allergies. It should also be stressed that if a child is found to be allergic, a risk management plan should be devised immediately.
- An awareness campaign also targeted at practitioners of homeopathy and naturopathy
- A management plan for all children at risk of anaphylaxis. Management plans should be the same for all children and not different plans devised by different doctors
- A Register of Deaths from Anaphylaxis to identify anaphylaxis as a cause of death and the circumstances of death

---

[9] An Australian support group similar to FAAN formed in 1993. (www.allergyfacts.org/au)

- A public awareness campaign devised and implemented to ensure the general community understands the problems associated with allergies and the possibility of severe reactions, especially anaphylactic shock
- Legislation similar to the Canadian "Sabrina's Law" be enacted to govern both schools and child-care centers in the public and private sector. The intention of the legislation would be to protect pupils at risk of anaphylaxis and to safeguard teachers and staff from prosecution if an act done to manage or save a child was undertaken in "good faith."

■ Emergency Lockdown Guidelines

School districts across the United States have developed emergency plans to deal with unexpected events that would shelter children and staff in place rather than evacuating them. Some schools refer to this as a "lockdown" or a "shelter-in-place program," where no one is permitted to leave the premises. Such emergencies may result from disasters involving hazardous materials, terrorism, earthquakes, tornados, or hurricanes.

The safety of all children during a lockdown is paramount. Parents have expressed concern that such emergency plans may not take into account the special needs of children with food allergies. One particular concern is the risk posed to children with food allergies when the main food source may be peanut butter sandwiches. FAAN has published emergency guidelines for managing students with food allergies during an emergency lockdown. The FAAN publication offers ways to address the medical concerns and ensure the safety of food-allergic children during the event of a lockdown situation. Contact FAAN to obtain a copy of this plan (see appendix).

■ How to Handle An Acute Allergic Reaction

Once an emergency situation arises in a school, college, or camp setting, the first responding staff member must assess the situation. The signs and symptoms of an allergic reaction can range from a mild skin or intestinal reaction to a severe life-threatening emergency. A delay in initiating treatment is the major reason for a near-fatal or fatal reaction. In many cases, the early signs are deceiving, as warning signs like hives are not apparent. The first sign or symptom may be a "funny feeling in the mouth" or abdominal discomfort.

The biggest decision for the first responder will be whether or not to administer injectable epinephrine. In my opinion, all too often there is hesitancy and a delay in administering epinephrine. When in doubt about whether to give epinephrine, better to give it immediately and then seek additional medical attention as most fatal reactions occur when epinephrine is delayed. Remember, there are no medical contraindications to giving epinephrine in a life-threatening emergency.

Complete guidelines for diagnosing, treating anaphylaxis, and administering injectable epinephrine are covered in the chapters on anaphylaxis. In my opinion, anyone who requires epinephrine in the school, camp, or college setting should be transported to an emergency room—not a doctor's office or local clinic—for additional evaluation and treatment. Remember a significant number of patients who experience an anaphylactic reaction may develop a delayed biphasic reaction. Table 18.1 on the facing page shows a ten-step protocol for first responders to life-threatening anaphylactic reactions in a school, camp, or college setting. ●

Table 18.1. Ten-Step Protocol for First Responders

1. Call 911 ASAP.

2. Summon the school nurse. If he or she is unavailable, ask a designated trained staff member to implement the emergency protocol.

3. Check symptoms: airway, respiratory rate, and pulse.

4. When there is more than just skin involvement (hives), administer an antihistamine like Benadryl and auto-injectable epinephrine per standing order or let the victim self-administer epinephrine.

5. If the victim has asthma, administer an asthma rescue medication like albuterol.

6. If the victim has collapsed, elevate the legs; do not sit the victim up!

7. Monitor vital signs—pulse and respiration rate.

8. Administer CPR if needed.

9. Contact parents and physicians ASAP.

10. Transfer victims treated with epinephrine to an emergency facility ASAP.

Chapter

19

Peanuts: To Ban or Not to Ban?

Should peanuts and tree nuts be banned from schools and public places? In my first draft of this book, I considered ducking this controversial question. However, after I "Googled" this subject and came up with more than 79,000 hits presenting valid arguments on both sides, I decided to add this chapter. Needless to say, I did not review all 79,000 sites. Some of the more interesting Internet entries that argue both the pro and con sides of this intense debate are presented below.

■ Pro Ban

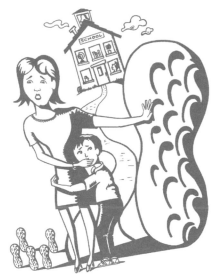

"As a parent of a child who is severely allergic, I totally agree with a complete and total peanut butter ban. Would you want your child to have to be home schooled? What if you didn't have the resources to do so? If my son smells peanut butter he will have a reaction and end up in the hospital. It's not just a matter of designating separate eating areas. Each child who eats peanut butter sandwiches would need to brush their teeth, wash their hands and the table would have to be scrubbed. How guilty would you feel if a child was sent to the hospital because you packed a peanut butter sandwich? Kids can go without peanut butter for a few hours a day.

"Your child being deprived of peanut butter between the hours of 9 to 3 is not life threatening. I hardly consider peanut consumption a need. Not eating peanut products during school is a fairly easy thing to do. Pretty selfish to have the allergic child treated like a leper just because folks like you refuse to make a small concession.

"My son is one of those children who are deathly allergic to peanuts or peanut-based foods. We have to carry an EpiPen everywhere we go. We do not eat in places where they have peanuts because his throat swells up and he can stop breathing. So yes, a peanut-free school is important to me."

■ Con Ban

"There is no such thing as a peanut-nut-free school. You can never guarantee that a school does not have peanuts or nuts without body searching everyone and everything all the time. Kids can have peanut butter on their hands from eating breakfast at home.

"The term, peanut-nut-free, gives everyone a feeling of false security, which in turn encourages complacency in the school about dealing with life-threatening allergies. Kids with allergies can become lax about the precautions they need to take because they think they are in a safe environment. Parents may think their job of educating and raising awareness is no longer necessary.

"When a ban goes into place, the energy and effort moves from educating and raising awareness to enforcing the ban. A ban can single out the children with allergies and make them susceptible to bullying. Children need to learn to fit in and have self-confidence, and not let their identity revolve around having peanut allergy.

"Telling people they can't have something because of a few is antagonistic to many parents and uncomfortable for the school. Generally our generation does not react well to the word 'ban.' When banning has been implemented, it usually takes about a year for the backlash to develop. By then, it becomes very difficult to retreat to a more middle-of-the-road approach because the parents who are upset are unwilling to listen or cooperate.

"Banning allergen-containing items is not the answer for dealing with life-threatening allergies. Peanut butter is not only a traditional food, but is an economic necessity for many families. We must prepare our children to live in the real world, while providing a safety cushion at school to help them learn the skills they need to live a long, healthy life with their allergy.

"If we ban peanuts because your child is allergic to them does that mean we should ban milk if a child was allergic to dairy? How many diabetics are in your child's class? They should not have concentrated sweets but we don't ban them.

"Any ban on peanut products would lead to resentment. The last thing any child needs is to be resented or ostracized by his peers, especially if he already feels different, which most food-allergic children do.

"A ban on peanut products would be too hard to monitor. Banning peanut products is more complicated than not allowing peanut butter at school. There are many products with hidden peanut ingredients, like peanut oil and peanut flour, not to mention the likelihood of cross-contamination in products like nuts, cookies, chocolate and other foods that may be processed on shared equipment with peanut products.

"Where do you draw the line? Granted, peanut allergy is an extremely serious allergy and should be handled very carefully. What about students who are allergic to bee stings? Would there be a ban on recess so that the allergic child would not get stung at school?

"Peanut butter is not cocaine. A number of schools are banning peanuts. Must we treat peanuts, peanut butter and foods with traces of peanuts in them as we do hard drugs or cigarettes? Must Jif and Skippy be subject to prohibition-like raids from law enforcement agencies? There is no question that a small percent of Americans react adversely to this substance, and to a handful of them, peanuts are fatal. But this targeted danger requires good judgment, not sweeping prohibitions.

"They have set a 'peanut-free zone' in the cafeteria which is great, but this is taking it too far. How about putting a big bubble dome over the entire school playground area to protect students who will die from bee stings—and what of all the asthma kids, what can we do for them and the diabetic kids—no kids can bring any foods with carbs or sugar. What about seed allergy—no foods with seeds and don't forget dairy allergies, everybody must drink soy milk sorry kids, everybody suffers for the few."

■ The Schools Respond

The principal of the Nickajack Elementary School outside Atlanta recently decreed that students would not be permitted to bring peanuts or peanut butter to school. According to the *Atlanta Journal-Constitution*, schools in at least nine states now ban peanuts and peanut butter. For this principal and the many other Americans who support a peanut ban, the issue is simple: peanut butter and jelly sandwiches on one side, the health of some students on the other side. Compassion obviously dictates a peanut ban. More and more Americans want American social policies from schools and government to be guided by compassion.

The Pleasant View Elementary School in Yorktown, Indiana, banned all peanut-based products. The policy was put in place to accommodate a first grader who had a severe life-threatening peanut allergy. Many parents were outraged. One parent said, "If the condition is so severe that it's considered life-threatening, then that child needs to be home-schooled." In response, the school has offered a compromise. Students are now able to bring peanut butter to school, but they must eat at designated tables separate from other students. The father of the allergic student said, "The compromise is what we asked for in the first place because of all the issues that go along with the peanut ban. We never asked for a complete ban, we just wanted them not to serve peanuts."

An Edmonton, Alberta, elementary school is looking at temporarily banning the sale of milk because of the allergies of two students. The superintendent of the school board said the students have potentially fatal dairy allergies, and the school board recommended stopping the milk program to protect them. The other 400 or so students would still be allowed to bring milk to school but would not be able to buy it at school. The sale of milk would resume once the children with allergies have moved on to another school.

My home state of Massachusetts has entered into this debate. The Massachusetts Bureau of Special Education Appeals ordered the Mystic Valley Regional Charter School to implement the following accommodation under a student's 504 Plan: "No peanut- tree nut-products are allowed in the student's classroom and all other accommodations accepted by parents shall continue to be implemented."

The idea of banning peanuts and tree nuts at a school in Charlotte, North Carolina, has triggered an intense debate.[1] Fearing for their children's safety, parents of children allergic to certain types of nuts at Antioch Elementary School want the school to ban them from the campus. One parent with an allergic child at Antioch said the Americans with Disabilities Act entitles children with life-threatening allergies to a safe school environment. "When you have a medical diagnosis from a doctor requiring a peanut- tree nut-free environment, it becomes very scary when school administrators ignore those facts and determine their way of managing is the best practice for the situation."

The school asked all parents to avoid bringing peanut- and tree nut-products to school to help the allergy sufferers. The school held an information session to educate parents about allergy dangers. Some parents argued they had a right to peanut butter and that some young finicky eaters

> *Compassion obviously dictates a peanut ban. More and more Americans want American social policies from schools and government to be guided by compassion.*

---
[1] *Charlotte Observer*, October 9, 2005.

refused to eat any other type of sandwich. Others felt children with allergies need to learn to manage them in all environments. Antioch principal Karen Anderson said specific classrooms with an allergic child are kept nut-free, and she estimates the school has a half dozen children with the allergy. "We're asking parents—for lunch, parties, refreshments—not to send it." Anderson said parents, overall, have responded well, and that she's become a label reader herself. "It's more difficult than you'd think. I no longer go to the grocery store without my glasses."

■ A Public Place Ban? I Doubt It!

What about banning peanuts in public places? A very sticky question indeed. I do not think you would last long in Boston if you tried to ban peanuts in Fenway Park. An amusing article by Gaylon H. White, "When the Peanut Was Banned From Baseball!"[2] should discourage anyone from mounting a campaign to ban peanuts in baseball parks or sporting arenas.

> Peanuts are as much a part of baseball as the seventh-inning stretch. They were around long before the San Diego Chicken. They preceded domed stadiums, artificial turf, body-hugging uniforms and multimillion-dollar contracts. But for one day in 1950, the peanut was banned from baseball.
>
> The place: San Francisco. The culprit: Paul Fagan, fastidious millionaire owner of the San Francisco Seals baseball team of the Pacific Coast League. Fagan was, in many ways, an early-day George Steinbrenner, always embroiled in controversy. At a time when there were only

[2] Gaylon H. White, "When Peanuts Were Banned from Baseball," in *The National Pastime*. Number 16 (Cleveland: Society for American Baseball Research, 1996)

16 major-league teams and none west of St. Louis, he agitated for the triple-A Pacific Coast League to become the third major league. Most appalling to baseball men, he criticized baseball's reserve clause that tied players to one team until they were traded or released, calling it "illegal" and "un-American."

> Fagan instituted new housecleaning rules. No more lucky sweatshirts or socks. Only the prescribed uniform. He had electric razors installed in the clubhouse for daily shaving, although most of the players had never seen electric razors. He even put in a barber chair for semi-monthly haircuts and a washing machine for the players to wash their personal belongings. The fans noticed that it was easier to read the numbers on the players' uniforms but, otherwise, watching the Seals lose was still the same. Fagan threatened to change that with his idea to ban the peanut. During a telephone conversation with C.L. (Brick) Laws, owner of the archrival Oakland Oaks, Fagan casually mentioned he was going to ban husked peanuts and sell salted peanuts instead. The official announcement followed on February 16, 1950. "We lose five cents on every bag of peanuts sold in the ballpark," Fagan complained. "That's $20,000 a year. It costs us $7\frac{1}{2}$ cents to pick up the husks and our profit on a dime bag is just $2\frac{1}{2}$ cents. The goober has to go!"
>
> That did it. San Francisco went nuts. A druggist groaned, "To me, baseball without peanuts would be like mush without salt." A beer vendor proclaimed, "I would as soon wrestle a tiger as take peanuts away from the baseball fans." An office girl sniffed, "Just like a man to think of something as nutty as that." Irate callers jammed the stadium switchboard, threatening to boycott Seals games. Oth-

er fans revolted by making plans to bring their own peanuts and scatter the shells. Radio newscasts lamented the depressing state of affairs. Newspapers up and down the West Coast editorially rushed to the peanut's defense. "To many deep, dyed-in-the-wool fans," the *Los Angeles Herald Express* commented, "it was just like ripping the heart out of baseball itself. The privilege of buying, shelling and eating peanuts at the ball game is just too sacred."

Fagan received support from hucksters who saw themselves reaping a harvest by selling peanuts outside the park. One of them even offered to supply the club with an electronic gadget guaranteed to detect concealed peanuts. The only backing Fagan's fellow owners gave him was the back of their hands. "I'd be lost at a ball game without a bag of peanuts," Oakland's Laws declared. "I'd as soon see a game without ball players as without peanuts. Why, the peanut is even part of baseball's theme song—'Take Me Out To The Ball Game.' You know how it goes...'Buy me some peanuts and Cracker Jacks...I don't care if I ever get back.' What's Fagan going to do about that? Change the lyrics? Fat chance!"

Within 24 hours, the uproar caused Fagan to concede defeat. "I give up," he said. "Mr. Peanut wins. It's the first time in my life I've been beaten and it had to be by a peanut." Fagan then made the grand gesture he hoped would make peace with the world. "I know when I'm wrong," he said. "The fans want peanuts and they'll get them. On opening day, I'm going to have 18,000 bags of peanuts passed out free among the fans." Fagan had to eat his words again. Some statistic-minded soul estimated Fagan's gift of 18,000 bags would result in 10 million peanut shell fragments. The boss of the local janitors union cried, "Foul!" and announced that the clean-up crew wanted a pay hike of 15 cents an hour. "It's worth more than we've been getting to clean up popcorn in the movies," the union leader said.

No sooner did Fagan make another reversal than the president of the National Peanut Council—a fellow appropriately named for the occasion, William Seals—called on Fagan to confess that his one-day war against the peanut was "just another publicity stunt to stimulate opening day business at Seals Stadium." Fagan pleaded innocent to the charge. And those closest to this one-man white tornado also denied that it was a publicity stunt. Manager O'Doul explained: "He had more crazy ideas per day than a dog has fleas. And I hope that doesn't libel a dog." A San Francisco sportswriter observed: "Fagan may have been puckish but not that puckish. What Fagan objected to was the peanut shells blowing in the San Francisco wind." In retrospect, Fagan would've had an easier time banning the wind instead of the peanut.

One baseball team has stepped up to the plate. The Bowie Baysox, the Class AA affiliate of the Baltimore Orioles, in partnership with FAAN, recently designated a separate section for food allergy sufferers and their families. On July 10, 2006, a special section was swept down and seats were wiped. Extra ushers were provided to keep the section nut-free, and EMTs were made available during that game. I would not be surprised if other sports teams follow this lead and create special seating sections for food allergy victims and their families.

Many communities, including my hometown, have banned peanuts and tree nuts in several schools and even in our public library. The recent studies on the risks posed by airborne peanut protein and contamination of eating surfaces would suggest that, in most instances, strict bans are unnecessary. Certainly, if there are no students in a given school with food allergies, there is no need to ban peanuts. On the other hand, if there are such students in the school, especially if they have asthma, some communities believe a total ban may be in order. Total bans might be more appropriate for younger, less responsible children attending day-care centers, nursery, or preschool settings. A lack of full-time school nurses or supervised lunch sessions may be another reason to consider a total ban.

Each school year, many school authorities seek guidance to assist them in developing policies to keep students with food allergies safe in the school environment. A total ban requires a long-term commitment and cooperation by the entire school community, including students, parents, teachers, school personnel, substitute personnel, and school cafeteria workers. A daily monitoring system would be needed to assure that the offending food never enters the school building, a nearly impossible task. Schools need to consider the ban's impact on children who rely on peanut butter as one of their major sources of daily calories and nutrients. Many parents prefer to prepare and send peanut butter sandwiches to school for their child's lunch as it is an economical source of protein that can be kept at room temperature.

■ The Bottom Line

After reviewing both sides of this debate, I tend to side with Anne Muñoz-Furlong, CEO and founder of FAAN, who in 1997 stated:

Over the past year, FAAN conducted an unprecedented number of interviews with radio, television, magazine, and newspaper reporters regarding the management of food allergy in schools. Sparking this activity and capturing the media's attention both in the U.S. and Canada was the decision by two elementary schools in Massachusetts to ban peanut products in order to manage students' food allergies. The results of this media frenzy were mixed.

As reporters interviewed various school personnel around the country, they found some school districts willing to ban peanuts, others refusing to do so; some making special considerations according to how demanding a student's parents were, others taking a 'we can't be responsible' position, requiring parents to sign liability waivers and come to the school to administer required medications in case of an allergic reaction. Rumors abounded that the school boards across the country were going to recommend a school-wide peanut ban. Further, "cafeteria personnel and classroom teachers of any student with a history of anaphylaxis should be trained to recognize the symptoms of anaphylaxis and be instructed in the administration of epinephrine."

Many parents feel that the only way to protect their child and prevent a tragedy at school is to demand that the school ban certain products, such as peanuts. The position of FAAN and our Medical Advisory Board is not to support this strategy. In order for a ban to work, one would need to have everyone in the school diligently reading ingredient labels and calling manufacturers to determine if that food contained any of the offending food. That's not a realistic expectation. Additionally, banning causes a number of problems. It may create a false sense of security that could be disastrous since diligence is key to preventing allergic reactions. Many parents believe banning peanut butter and jelly sandwiches will take care of the peanut allergy problem, but peanuts are used in many ways in many products. One school where peanuts were banned last year reported two accidental ingestions of peanuts used in baked goods and candies.

A ban may pit parents against parents. When the peanut ban was declared in North Andover, Massachusetts, the media had a field day showing how emotionally charged this issue can be. Some parents declared peanut butter was all their children would eat and they would starve without it. Others protested that their children might die if exposed to peanut butter. Several parents of allergic children complained that they wanted their children to be treated as "normal" people and that creating a ban stigmatizes them and fails to teach the children how to live with their allergy. Some parents in the North Andover schools whose children have peanut allergy actually took that information off the school health forms so their children would not be singled out. This action illustrates the problem with extreme measures. The children were left with the most dangerous of all possibilities— no one besides the parents of these children knew they were at risk for a potentially fatal allergic reaction. While peanuts are a big factor in the field of children's allergies, it should not be forgotten that milk, tree nuts, and eggs also present problems. One way to minimize these problems is through education. It is the key to avoiding an allergic reaction and successfully living with peanut or other food allergies."

■ Taking It to Extremes[3]

How far can we take the banning of exposure to peanuts or tree nuts? In July 2006, the seaside city of Milford, Conn., agreed to cut down three 60-foot-high hickory trees that were growing on a city-controlled easement over the backyard pool of the grandmother of a three-year-old child with nut allergy. Not everyone in the city was happy with the ruling that the trees had to go. If you take this example to the extreme, you could make an argument for cutting down any nut-bearing tree that such a youngster would be exposed to at a playground or at school. Common sense and education of child caretakers should prevail in such bizarre cases. ●

---

[3] Douglas Healey, "Boy with an Allergy Wins in Battle over City Trees," *The New York Times,* July 18th, 2006.

Chapter 20

Can Food Allergy Be Prevented?

Presently, the only way to prevent a food allergy reaction is to avoid the offending food. The ultimate goal of research is to stop the "allergic march" before it starts or soon after it begins. The three basic approaches in prevention are: 1) modifying gene structure, 2) controlling the environment during pregnancy, early infancy, and childhood, and 3) diverting the immune response to allergens. While genetic modification is being studied in animals, it does not appear that gene therapy will be available to humans any time in the near future. Other methods of prevention include changing the mother's diet during pregnancy and while breast-feeding, avoiding allergenic foods in infancy and early childhood, administrating friendly bacteria (probiotics) to mothers and/or infants, changing the way foods are processed, and lastly, reprogramming the immune system with vaccines or anti-allergic antibody therapy to make it follow a non-allergic pathway.

■ Maternal Diet in Pregnancy

A mother plays a vital role in the development of her infant's immune system. During pregnancy, she is the

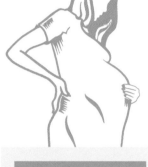

As previously discussed, the fetus's immune system is set up to favor an allergic response to allergens. The only reason why everyone does not have an allergy is that our immune system usually switches over to a Th-1, or non-allergic response, shortly after birth.

infant's only environment; and while breast-feeding, she is the infant's sole food source for the first six months of life. Can food allergy begin in pregnancy? The unborn child (fetus) is able to make allergic, or IgE antibodies, as early as the eleventh week of pregnancy. Maternal allergens are present in amniotic fluid as early as sixteen to eighteen weeks of pregnancy. A fetus can be exposed to allergens through the amniotic fluid or the placenta.

As previously discussed, the fetus's immune system is set up to favor an allergic response to allergens. The only reason why everyone does not have an allergy is that our immune system usually switches over to a Th-1, or non-allergic, response shortly after birth.

At the present time, there are no solid data to support a recommendation that mothers should avoid allergenic foods in pregnancy to prevent food allergy in their offsprings. Numerous studies have looked at the short-term and long-term effects of eliminating potentially allergenic foods during pregnancy. In one study, pregnant women with at least one allergic family member eliminated cow's milk and egg during the last twelve weeks of pregnancy. The control mothers in the study ate a normal diet. At age five, there was no difference in eczema, allergic rhinitis, asthma, or food allergy between the two groups. Several other studies found that the only benefit derived from eliminating allergenic foods during pregnancy was less eczema in infants during the first four years of life.

Dr. Gideon Lack from St. Mary's Hospital in London found no difference in peanut consumption during pregnancy in mothers whose children developed peanut allergy compared with children who did not develop a peanut allergy. While the American Academy of Pediatrics currently recommends that high-risk mothers avoid allergenic foods in pregnancy, European organizations do not.

The bottom line: data from more than 4,000 articles imply that breast-feeding appears to protect against eczema and a wheezing illness only up to age four.

Does fish oil supplementation in pregnancy reduce the risk of allergic diseases in infants? Australian pediatricians reviewed studies suggesting that fish oil could prevent allergy. Their paper makes a strong case that supplementation with foods rich in Omega-3 fatty acids may protect against allergic disease. But more studies are needed before making a recommendation on this question.

An Italian study of nearly 900 nonallergic and allergic mothers investigated whether the consumption of fish, butter, or margarine by pregnant mothers might influence the development of allergies in their offspring. They found that eating fish two to three times a week might be protective for the offspring of non-allergic mothers. There was no effect regarding butter or margarine consumption in either group.

■ Is Breast Best or Not So Best?

There is no doubt that breast milk is the best food source for infants. Breast-feeding provides ideal nutrition and protects against viral and bacterial infection and promotes a close relationship between the baby and mother. Breast milk contains protective antibodies and living cells that ensure a healthy immune response for most infants. Forty-one breast-feeding women were randomly allocated to receive a test breakfast, identical except for the egg content (no egg, one raw egg, half a cooked egg, or one cooked egg). Breast milk samples were collected at two-hour intervals for eight hours, and egg protein was measured. There was a direct dose-response between the amount of ingested egg and the egg protein levels in breast milk. The study concluded that egg protein was present in the breast milk of lactating women up to eight hours after egg intake. The excretion of egg protein in human milk appears to be a normal phenomenon and seldom causes adverse symptoms. However, further studies are needed to determine the threshold of egg protein that leads to symptoms in egg-allergic breast-fed infants.

In 1939, a review of the feeding patterns of 20,000 infants found that breast-feeding lowered the incidence of eczema. Over the next 60 years, thousand of studies have attempted to verify this finding. Studies in the 1970s and 1980s found that breast-fed infants had less eczema, fewer bouts of wheezing, and lower allergic antibody (IgE) levels. A recent study of 3,619 Swedish children who were breast-fed for at least four months found a reduction in the incidence of asthma and eczema in later childhood. The best outcomes were observed in children who had no family history of allergy. One United Kingdom study found less egg and inhalant allergy at eighteen months of age when mothers avoided eggs in the last two trimesters of pregnancy and while breast-feeding. The bottom line: data from more than 4,000 articles imply that breast-feeding appears to protect against eczema and a wheezing illness only up to age four.

In June 1998, *The British Medical Journal* published a letter entitled, "Women Warned to Avoid Peanuts During Pregnancy and Lactation." According to Dr. John Warner, professor of Child Health at Southampton University and a member of the government's working group on peanut allergy, there may be a link between maternal consumption of peanuts and peanut products and the early onset and rising prevalence of peanut allergy. Lactation is the more likely route of primary sensitization. Pregnant mothers who ate peanuts more than once a week were more likely to give birth to a peanut-allergic child than mothers who consumed peanuts less than once a week. In the June 2000 newsletter of the Anaphylaxis Network of Canada, Dr. Peter Vadas, past president of the Anaphylaxis Foundation stated:

A study just completed in my laboratory has shown that peanut protein does pass from the maternal diet via the bloodstream into breast milk. Using a sensitive assay for peanut allergens, we tested samples of breast milk for the presence of peanut protein after consumption of dry roasted peanuts by a group of volunteers. Major peanut allergens were detected in breast milk within one to three hours after ingestion in approximately 50 percent of the volunteers. These data confirm the previously unproven notion that some infants are sensitized by exposure to peanut protein through breast-feeding.

However, the story is not quite so simple. The concentration of peanut protein, timing of exposure and frequency of exposure may lead to either allergic sensitization or tolerization. The latter process actually protects against allergies. In some cases, exposure to peanut protein in breast milk may actually protect against later development of peanut allergy. At this stage, it would be overly simplistic to suggest that all lactating women avoid peanut products during breast-feeding. While this may protect some children from peanut sensitization, it may predispose other children to acquiring peanut allergy by preventing the process of tolerization. Instead, it may be more prudent for lactating mothers to avoid peanut products while breast-feeding high-risk infants, namely those who have a strong family history of allergy.

Presently, there is no solid evidence that breast-feeding protects against food allergy. Double-blind studies at this point in time would be unethical due to the beneficial effects of breast-feeding. Studies on the protective effects of breast-feeding are clouded by other factors, including higher socioeconomic levels, less exposure to tobacco smoke and household pets, and delayed introduction of solid foods.

Dr. Robert Zeiger has put the best spin on this issue. "Breast-feeding is the preferred method of infant nutrition for numerous reasons. However, its role in the prevention of allergic disease remains controversial. Reasons for this controversy include differences and flaws in the studies performed to date, the immunologic complexity of breast milk itself and, possibly, genetic differences among patients that would affect whether breast-feeding is protective against the development of allergies or is, in fact, sensitizing. The preponderance of evidence does suggest, however, that there would be much to lose by not recommending breast-feeding. In general, studies reveal that infants fed formulas of intact cow's milk or soy protein compared with breast milk have a higher incidence of atopic dermatitis (eczema) and wheezing illnesses in early childhood. Consistent with these findings, exclusive breast-feeding should be encouraged for at least 4 to 6 months in infants with both a high and low risk of atopy, irrespective of a history of maternal asthma.

New research has shown that extending exclusive breast-feeding beyond six months may increase the risks for allergy. Research was started 20 years ago when scientists at the Helsinki Skin and Allergy Hospital in Finland asked 200 mothers to breast-feed their newborns for as long as possible. The children were assessed for allergies at the ages of five, eleven and twenty years of age. Feeding children exclusively on breast milk for nine months or more appeared to increase their risk of developing allergic conditions, such as eczema and food hypersensitivity.

The researchers noted that children who developed allergies after prolonged exclusive breast-feeding were most likely to do

> *Another reason to breast-feed for six months versus four months is a February 2006 study in Pediatrics that found that when breast-feeding was stopped at four months, infants had a two-fold increased risk of ear infections and a fourfold increased risk of pneumonia.*

so during the first years of life. The study suggests that environmental factors such as pollen exposure, diet and disease play a more important role in the onset of allergies in later childhood and adulthood. Prolonged exposure to breast milk may provide too much early protection against these triggers. There may a critical time window when the immune system needs to be exposed to foreign proteins to develop a tolerance to these antigens

Consider one final thought on breast-feeding. Studies showing that prolonged breast-feeding may increase the risk of allergy might be skewed, as mothers whose infants show early signs of an allergy, like eczema, might be more inclined to breast-feed for longer periods of time. Another reason to breast-feed for six months versus four months is a February 2006 study in *Pediatrics* that found that when breast-feeding was stopped at four months, infants had a twofold increased risk of ear infections and a fourfold increased risk of pneumonia.

■ An Old Disease Reappears

Once a rare disease, rickets is on the rise. Rickets is caused by a vitamin D deficiency resulting in soft, poorly formed bones. The primary source of vitamin D is sunlight. Due to risks associated with sunlight exposure, such as skin cancer, cataracts, and melanoma, children today may have less sun exposure and are therefore at greater risk for vitamin D deficiency.

In an effort to provide an alternative to sunlight, foods commonly eaten by infants and children (such as infant formulas and cow's milk) are fortified with vitamin D. Human milk is one of the few foods that naturally contains vitamin D, but human milk was not intended to be a replacement for sunlight as the primary source vitamin D. In 2003, the American Academy of Pediatrics recommended that starting around two months of age breast-fed infants be given a supplement of 200 international units of vitamin D each day. Most new cases of rickets occur in inner-city, breast-fed black children. The reason for the surge in rickets is due to the boom in breast-feeding, a lack of sun exposure, and the fact that many doctors neglect to tell breast-feeding mothers to administer vitamin D to their infants. Lack recently described a fourteen-month-old cow's milk-allergic boy who developed rickets. Dr. Michael Holick from Boston Medical Center has stated that his center now sees about ten to fifteen new cases of rickets cases a year.[1]

Current Guidelines for Infant Feeding—A Right or Wrong Approach?

In 2000, the American Academy of Pediatrics published dietary recommendations for at-risk pregnant and breast-feeding mothers and their infants. At-risk mothers, defined as having one immediate family member with an allergy, were advised to avoid peanut- and tree nut-products in pregnancy and while breast-feeding. They were also advised not to feed their infants milk products until age one; egg products until age two; and peanuts, tree nuts, and seafood until age three. British authorities have made similar recommendations. At this time, other than the use of the extensively hydrolyzed formulas, there are no conclusive studies that restriction of allergenic foods from infants' diet prevents food allergy.

Data on diet and the diagnoses of eczema were collected semiannually, and allergy antibody (IgE) levels were measured at two years of age in 2,612 German infants. There was no evidence for any protective effect of a delayed introduction of solids on eczema and allergic symptoms in children of allergic parents. In fact, the introduction of several solid foods by six months of age reduced the chances of having doctor-diagnosed eczema. This study is in contrast to a New Zealand study of 1,210 children who had a positive association between introduction of solid foods at four months of age and eczema at ages two and ten years of age. An English study that recruited 642 children from 1993 to 1995 found no evidence that a delayed introduction of solids prevented eczema at age five years. Results from a Finnish study found a protective effect of solid food avoidance during the first six months of life on eczema at age one year, but not at age five years.

In summary, most of the medical literature fails to provide any evidence that delayed introduction of solid foods beyond age six months prevents the development of allergic diseases. These studies have fostered a growing concern that stringent feeding guidelines that delay the introduction of solid foods may be the wrong approach for some at-risk infants.

These studies have fostered a growing concern that stringent feeding guidelines that delay the introduction of solid foods may be the wrong approach for some at-risk infants.

Th-1 Soup?

In 2003, I conducted a study that compared the prescription rate of auto-injectable epinephrine devices in school settings for peanut- and tree nut-allergy in two affluent suburban towns with over 90 percent white students and an urban city with a 60 per-

[1] *Boston Herald,* January 29, 2006.

cent minority enrollment. My survey found a fivefold to eightfold higher use of auto-injectable epinephrine for nut allergy in white suburban school children compared to the minority, urban-based school children, suggesting that minority children had a much lower incidence of peanut- or tree nut-allergy. An informal survey of Hispanic and Asian mothers in the urban setting revealed that many mothers fed their infants a "blenderized" mix of table foodstuffs containing rice, beans, and seafood; whereas, white suburban mothers were more likely to feed their infants individualized jars of store-bought, non-allergenic baby foods. My good friend Dr. Michael Mellon likes to call the blenderized mix "Th-1 soup."

> *Dr. Lack's group is starting an important seven-year study that will follow children fed solid foods at an early age to determine if early introduction of solid foods in infancy, including the more allergenic foods, is detrimental or helpful.*

One possible explanation for this striking disparity in the peanut- and tree nut-allergy in suburban versus urban schools is that early introduction of the blenderized "Th-1 soup" in minority infants and young children, especially Hispanic and Asian schoolchildren, may induce a state of immune tolerance that leads to a lower incidence food allergy.

Confirmation of such an association would raise the possibility that alterations in present-day maternal and infant feeding (and non-feeding) habits, like those presently proposed in the United States and the United Kingdom, might prevent the development of peanut- and tree nut-allergy in at-risk infants and children. Could a delay in introducing allergenic foods like peanuts, tree nuts, or seafood prevent the development of immunological tolerance? These strict avoidance measures might, paradoxically, be favoring allergic sensitization in at-risk infants and children. This may also be the reason that that exposure to inhaled allergens, such as dogs and cats, in early infancy prevents the development of inhaled allergies later on in childhood.

Additional support for this concept comes from a prospective study of 4.089 newborn infants in Sweden followed for four years using parental questionnaires at ages two months, one, two and few years to collect information on exposure and health effects. Regular fish consumption during the first year of life was associated with a reduced risk for allergic disease by age four. Regular fish consumption before age one was associated with a reduced risk of allergic disease and sensitization to food and inhalant allergens during the first four years of life. The lower risk for sensitization was only seen in children without heredity for allergic disease.

In one study of sixteen children with reported wheat allergy, children who were first exposed to cereals after six months of age had an increased risk of wheat allergy compared with children first exposed to cereals before six months of age.

Dr. Lack has noted that in places like Thailand, where children are given peanut products at a young age, virtually no peanut allergies are reported. In his practice, he sees mothers who breast-feed for nine months or more and then feed their infants a very limited range of foods. Yet, many of these children develop all sorts of food allergies. Dr. Lack's group is starting an important seven-year study that will follow children fed solid foods at an early age to determine if early introduction of solid foods in infancy, including the more allergenic foods, is detrimental or helpful.

"Forget Cereal—Feed Your Baby Enchiladas!"

An interesting article by J. M. Hirsch, entitled "Forget Cereal—Feed your Baby Enchiladas!" appeared in the *Montreal Gazette* on October 10, 2005. Some highlights from the article include the following.

Most of the advice parents get about weaning infants to solid foods, even from pediatricians, is more myth than science. "There's a bunch of mythology out there about this, there's not much evidence to support any particular way of doing things," said Dr. David Bergman, a Stanford University pediatrics professor. Yet, experts say children over six months of age can handle most anything, with a few caveats: Be cautious if you have a family history of allergies; introduce one food at a time; and watch for any problems.

Dr. Nancy Butte, a pediatrics professor at Baylor College of Medicine, found that many strongly held assumptions, such as the need to offer foods in a particular order or to delay allergenic foods have little scientific basis. Butte's review found no evidence that children without family histories of food allergies benefited from this approach. Others suspect avoiding certain foods or eating bland diets actually could make allergies more likely.

Dr. David Ludwig of Children's Hospital in Boston, a specialist in pediatric nutrition, said some studies suggest that rice and other highly processed grain cereals actually could be among the worst foods for infants. "These foods digest very rapidly in the body into sugar, raising blood sugar and insulin levels, and could contribute to later health problems, including obesity."

The Westernized Diet

Could a westernized diet be responsible for the allergy epidemic? Starting in the 1960s, industrialized societies turned away from the consumption of locally grown fruits and vegetables, cow's milk, oily fish, and meat. We now eat processed foods raised in many parts of the world. Today's typical diet contains more salt and unsaturated fatty acids like margarine and vegetable oil. Such a diet has less fiber; fewer fruits, vegetables, and oily fish, like tuna and salmon; and fewer minerals and antioxidants, such as vitamins C and vitamin E.

Several cultures that have not adopted a westernized diet have been studied. Asian children who eat westernized food after moving to the United States have more asthma and allergy than those who stick to their native Asian diet. Australian children and Eskimos who consume large quantities of oily finfish have fewer allergies and asthma. One interesting study found that desert-raised Saudi Arabian children who eat a native Arabian diet of non-pasteurized milk and fresh vegetables, have less asth-

One interesting study found that desert-raised Saudi Arabian children who eat a native Arabian diet of non-pasteurized milk and fresh vegetables, have less asthma than Saudi children living in cities where they have adopted a traditional westernized diet.

ma than Saudi children living in cities, where they have adopted a traditional westernized diet.

Dr. Anthony Seaton is a big proponent of vitamin E. After tracking 2,000 women during and after pregnancy, he found that the risk of asthma and Type I diabetes was higher in smoking mothers who consumed less vitamin E. Male sex and early use of antibiotics in infancy were additional risk factors. In a survey of nearly 80,000 nurses in the United States, nurses who took in less vitamin E had more asthma, especially if they were overweight. As previously discussed, farm-raised children who drink non-pasteurized milk and eat farm-fresh produce and meats have less asthma and allergy.

These observations suggest that a deficiency in dietary antioxidants may be contributing to the rising allergy prevalence by polarizing the Th-2 immune response.

A new rice-based formula available in Europe may be another alternative for milk-allergenic infants, as only one of ninety milk-allergic Italian children who ingested a rice-based hydrolysate formula had a reaction to it.

The intake of Omega-3 fatty acids present in high amounts in fish oil has diminished in many societies. The once common practice of giving children unpalatable cod liver oil (ugh!) as a source of fat-soluble vitamins is nonexistent. Compelling studies suggest that consumption of fish oil may lower lung inflammation in elite athletes. Infants born to mothers who consumed fish oil in pregnancy had a lower risk of egg allergy and eczema.

Hypoallergenic Formulas

Hypoallergenic formulas have been around for more than sixty years. They are produced by subjecting milk to heat, enzyme exposure, and filtration to produce a less allergenic formula. While these products still may contain trace amounts of milk protein, they are quite safe for over 90 percent of milk-allergic infants. The three products available in the United States (Alimentum, Nutramigen, and Pregestimil) can be used in high-risk infants who cannot breast-feed. Their drawbacks are their high cost and poor taste. Milk-allergic infants and children who do not tolerate these formulas may have to resort to elemental amino acid-based formulas, like Neocate and EleCare, that are also very expensive and have a poor taste.

There is no evidence that hypoallergenic formulas, except for the elemental amino acid-based formulas, prevent food allergy. A new rice-based formula available in Europe may be another alternative for milk-allergic infants, as only one of ninety milk-allergic Italian children who ingested a rice-based hydrolysate formula had a reaction to it.

Eat Some Bugs?

Man's intestinal tract contains millions of friendly and unfriendly bacteria that control the delicate balance between a healthy or unhealthy intestinal tract. The impact of intestinal bacteria is most pronounced in infancy. Before birth, the fetus's intestinal tract is sterile—it has no bacteria. The first exposure to bacteria occurs during a vaginal delivery when infants swallow bacteria-laden fluid from the mother's vaginal birth canal during delivery. Over the next several months, these bacteria multiply and, by age two, the intestine harbors millions of bacteria. Most infants become tolerant of these bugs that are potent stimulators of the nonallergic immune response. In contrast, infants delivered by cesarean birth are not exposed to birth canal secretions laden with bacteria. In Norway, cesarean birth babies were seven times more likely to be allergic to eggs, fish, or nuts if their mother was allergic. There was no increased risk to the children of nonallergic moms. A more recent study refutes this observation. A United Kingdom group that looked at the incidence of food allergy in 1,387 infants born by cesarean birth and 980 vaginal deliveries found no difference in food allergy in either group. Stay tuned, there will be more studies on this interesting question.

Ongoing research is looking at ways to divert the immune system away from an inflammatory, or allergic, response by administering friendly bacteria called probiotics. As previously discussed, a probiotic is a live bacterium that provides beneficial effect to the host by crowding out bad bacteria in the intestinal tract. Probiotics have been used for thousands of years in fermented milk. Persian tradition has it that Abraham owed his fertility and longevity to yogurt. In the early 20th century, Russian immunologist Elie Metchnikogg proposed that lactic acid bacteria might have beneficial health effects. The concept of preventing allergic disease by administering probiotics arose out of the hygiene hypothesis that proposed that the allergy epidemic of the late twentieth century was due to a lower exposure to infectious agents.

Interest in probiotics surged when it was found that allergic children had lower levels of friendly bacteria in their intestinal tract and higher levels of pathogenic bacteria, like staphylococcus and *E. coli*. Studies looking at the effects of administering *Lactobacillus* (a member of the lactic acid family of bacteria found in many foods like yogurt) to pregnant and breast-feeding mothers found a modest reduction in eczema with no change in the incidence of asthma, hay fever, or food allergy. The best results with probiotic therapy are reported in antibiotic-induced diarrhea, traveler's diarrhea, and rotavirus infection.

A recent French report described an eleven-month-old infant allergic to cow's milk who experienced flushing and throat fullness fifteen minutes after ingesting the probiotic Bacilor. Skin tests to Bacilor and cow's milk were both positive. Three other children with cow's milk allergy tested positive to Bacilor and another the probiotic Imgalt. The manufacturers of these products admitted using lactoserum proteins and casein to grow the bacteria used in these probiotics. Another probiotic, Ditopy, uses hydrolyzed soy protein as a growth medium. Thus, patients allergic to cow's milk and soy should avoid probiotics that can contain residual milk or soy protein. Some disturbing papers have described sepsis and severe immune suppression in infants given probiotics. Thus, at this time more studies are needed before I endorse probiotic therapy.

> *Some disturbing papers have described sepsis and severe immune suppression in infants given probiotics. Thus, at this time more studies are needed before I endorse probiotic therapy.*

▪ Secondary Prevention of Food Allergy

The previous section discussed primary ways of preventing food allergy before symptoms begin. Any attempt to block an allergy once it starts is called secondary prevention. Could you lower the allergic potential of a food protein by genetically modifying the food; by blocking the allergic reaction with anti-allergic-IgE antibody; by administering drugs or herbal therapy; or by changing the way our immune system responds to a food allergen with the age-old allergy treatment known as immunotherapy?

■ Genetic Modification of Foods

Genetic engineering may one day make the plants and animals we eat more abundant and more nutritious. Genetic engineering also has the potential to eliminate allergens from foods. Genetically engineered foods increase crop production, reduce pesticide use, lower levels of unhealthy fatty acids and starches, lower animal feed requirements, and reduce animal waste. Such crops are more resistant to weather extremes and provide inexpensive foods for the world's growing population. Foods that have been genetically engineered include soybeans, corn, squash, potatoes, canola, and tomatoes. Oranges and tangerines have been combined to produce the tangelo.

However, many genetic researchers feel the wide array of allergenic proteins in foods will make it extremely difficult to genetically produce non-allergenic foods.

One of the first products of genetic alteration was a softer tomato with a longer shelf life. Such foods are extensively studied before they reach the marketplace, and, to date, there is no evidence that genetic engineering either decreases or increases the allergenic potential of foods. Several centers are attempting to develop non-allergenic peanut and seafood products. A team led by Dr. Samuel Lehrer at Tulane University in New Orleans is studying a shrimp species that lacks the protein responsible for nasty and potentially fatal reactions to shrimp. Allergy-free peanut and soybean products are also under study. However, many genetic researchers feel the wide array of allergenic proteins in foods will make it extremely difficult to genetically produce non-allergenic foods.

■ Anti-IgE Therapy

As previously discussed, the allergic, or IgE, antibody plays a pivotal role in allergic disease. In 1987, Dr. T. W. Chang came up with the idea of trying to block this influential antibody with an anti-IgE antibody protein. Chang astutely theorized that if you could shut down IgE production, you might prevent asthma and other allergic disorders. In 2003, after successful trials (in both mice and men), the anti-IgE antibody Xolair (omalizumab) was approved by the FDA for the treatment of moderate-to-severe asthma. Xolair injections induced a dose-related decrease in serum IgE levels and improvement in asthma symptoms. Studies in San Francisco and Denver found that serum IgE levels were lowered by 99 percent after receiving Xolair. That's the good news.

The bad news is that when the study subjects stopped taking Xolair, IgE levels bounced back to the same as or higher than pretreatment levels. The rebound reaction is somewhat disturbing, as it looks like Xolair has to be administered at regular intervals on an indefinite basis for it to be effective. Xolair is the first new biological (non-drug) therapy for asthma since allergen immunotherapy was introduced in 1911. It has been studied in thousands of children and adults with asthma, allergic rhinitis, anaphylactic reactions to peanuts, allergic reactions to latex, and, most recently, in patients undergoing allergy injections, or immunotherapy.

Several food-allergy research centers started preliminary clinical trials with this drug (renamed TNX 901) in patients with severe peanut allergy. Preliminary results found that TNX 901 raised the threshold of the number of peanuts that induced a reaction from two peanuts to twenty-four peanuts. Thus, TNX 901, while, not curative, may provide protection for patients with a severe life-threatening peanut allergy. This drug was given a fast-track status by the FDA, and, in 2005, clinical trials were started in several centers in the United States. The study required injections for twenty-four weeks in patients with a positive oral challenge to peanuts.

It was planned to take two to four years to complete these studies. Unfortunately, in early 2006, Genentech Inc., the producers of TNX 901, announced that clinical trials were being suspended due to safety concerns. In the process of qualifying for the study, two children experienced life-threatening allergic reactions when they were given trace amounts of peanut protein to evaluate the severity of their peanut allergy. Neither child had been started on TNX 901. Once a safer study design is approved by the FDA, I believe these important trials will resume.

Immunotherapy

In 1911, two ingenious pioneers in allergy research, Doctors Leonard Noon and John Freeman, discovered that hay fever victims injected with an extract of grass pollen before the grass pollen season suffered fewer symptoms once grass pollinated in early summer. Modern research has documented their astute observations, and allergy injections, or immunotherapy, is now an accepted therapy for many allergic conditions, including asthma, allergic rhinitis and sensitivity to stinging insects. In immunotherapy, a very diluted dose of an allergen is injected once or twice a week for three to four months. Each succeeding dose delivers a higher concentration of the allergen. These weekly injections build up to a maintenance dose that is usually the highest dose the patient can tolerate without risking an allergic reaction. Once this maintenance dose is reached, injections are given every two to four weeks and continued for at least three to five years on a year-round basis. The good news is that when patients are properly chosen, allergy injections work quite well. The bad news is that immunotherapy takes a long time to work, can cause allergic reactions, and is expensive. Early immunotherapy trials in patients with peanut allergy proved to be too dangerous, as several subjects had a high rate of allergic reactions to the injections. Ongoing clinical trials are now studying engineered vaccines using less allergenic proteins called peptides.

Dr. Hugh Sampson is currently studying a peanut allergy vaccine based on a modified peanut protein. The future treatment of food allergy may involve an expensive combination of anti-IgE therapy and peptide immunotherapy injections.

Oral Desensitization

In 1829, a French physician, R. Dakin, reported that poison oak and poison ivy reactions were prevented by eating the leaves of these toxic plants. This first (and very dangerous) example of oral tolerance was duplicated in many animal models. Oral desensitization has had some success in pollen-allergic patients. Several worldwide allergy centers are studying the effects of placing small amounts of an allergen under the tongue at regular intervals in what was once called sublingual immunotherapy. In March 2006, researchers at the annual meeting of the American Academy of Allergy, Asthma and Immunology reported the results of sublingual treatment trials. Ninety-one patients took roughly 4,500 doses of cat dander, grass, ragweed pollen, and house dust mite-allergen over eight weeks. Investigators were able to achieve safe doses of allergens that would have taken months to achieve by allergy injections. If this approach works, painful allergy injections may become a thing of the past.

Preliminary studies suggest that food-allergic children and adults can be safely administered small amounts of cow's milk, egg, or peanuts. Dr. B. Neggermann reported over 80 percent of German adults fed increasing amounts of milk and hens' eggs for three to twelve months achieved oral tolerance. In most cases, it took a long time (up to nine months) to achieve a maximum tolerated dose. In one patient, allergy symptoms to hens' eggs returned after stopping egg intake for only two days.

One argument for oral desensitization is that some children who have outgrown their peanut allergy become re-sensitized if they do not eat peanuts on a regular basis.

Thus, you may need regular intake of the offending food to maintain a state of tolerance. One argument for oral desensitization is that some children who have outgrown their peanut allergy become re-sensitized if they do not eat peanuts on a regular basis. Spanish allergists administered small amounts of hazelnuts and a placebo to twenty-two adults. Five of eleven who received hazelnuts over four days were able to tolerate fifteen to twenty hazelnuts.

Several United States centers are examining the effectiveness and safety of sublingual immunotherapy in egg-allergic and peanut-allergic patients. One preliminary trial by Dr. Wesley Burks at Duke University found that a small amount of egg protein shut down IgE production and induced T-cell suppression in three egg-allergic children. Burks is also studying a new method for fighting peanut allergy in children. His research group is taking small amounts of peanut protein and gradually giving increasing amounts to peanut-allergic children over an initial day and then over a period of three-and-a-half to four months. The children receive a larger dose every other week. At the end of that period, they're getting about 300 milligrams of peanut protein— the equivalent of one peanut. What Burks is finding is that the children are less sensitive when they accidentally eat a peanut. By the end of this study, it is hoped that the subjects will have "outgrown" their peanut allergy.

The attractive premise that food allergy might be prevented by feeding at-risk infants and children small amounts of allergenic foods is borne out by the observation that children raised in countries and cultures where infants are fed allergenic foods in early infancy have fewer food allergies. Israeli children fed peanut snacks at an early age have far less peanut allergy than children from the United Kingdom and the United States where peanut avoidance is the norm. Oral desensitization was performed in twenty-one children with cow's milk allergy in increasing doses, starting from 0.06 milligrams of cow's milk proteins. Overall, fifteen of twenty-one children (71 percent) achieved an average daily intake of 200 milliliters (about 6 to 7 ounces) during a six-month period. Three of twenty-one children (14 percent) failed the desensitization trial, as they developed allergic symptoms after ingesting minimal amounts of diluted cow's milk.

Dr. Lyndon Mansfield recently described two children with severe peanut allergy, a seven-year-old female and a seven-year-old male. He bravely, I might add, administered very small amounts of peanut every fifteen minutes until they tolerated eight grams or the equivalent of two peanuts. These two children are now reportedly safely eating two peanuts a day. This is an exciting finding. I would caution that both sublingual immunotherapy and oral desensitization therapies are experimental approaches and should only be conducted under well-controlled conditions in food allergy research centers.

Oral administration of the offending food, also called specific oral tolerance, starts with very low doses and gradually increases the daily dosage up to an amount equivalent to a usually relevant dose for daily intake. This is followed up by a daily maintenance dose. Unfortunately, the body of scientific evidence concerning this approach is limited. Only a few studies on a limited number of patients including different allergens are available. So far, no placebo-controlled, long-term study has been published. More studies are needed before I endorse such therapies.

■ One Last Thought

Arc there any drugs out there that could prevent an at-risk infant from developing an allergic disease? One group of drugs that might do the trick are the cortisone or steroid drugs, but their toxicity prevents using them over a long period of time. One report from Europe is quite interesting. Investigators studied 750 infants with a positive family history of allergy and eczema. Half the group took the antihistamine cetirizine (Zyrtec) and the other half took a placebo for eighteen months. Both groups were followed for another eighteen months. The group who took cetirizine, which has some anti-inflammatory properties, had less asthma at the end of thirty six months. This is the first study to suggest taking a relatively innocuous antihistamine could prevent asthma. Additional studies are planned with a derivative of cetirizine called levocetirizine. To date, there are no studies of this nature dealing with food allergy.

The bottom line: at the present time, there is no way to prevent food allergy other than by avoiding the offending food. Gene therapy is a long way off. Controlling food intake during pregnancy, while breastfeeding, and in early childhood does not seem to be the answer. Probiotic therapy needs more study. The most promising approaches might be to tweak the immune system away from the "allergic march" with an earlier introduction of solid foods, anti-IgE therapy, peptide injections, oral desensitization, or Chinese herbal therapy. ●

Chapter

21

Alternative Therapy

The terms alternative and complementary therapy refer to non-traditional medical treatments that have neither been approved nor been shown to be effective in controlled studies by the established western medical community. Alternative treatment and products include phytopharmaceuticals (herbal agents), homeopathic remedies, nutraceuticals, and anthroposophics. While these products are governed by legislation (United States Dietary Supplement and Health Education Act or DSHEA), they do not require proof of safety or efficacy by the Food and Drug Administration (FDA). As there is no financial incentive to test or study these products, new FDA-required drug applications (NDAs) are not needed.

The only way the FDA can remove an alternative medicine or herbal remedy from the marketplace is to prove that it is unsafe. This is in marked contrast to the United Kingdom, Germany, and Canada, where governments closely regulate herbal or alternative therapy.

The only way the FDA can remove an alternative medicine or herbal remedy from the marketplace is to prove that it is unsafe. This is in marked contrast to the United Kingdom, Germany, and Canada, where governments closely regulate herbal or alternative therapy.

■ A Popular Approach

Over the past decade, the popularity of alternative therapy has grown immensely. It is estimated that 40 percent of allergy sufferers in the United States use some form of alternative medicine. Fourteen percent of 118 families surveyed at a FAAN food allergy conference admitted using complementary medicine or an herbal product. Millions of American health-care consumers spend more than $20 billion per year on natural herbal supplements, and $30 billion go to providers of alternative health care. More people visit alternative medical practitioners than primary care physicians—600 million visits to alternative care providers versus 400 million visits to primary care physicians.

When you look back on the history of pharmacological products in medicine, natural drugs are not all that new. The asthma drug cromolyn sodium (Intal) was derived from *Ammi visnaga*, a Mediterranean plant used by Arabic physicians to treat intestinal colic 100 years ago. Theophylline was extracted from tea leaves and coffee beans. The heart drug digitalis comes from the foxglove plant. Aspirin comes from the bark of the willow tree. Penicillin was discovered when Sir Alexander Fleming accidentally noted that penicillin-like molds were killing bacteria on culture plates in his laboratory.

Why is alternative therapy becoming more attractive? Such remedies offer a ray of hope for many patients who are confused by complicated drug programs. As conventional prescription drugs kill more than 100,000 Americans each year, patients fear traditional medicine and its outcome. Dissatisfied patients constantly surf the Internet to consult herbalists and seek alternative therapies. Courses in alternative therapy are now offered in medical schools and teaching hospitals. Most physicians, including myself, have underestimated the potential benefits of alternative therapy.

The United States Congress has responded to this explosion in alternative therapy by creating the Office of Alternative Medicine (OAM). In 1998, the National Institutes of Health launched the National Center for Complementary and Alternative Therapy, which has a yearly budget of $100 million. Alternative therapies now being investigated by the NIH include herbal remedies, nutritional supplements, acupuncture, hypnotherapy, relaxation techniques, and chiropractic therapy. Ongoing clinical trials are evaluating the use of St. John's Wort in depression, shark cartilage in lung cancer, and ginkgo biloba in dementia. The development of modern-day herbal remedies is based on the philosophies and beliefs dating back to ancient Greek, Roman, Arabic, and Chinese cultures.

The basic components of herbal remedies are botanical products derived from natural plant life. Herbs are any part of a plant—including the leaf, flower, root, stem, fruit or bark—used to make a medicine, fragrance, or food flavoring. Herbal medicines are touted as a safer and more natural approach to health care. Herbal supplements are packaged in teas, powders, tablets, liquids, and capsules.

The traditional Chinese medicine branch of herbalism relies on maintaining a balance between two forces, the yin and the yang, and the five major elements: fire, earth, water, metal, and wood. Many Chinese asthma herbs are derived from *ma huang*, a herb extracted from the ephedra bush. Chinese physicians and healers have used *ma huang* for more than 4,000 years to treat asthma. The study of *ma huang* led to the development of a western drug called ephedrine, a major ingredient of asthma medicines since the early twentieth century. Other popular herbal remedies include ginko biloba, believed to improve memory and thinking ability. St. John's Wort is widely used by people with mood disorders. Glucosamine and chondroitin sulfate are popular alternative treatments for joint pain and arthritis. Herbal research is in its first trimester. Only 5,000 of the world's 500,000 plants have been studied. While the majority of herbal papers are written in Chinese or Japanese, millions of Americans with allergies and asthma utilize these unproven products. The typical herbal user is a well-educated, middle-aged individual with a higher income. In other words—baby boomers are into herbal medicine big time.

> *While the majority of herbal papers are written in Chinese or Japanese, millions of Americans with allergies and asthma utilize these unproven products. The typical herbal user is a well-educated, middle-aged individual with a higher income. In other words—baby boomers are into herbal medicine big time.*

■ Herbal Side Effects

Presently, there are no standards in the United States that regulate the quality or strength of herbal products. The United

States lags far behind many European countries where herbal products are classified as drugs. It has been suggested that the FDA classify herbal products as over-the-counter medications. This would require manufacturers to provide proof of safety and effectiveness. There are several obstacles in the way of controlling herbal products. Many herbs will never be investigated as the cost of bringing a new drug to the marketplace approaches $500 million. Even if such a product were developed, patent rights would not protect it. The general public suffers under the misconception that all herbal products are safe. Since they have a decided pharmacological action, they do have risks.

Presently, there are too many unanswered questions regarding the rate of absorption in the body, dosages, and contaminants of herbal products. All users of herbal products should buy reliable brands and monitor publications dealing with the potential side effects and drug interactions of herbal medicines. Reliable sources for such information include *Consumer Reports*; NIH publications; *Prevention* magazine; and MEDLINE, a bibliographic database from the National Library of Medicine.

Many health-care providers have been too bewildered to thoroughly learn about alternative herbal products. Much of the care in this area is self-experimentation, where patients are more willing to rely on an unregulated herbal remedy than take a prescription drug. There is a growing need for educational efforts in the field of herbal medicine that will allow physicians to partner with their patients to help them make informed choices. A recent article in *Consumer Reports* noted that conventionally trained doctors were learning to be more sympathetic and less scornful. Most studies of herbal remedies for asthma and allergic disorders are poorly controlled and done in only a few patients. The bottom line: at the present time, I cannot recommend any herbal medicine as a form of alternative care in the treatment of food allergy or any other allergic disorder.[1]

> *The bottom line: At the present time, I cannot recommend any herbal medicine as a form of alternative care in the treatment of food allergy or any other allergic disorder*

■ Chinese Herbal Therapy— the Wave of the Future?

The first exciting study in Chinese herbal medicine and allergy was performed in mice. Researchers at Johns Hopkins and Mount Sinai schools of medicine found that the Chinese herb MSSM-002 contained fourteen herbal extracts that had significant anti-inflammatory and anti-asthmatic properties. Using a mouse-asthma model, the investigators found that the herbal preparation was comparable to cortisone drugs used to treat asthma. While a mouse is not a man, this promising study suggested that herbal preparations could have potent anti-inflammatory properties. In a follow up to this study, Dr. Xiu-Min Li from the Jaffe Food Institute found that a complex mixture of Chinese herbs

---

[1] For additional information and reading materials on alternative therapy, I recommend Natural Medicines Comprehensive Database, 3120 W. March Lane, P.O. Box 8190, Stockton, CA 95208, Telephone: 209-472-2244, and Fax: 209-472-2249. Also check out these Web sites: www.NaturalDatabase.com and Galaxy.com, a directory that lists the top ten places on the Internet for alternative health-care information.

turned off the anaphylactic response in peanut-allergic mice. Li overcame the hurdle of being able to duplicate this complex mixture of herbs (now called FAHF-2) by eliminating toxic herbs from the original formula.

Recent studies found that pretreatment of peanut-allergic mice with the Chinese herbal formula completely blocked peanut-induced anaphylaxis for up to six months—about 25 percent of a mice's life span. So far, the mice have not experienced any toxic side effects. Dr. Kamal D. Srivastava from Mount Sinai School of Medicine in New York states, "This is a significant finding in terms of the duration of protection with a single course of treatment that can be taken orally, making it an effective and convenient treatment that can be administered at home.

"We will also be working to identify the bioactive compounds present in the formula. The mechanism(s) underlying the effects of FAHF-2 remain to be elucidated. Our preliminary findings indicate that FAHF-2 may target multiple cell types like mast cells and T-cells."[2] Plans for human trials with this herbal preparation are now underway at the FDA. If man responds like a mouse, safe and inexpensive herbal therapy may ultimately provide an entirely new class of drugs to treat allergic disorders.

■ Controversial Food Allergy Therapy

All new drugs and procedures should be well studied in animals and humans to determine if they are safe and effective before being approved for general use. During clinical trials, a new drug or experimental procedure is administered to patients who have given their informed consent. The FDA and institutional review boards (IRBs) must approve these clinical trials. Unfortunately, these strict guidelines only apply to new drugs and medical procedures. Many older, outmoded, and controversial techniques have not been subjected to these stringent regulations. As a result, thousands of allergy and asthma sufferers are unknowingly victimized by unproven and controversial medical treatments.

Most medical and surgical specialists rely heavily on hospital support to practice medicine. When a doctor is judged to be incompetent or engages in unethical or questionable practices, the hospital can censure the offender or even suspend the doctor's hospital privileges. Regrettably, there are no such controls for some specialists or self-proclaimed allergists operating out of their private offices or clinics. The FDA and most state medical societies do not regulate medical practice in a private office setting unless the doctor is negligent or prescribes dangerous drugs.

If man responds like a mouse, safe and inexpensive herbal therapy may ultimately provide an entirely new class of drugs to treat allergic disorders.

Some popular approaches that have no scientific validity whatsoever include: kinesiology, where a patient holds foods in one hand and the practitioner tests muscle strength in the other hand; cytotoxic tests, which look at changes in white blood cells when they are exposed to foods; and electrodermal testing, where the subject is connected to a machine that measures a drop in electrical conductance.

---

[2] Megan Rauscher, "Chinese Herbal Formula Silences Peanut Allergy in Mice," *Reuters Health*, March 8, 2006.

■ Conditions Often Falsely Attributed to Food Allergy

Many practitioners would lead you to believe that many common medical disorders are due to a food allergy or a food intolerance. Chronic fatigue syndrome is defined as the onset of fatigue that reduces activities by more than 50 percent for more than six months without evidence of any other disease. Other symptoms include low-grade fever, headaches, joint pain, depression, sleep disorders, and visual problems. While some studies have attributed chronic fatigue syndrome to chemical sensitivities, there are no data that link chronic fatigue syndrome to food allergies or food intolerances.

Irritable bowel syndrome, which affects up to 25 percent of the population in western countries, is defined as a functional bowel disorder where abdominal pain is associated with changes in bowel habits. The diagnosis of irritable bowel syndrome is usually made when no other cause can be found for the patient's symptoms. In one study, two-thirds of irritable bowel syndrome victims reported their symptoms were triggered by foods. Additional studies have not linked food allergy to the irritable bowel syndrome.

Allergy specialists are often asked to evaluate patients with migraine headaches to rule out food allergies. Many foods and food additives can trigger vascular or migraine headaches, especially foods that contain additives like MSG, sulfites, and tyramine. Such foods include aged cheese, fresh yeast, fermented foods (such as pickles), legumes, chocolate, processed meats, sardines, anchovies, alcohol (especially red wine), and chicken. These reactions are not true allergic responses but are typical chemical intolerances or sensitivity reactions. An elimination diet for four weeks and an oral challenge may help to identify offending foods and chemicals in patients with migraine headaches. Many foods and chemicals have been implicated in diseases involving inflammation of joints and blood vessels. With the exception of gluten- or wheat-intolerance, there are no convincing studies indicating that foods or chemicals trigger these diseases.

More than eighty years ago, the notion that hyperactive behavior in children was due to food allergy was proposed. In the 1950s and again in the 1970s, hyperactivity, poor sleep patterns, and anxiety disorders were attributed to various food and food additives. In 1973, Dr. Ben Feingold reported that 30 to 50 percent of hyperactive children improved when they were placed on a sugar-free and additive-free diet. This diet, known as the Feingold diet, has not stood up to rigorous, well-conducted scientific studies. Thankfully, the Feingold diet, once very popular in the 1970s and 1980s, has faded out of the picture. However, some practitioners continue to employ similar unproven techniques that are often popularized by the media and talk shows.

A recent study looked at whether food additives, specifically food dyes and preservatives, had any effect on behavior in 277 children from the Isle of Wight, United Kingdom. This was a four-week study that followed a lead-in week in which the diet was free of artificial colorings and sodium benzoate. During the second or fourth week, children received either the placebo or the food additive, and they drank a fruit juice that was a placebo or one that contained various dyes, colorings and sodium benzoate. The children's behavior was assessed weekly by the clinic, and the parents also rated behavior. There was no difference in the activity scores measured in the clinic during the study. However, the parents' ratings showed a reduction in hyperactive behavior when the food additives were removed from the diet. One reviewer commented on the difficulty of reviewing this study:

"The authors have taken the gold-standard model of 'testing' and applied it with behavior as the outcome. A potential problem is the fact that this study was done at home and over an extended period of time and was not done solely in the clinic. Also of note is that the dyes and preservatives are not available for skin testing. Another message in this study is that the tools and the situation that is offered in the office to assess behavior do not match the parental observations. In summary, while there may be a subpopulation of children who exhibit bizarre behavior when exposed to food additives or colorings, there is absolutely no evidence that food allergy is involved in hyperactivity or attention deficit disorders." ●

Appendix

■ Food Allergy Organizations

The Food Allergy and Anaphylaxis Network

In 1991, Anne Muñoz-Furlong founded the Food Allergy and Anaphylaxis Network or FAAN. Her foresight created the world's most outstanding, nonprofit organization that provides support and educational materials for food allergy victims, their families, and anyone involved with food allergy. FAAN's primary mission is to raise public awareness, provide advocacy and education, and advance research for those affected by food allergy and anaphylaxis. FAAN's proactive programs and publications are referenced throughout this book.

Its membership includes patients, families, dietitians, nurses, physicians, school staff, and representatives from government agencies and food and pharmaceutical industries. FAAN is the world's leader in food allergy, anaphylaxis awareness, and the issues surrounding this disease. FAAN publishes a number of newsletters and dozens of books, booklets, and videos. The organization conducts seminars and training sessions on food allergy and anaphylaxis for patients, families, government officials, and industry leaders. FAAN works with policymakers on the federal, state, and local levels in such areas as food labeling, schools, emergency medical services, camps, restaurants, and airlines.

FAAN's bimonthly newsletter, *Food Allergy News*, provides the latest updates on food allergy research, legislative activities, dietary guidelines, and practical tips for managing food allergies. *Food Allergy News for Teens*, a bimonthly newsletter, offers information about food allergy and anaphylaxis, highlights the importance of carrying medications, and provides tips for managing food allergies in social settings, school, restaurants, and at work. Its youngest members receive *Food Allergy News for Kids*, a newsletter written for kids. *Food Allergy News for Physicians* is mailed quarterly to approximately 19,000 health-care professionals. Annual dues, sales of materials, grants, and donations help support FAAN. I strongly urge any patient, family, or organization impacted by food allergy to contribute to and join FAAN. For additional information contact FAAN at:

11781 Lee Jackson Highway, Suite 160
Fairfax, VA 22033
Phone: 800-929-4040 or 703-691-3179
Fax: 703-691-2713
Web site: foodallergy.org

The Food Allergy and Anaphylaxis Alliance Network

The Food Allergy and Anaphylaxis Alliance was established by FAAN in 1999 to exchange information among international nonprofit food allergy organizations. Its mission is to unite and share information among worldwide nonprofit FAAN-like organizations working in the field of food allergy and advance key issues in food allergy and anaphylaxis. International members of the Food Allergy and Anaphylaxis Alliance Network include:

Anaphylaxis Canada
2005 Sheppard Avenue East, Suite 800
Toronto, Ontario M2J 5B4
Phone: 416-785-5666
Fax: 416-785-0458
E-mail: info@anaphylaxis.ca

Association Quebecoise
des Allergies Alimentaires
445, boul. Sainte-Foy, Bureau 100
Longueuil, Québec J4J 1X9
Phone and fax: 514-990-2575
E-mail: info@aqaa.qc.ca
Web site: aqaa.qc.ca

Allergy New Zealand
PO Box 56 117
Dominion Road
Auckland, New Zealand
Phone: (09) 303-2024 or (09) 623-3912
Fax: (09) 623-0091
E-mail: mail@allergy.org.nz

Anaphylaxis Australia
21 Robinson Close
Hornsby Heights, NSW 2077, Australia
Web site: allergyfacts.org.au

The Anaphylaxis Campaign
PO Box 275
Farnborough Hampshire GU14 6SX
Phone: 01252 546100
Helpline: 01252 542029
Fax: 01252 377140
E-mail: info@anaphylaxis.org.uk

Food Allergy Italia
Via Paolotti
735121 Padova, Italy
Web site: foodallergyitalia.org

Nederlands Anaphylaxis Network
Oranjelaan 91 3311 DJ
Dordrecht, Nederland
Fax: 0031 (0)78 639 02 43
E-mail: info@anafylaxis.net

The Food Allergy Initiative
The Food Allergy Initiative, or FAI, is a nonprofit organization based in New York, dedicated to raising funds to support food allergy research. Established by concerned parents and grandparents, FAI's goal is to support research to find a cure for food allergies and anaphylaxis by 2010. In addition to funding research and clinical activities to identify and treat those at risk, FAI supports programs to create a safer environment for those afflicted by food allergy and heighten awareness of food allergy among health- and child-care workers, schools, camps, and members of the hospitality and food service industry. FAI provides grants to support food-allergic patients and their families at several research centers throughout the United States. In addition, they have established an international council to increase communication among leading scientists in Asia, Australia, Europe and the United States. FAI has established a medical advisory board to identify and recommend support for the most promising research projects in the United States and around the world. If you would like more information about this worthwhile organization, contact them at:

    41 East 62nd Street
    4th Floor
    New York, NY 10021
    Phone: 212-572-8428
    Fax: 212-572-8429
    E-mail: info@foodallergyinitiative.org
    Web site: foodallergyinitiative.org

The Asthma and Allergy Foundation of America

The Asthma and Allergy Foundation of America (AAFA) is a national, nonprofit organization dedicated to improving the quality of life for people affected by asthma and all allergic diseases. AAFA provides practical information, community-based services, educational programs, support, and referrals through a national network of chapters and educational support groups. AAFA's programs are designed to improve the quality of life and care for people with asthma and allergies in communities across the country. Its advocacy and outreach efforts have played an important role in establishing guidelines for the diagnosis and management of asthma and allergies; setting national standards to improve quality care for patients; obtaining federal funding for prevention programs; and strengthening laws that protect patient rights. To obtain more information on its programs or locate an AAFA chapter in your area, contact AAFA at:

1233 20th St. NW, Suite 402
Washington, DC 20036
Phone: 800-7-ASTHMA or
202-466-7643
Web site: aafa.org

The American Academy of Allergy, Asthma & Immunology (AAAAI)

The AAAAI is the largest professional specialty organization in the United States that represents allergists, asthma specialists, clinical immunologists, allied health professionals, and others with a special interest in the research and treatment of allergic disease. Established in 1943, AAAAI has more than 6,300 members in the United States, Canada, and 60 other countries. AAAAI's mission is the advancement of the knowledge and prac-

tice of allergy, asthma, and immunology for optimal patient care. AAAAI serves as a public advocate by providing educational information and publishing newsletters, pamphlets, and booklets for medical professionals and laypeople to keep them abreast of the latest news about allergies, asthma and immunology. AAAAI's Web site offers such information as pollen counts, a listing of asthma camps, timely press releases, the latest research on asthma and allergy, and a physician referral guide. Contact AAAAI at:

611 East Wells St.
Milwaukee, WI 53202
Phone: 800-822-2762 or 414-272-6071
Web site: aaaai.org

The American College of Allergy, Asthma & Immunology (ACAAI)

The ACAAI is a professional association of 4,900 allergists and immunologists. Established in 1942, ACAAI is dedicated to improving the quality of patient care in allergy and immunology through research, advocacy, and professional and public education. ACAAI's goals include improving the quality of patient care in allergy, asthma and immunology; maintaining and advancing the diagnostic and therapeutic skills of members; and fostering their appropriate application.

ACAAI serves as an advocate to the public by providing educational information, newsletters, pamphlets, and booklets for both medical professionals and laypeople to keep them abreast of the latest news about allergies, asthma and immunology. To contact ACAAI:

85 West Algonquin Road, Suite 550
Arlington Heights, IL 60005
Phone: 847-427-1200
Fax: 847-427-1294
Web site: acaai.org

Allergy & Asthma Network-Mothers of Asthmatics or AANMA

The organization, founded in 1985 by Nancy Sander, is a national nonprofit network of families whose desire is to overcome, not just cope with, allergies and asthma. The shortest route to that goal is knowledge— that's why AANMA produces accurate, timely, practical, and livable alternatives to suffering. AANMA's *Allergy & Asthma Today* magazine, *The MA Report* newsletter, e-news updates, toll-free help line, community awareness programs, and Breatherville, USA are valuable programs offered by AANMA. Its staff addresses questions and concerns, advocates for patient access to specialty care and appropriate treatments, promotes the importance of a school nurse in every school, and supports children's rights to carry inhalers while at school.

Allergy & Asthma Today is the newest member of AANMA's family of award-winning publications. This quarterly magazine is the ultimate consumer publication for people looking to build a healthier future free of allergy and asthma symptoms. Inside each issue you will find the latest news, practical how-to articles, real-life stories, and winning strategies for the whole family. To join or donate to AANMA:

2751 Prosperity Ave., Suite 150
Fairfax, VA 22031
Phone: 800-878-4403
Web site: breatherville.org

Anaphylaxis Canada

The Anaphylaxis Canada Registry is a Canadian information service for people who are allergic to food, insect stings, or medications; or who experience anaphylaxis with latex exposure or during exercise. Patients and families provide information about their allergies and then choose which information they want to receive, including updates on food labeling and product alerts, latest research findings, tips for staying safe, and school-related issues. Anyone with an interest in anaphylaxis can also sign up for this information service, including school and camp personnel, media, and medical professionals. Data from the Anaphylaxis Canada Registry, which is used to advance education about the scope of serious allergies in Canada, help the registry raise public awareness about anaphylaxis. Contact the registry at:

2005 Sheppard Avenue East, Suite 800
Toronto, Ontario M2J 5B4
Phone: 416-785-5666
Fax: 416-785-0458
Web site: anaphylaxis.ca

The Food Allergy Project

Founded by businessman David Bunning and his wife Denise, a former elementary school teacher who runs a support group for more than 200 Chicago families, the Food Allergy Project is a national coalition of parents, researchers, educators and experts who have come together to demand more federal resources dedicated to food allergy research and spur the scientific studies necessary to save children's lives. The Food Allergy Project has already raised more than 15 million dollars for food allergy research for the sake of millions of American children like their sons Bryan and Daniel, who have life-threatening allergies to milk, eggs, nuts and shellfish.

The Food Allergy Project has supported important research projects at Duke University, Children's Hospital Boston, Mt. Sinai Hospital in New York, Children's Memorial Hospital in Chicago, Northwestern University's Feinberg School of Medicine, and the University of Chicago Comer Children's Hospital. To contact or contribute to this worthwhile organization contact them at:

Phone: 212-681-1380
Email:
FoodAllergyInfo@FoodAllergyProject.org
Website: www.foodallergyproject.org

Allergy Asthma Information Association of Canada

The Allergy Asthma Information Association is a Canadian-registered charity dedicated to helping allergic individuals and their families cope with everything from the sniffles and sneezes of hay fever to life-threatening food allergies and asthma. It was founded as a voluntary organization in 1964 by concerned parents of allergic children who set out to get labeling on foods. Patient information is provided to 6,000 members across Canada in the form of counseling, seminars, and publications. A quarterly magazine keeps members informed of new research discoveries, new treatments, new products, and the successes of advocacy activities. Members have access to more than forty different "info letters" dealing with various aspects of asthma or allergy, as well as restaurant cards, warning buttons for children, cookbooks, videos, and presentation packages for parents. Contacts:

Box 100
Toronto, Ontario, Canada M9W 5K9
Phone: 416-679-952
Fax: 416-679-9524
Web site: calgaryallergy.ca/aaia

F.A.C.T.S. Association—Australia

The Food Anaphylactic Children Training and Support Association (FACTS) has operated as a nonprofit organization in Australia since 1993. Its award-winning Australian Web site has outstanding information for food-allergic children. It contains a wealth of reliable and up-to-date information on food allergies, food ingredients, food product alerts, product labeling, and resources. One highlight is its presentation of an animated cartoon for kids. This site will appeal to parents and allergic children.

Web site: allergyfacts.org.au

The Anaphylaxis Campaign— United Kingdom

In October 1993, seventeen-year-old Sarah Reading died after eating a lemon meringue pie served to her in the restaurant of a well-known department store. The dessert contained peanuts to which Sarah was fatally allergic. It soon became clear to Sarah's family that the condition from which she died was by no means rare. Consequently, a small group of parents in the United Kingdom, including Sarah's father, launched the Anaphylaxis Campaign in January 1994. Immediately, the newly formed campaign became inundated with calls for advice and information. The vast majority of these inquiries came from the parents of children who suffered serious reactions to peanuts, tree nuts, and other foods.

The Anaphylaxis Campaign is a membership-based organization that provides information and guidance primarily to its members and to potential members, but also to the media, health professionals, and food companies. By spring 2005, the Campaign had attracted nearly 8,000 members. The goals of this campaign are to preserve the health of those persons who suffer anaphylactic reactions and associated disorders. It does this by advancing research into the cause and care of such conditions and publishing the results of research to advance the education and general understanding of the public concerning anaphylaxis and associated disorders. The Anaphylaxis Campaign has a range of educational products, including information sheets, videos and a children's book.

Web site: anaphylaxis.org.uk

Asthma and Allergy Information and Research (AAIR)—United Kingdom

Asthma and Allergy Information and Research (AAIR) is the name for the

Leicester Branch of Midlands Asthma and Allergy Research Association (MAARA), a registered charity. Its medical advisor is Dr. Martin Stern, Consultant Clinical Immunologist at Leicester General Hospital.

12 Vernon St
Derby, U.K
Phone: 116 270-7557
Web site:
users.globalnet.co.uk/~aair/index.htm

Allergy Awareness Association— Everybody New Zealand

The Allergy Awareness Association is a national group that aims to assist individuals and families who need to cope with allergies and related illnesses. Presently, the Association provides an informative quarterly magazine, *Allergy News*, supports groups throughout New Zealand, and holds public meetings and panel discussions. It also provides access to medical and health professionals with expertise and experience in allergy. Contacts:

Box 56 117 Dominion Road
Auckland, New Zealand
Phone: 09-623-3912
Fax: 09-623-0091
Web site: everybody.co.nz/index.html

■ Other Internet Sites

Allergyadvisor.com

This is the hidden gem on the Internet. For the first time anywhere on the Web, one site consolidates worldwide, allergy-related journals (both printed and online versions) in a single site for rapid scanning by those interested in this field. Interesting articles, changes, and information are added to the site on a monthly basis. Its Internet newsletter, *The Allergy Advisor Digest*, highlights some of the more interesting articles. The site offers educational

reviews of food allergy and food intolerance aimed at supporting health professionals in their endeavor to assess and manage food allergies and food intolerances. The Web site and newsletter are compiled by Karen du Plessis, a registered dietitian, and edited by Dr. Harris Steinman (South Africa), Professor Janice Joneja (Canada), and Sabine Spiesser (Australia). To subscribe:

E-mail: info@zingsolutions.com.

Peanut Allergy: Where Do We Stand? allerg.qc.ca/peanutallergy.htm

If you want to review of all the important publications in the world's medical and lay press on peanut allergy, go to this informative Web site. The Web site is maintained by Dr. John Weisnagel, a pediatrician and allergist in private practice at Polyclinique Médicale Concorde, 300 est boul. de la Concorde, Laval, Qué. H7G 2E6. Weisnagel's comprehensive review of peanut allergy dates back to 1998. A great read and resource.

Kids With Food Allergies, Inc. kidswithfoodallergies.org

An informative site founded by Lynda Mitchell, Kids With Food Allergies provides online programs for families raising children with food allergies and anaphylaxis. Parents of Food Allergic Kids (POFAK) is its most popular and active feature, where parents connect with each other for support in a 24-hour chat room. POFAK Child of the Month is a new section that features children's food allergy stories submitted by their parents. Resources provide practical, been-there tips from other parents, articles, and frequently asked questions (FAQs) developed by its medical advisory team. The recipe database offers hundreds of allergy-friendly recipes for your family in a searchable format. Family memberships are $25 per year. Contact:

Phone: 215-230-5394
Fax: 215-340-7674
E-mail:
lmitchell@kidswithfoodallergies.org

Allergic Child USA
Allergicchild.com

This is the creation of Robert and Nicole Smith, the parents of two children with allergies. Their experience, and thereby expertise, in raising two children with severe allergies spawned this Web site. The Smiths share their experience with you to help you keep your food- allergic child safe, healthy, and living as close to a "normal life" as possible. Contact:

425 W Rockrimmon Blvd, Suite 202
Colorado Springs, CO 80919
Phone: 800-444-4094.

Access4allergickids.com

This informative site for parents of children with severe food allergies, asthma, and other allergic conditions is maintained by Nadine O'Reilly, a practicing school psychologist and mother of a peanut-allergic and asthmatic toddler. This site offers excellent advice on how to get the most out of your food-allergic child's experience in the American school system.

■ Food Allergy Publications for Adults

There are more than 300 publications on food allergy and food intolerance and thousands more on diet and nutrition. In the following sections, I will review what I consider to be the more informative (non-medical) books on food allergy and food intolerance. Some of the reviews are mine.

Other reviews, especially on cookbooks, were gathered from Internet sites, such as Amazon and Barnes and Noble. For additional information and reviewers' comments on these publications, I suggest you Google each title. FAAN is the best overall source for books, publications, and pamphlets on food allergy.

Caring for Your Child with Severe Food Allergies: Emotional Support and Practical Advice from a Parent Who's Been There. John Wiley and Sons, 2000, by Lisa Cipriano Collins, MA, MFT.

A *Library Journal* review states, "Lisa Collins, a family therapist and the mother of a child with severe nut allergies, outlines the management of life-threatening childhood allergies and the stresses they create within the family. She presents a short, concise manual for parents and other family members and caregivers. Most of the text is devoted to providing techniques for maximizing safety and minimizing the risk of anaphylactic shock. The book explores the emotional family context as well as the complexities of allergy management outside the home, in school settings, in restaurants, and on trips. The medical components of the book are well documented, and a short resource guide accompanies the text."

CDC Travel Health Book

In my Internet and bookstore perusals, I came across this informative publication. While it does not specifically address food allergy, "The Yellow Book," which is named for its traditionally yellow cover, is officially entitled *Health Information for International Travel*. It serves as an authoritative guide for pre-travel health-care recommendations and essential information about health risks abroad. It is a resource for travel medicine specialists as well as primary health-care providers who need to provide travel advice. The book offers vaccination and medication information for disease risks by destination as well as helpful health hints for cruise ship travel, international adoptions, and a wide range of common travel problems. The new edition of the "Yellow Book," the Centers for Disease Control and Prevention's definitive guide on healthy travel, is now more accessible than ever to the traveling public. It is available at bookstores, through Internet booksellers, or from Elsevier Book Order Fulfillment at 800-545-2522 or on its Web site: us.elsevierhealth.com.

Dealing With Food Allergies. A Practical Guide for Detecting Culprit Foods and Eating a Healthy, Enjoyable Diet. Bull Publishing, 2003, by Janice Vickerstaff Joneja, PhD, RDN.

This book targets food sufferers and their families. Up-to-date medical and scientific research helps the reader understand the differences between food allergy and food intolerance. It features practical methods for uncovering hidden food culprits and provides a step-by-step guide for elimination and challenge procedures. It is one of the best sources I found for elimination diets, recipes, and meal plans for food allergy and intolerance. If you have a food allergy or food intolerance and need to go on an elimination diet, this is the book that tells you what you can and cannot safely eat.

Dietary Management of Food Allergies & Food Intolerances. A Comprehensive Guide. J.A. Hall Publications, 2003, by Janice Vickerstaff Joneja, PhD, RDN.

Another extremely informative book by Joneja that is designed to provide the information and tools required to detect food sensitivities and advise on nutritionally adequate diets. This reference book is targeted to allergy specialists, primary care providers, and nutritionists involved in treating patients with food allergies and food intolerances.

FAAN's Cookbooks

The Food Allergy News Holiday Cookbook. **FAAN,** 2005.

This FAAN cookbook offers more than 150 tempting recipes and helpful tips for substituting foods, cooking, and hosting safe celebrations throughout the year. All recipes feature easy directions and simple ingredients and are marked to indicate which of the eight major food allergens they exclude. Whether you are hosting a Super Bowl party at your home or traveling to an Independence Day barbecue, this book will be a great reference for festive, allergy-free recipes for every occasion. It includes a recipe index and 12 black-&-white photos. FAAN also publishes *The Food Allergy News Cookbook: A Collection of Recipes from Food Allergy News and Members of the Food Allergy Network.*

5 Years Without Food: The Food Allergy Survival Guide. Allergy Adapt, 1997, by Nicolette M. Dumke.

This book helps those with food allergies get to the root of the daily problem of what to eat while on an allergen-free diet. The book includes an easily personalized rotation diet for allergies and 500 recipes. For those who don't have time to cook, there are sources of commercially prepared foods for people with allergies. Health journalist Marjorie Jones, RN, says, "If you are serious about turning your health around, this book belongs in your health library—or more accurately, at your fingertips for daily use."

***Foods That Harm, Foods That Heal—
An A-Z Guide to Safe and Healthy
Living.*** Reader's Digest Association, 2004.

Being neither a dietitian nor a cook, I
have not researched all the important
books in this specialty. However, of those
food books that I have read, this is by far
the best of the best. Leading nutrition
experts shatter many long-held beliefs
about what it means to eat healthily, fight
disease, look better, live longer and feel
stronger. No wonder 6 million copies of
the original book have been sold worldwide. Totally revised and updated with the
latest scientific findings and time-honored
natural remedies, *Foods That Harm, Foods
That Heal* offers important information on
the role diet plays in the struggle against
heart disease, cancer, diabetes, and other
serious illnesses, as well as the impact of
food on stress, insomnia, and other common complaints.

This coffee table publication dispels
many myths and gives the reader a useful
and comprehensive look at food, nutrition,
and health. It analyzes many different kinds
of foods, telling you what is good and bad
about each one. The information is well-
organized, making it easy to skim through
for quick reading if your interest is specific to a certain food or what to eat if you suffer from a specific disease. Lastly, the book
is also a visual treat filled with incredible
color photographs and easy-to-read text
and charts. A great reference book and a
valuable addition to anyone's library who
has an interest in foods and nutrition.

***How to Manage your Child's Life-threat-
ening Food Allergies: Practical Tips for
Everyday Life.*** Plumtree Press, 2004, by
Linda Marienhoff Coss.

The author has over ten years of experience raising a child with severe food allergies and leading a support group for parents of children with food allergies. She is
also the author of a popular food allergy
cookbook. Topics covered include preparing for and treating allergic reactions; pur-
chasing and cooking food; making your
home a "safe haven;" teaching others about
your child's allergies; handling parenting
issues; creating a safe school and day-care
environment; and having a social life and
dining in restaurants.

***Food Allergies and Food Intolerance.
The Complete Guide to Their Identification and Treatment.*** Healing Arts Press,
2000, by Jonathan Brostoff, M.D. and
Linda Gamlin.

This book clearly defines the difference
between food allergy and food intolerance
with numerous case studies. Brostoff, a
professor of allergy at University College
London Medical School, is a leading international authority on food intolerance.
Gamlin is a biochemist and acknowledged
expert on food allergy. While most conventional allergists like myself may not
always agree with many of the food intolerance concepts, this book is a very
informative source on these issues. An
excellent read for those who seek more
information on food intolerances.

***Understanding and Managing Your
Child's Food Allergies.*** Johns Hopkins
University Press, 2006 by Scott H.
Sicherer, M.D.

This guide gives parents the information
needed to manage their children's health
and quality of life. Parents will learn how
to recognize emergency situations, how to
get the most out of a visit with an allergist,
what allergy test results mean, and how to
protect their children—at home, at school,
at summer camp, and in restaurants.

"Provides families with state-of-the-art
education about food allergy."—Robert A.

Wood, M.D., Director, Division of Pediatric Allergy and Immunology, the Johns Hopkins Children's Center

"Dr. Sicherer is a rare combination of brains, compassion, understanding, and practicality ... A reference tool that belongs in everyone's bookcase."—from the foreword by Anne Muñoz-Furlong, the Food Allergy & Anaphylaxis Network.

Food Allergy Survivors Together Handbook. iUniverse, 2002, by Melissa Taylor.

This book is geared toward teenagers and adults who are newly diagnosed with food allergy. The book takes the reader on a journey through the various skills needed, such as learning to make food fun again, reading labels, shopping, dealing with others, and much more. Not a recipe book nor a cookbook, this upbeat guide offers practical tips for living with food allergies.

With participation from nearly two dozen individuals, this innovative book contains a little bit of everything. You'll find articles, cooking tips, extracurricular activity suggestions, humor, jokes and cartoons, photographs, travel tips, and profiles of people with allergies. Best of all, the book is informal and uplifting, not heavy and weighty as health literature can tend to be. This book has received five-star reviews on both the Amazon and Barnes-Noble Web sites.

Great Foods Without Worry. Aventine Press, 2003, by Cindy Moseley.

Some Internet reviewers' comments: "The recipes are written for those with multiple food allergies (wheat, dairy, egg and nuts). For the first time (and after four years of trying!) we have baked goods that are safe for our daughter and we feel are actually as good as the normal ones. We love this book! Finally, a good book for multiple allergies."

"We have several other food allergy cookbooks, and the recipes are OK. Cindy's recipes are fantastic! Not only are they truly delicious, but extremely helpful when dealing with a diet limited by food allergies. Her recipes are the first wheat-free recipes I have tried that aren't taste-free! Something I also found helpful was the fact that almost all the recipes use the same basic ingredients, so once you have a few of the different flours, you can pretty much make almost any recipe in the book. I highly recommend this book!"

Stories from Parents' Hearts: Essays by Parents of Children with Food Allergies. by Anne Muñoz-Furlong, CEO and founder of FAAN.

This book is a collection of stories from families with different approaches to food allergy. It is an excellent source to better understand family dynamics. Other valuable books in this series include, *Stories from the Heart: A collection of Essays from Teens with Food Allergies*, Volumes 1 and 2.

The Allergy Self-Help Cookbook. Rodale Press, 2001, by Marjorie Hurt Jones, RN.

This manual contains over 325 natural foods recipes, free of all common food allergens. One reviewer states, "This book stresses eating a variety of foods. Many of the recipes are fine, no-nonsense recipes for family eating. Most of the ingredients are readily available. I haven't followed the recipes exactly, just borrowed ideas as I saw fit." The book includes a very comprehensive guide to mail-order companies.

The Complete Food Allergy Cookbook: The Foods You've Always Loved Without the Ingredients You Can't Have. Prima Press, 1997, by Marilyn Gioannini.

The author provides information on detecting food allergy symptoms, avoiding problems at dinner parties and restaurants, substituting foods, and altering recipes. This book makes the difficult task of changing your diet amazingly easy. Avoiding such common foods as wheat, corn, and dairy products doesn't have to be a hassle or mean giving up favorites like, bread, pizza, or even ice cream!

At the heart of *The Complete Food Allergy Cookbook* are more than 150 appetizing recipes incorporating substitutions that make it possible to eat what you want without adverse reactions. In addition to hundreds of great ideas for delicious allergen-free cooking, you'll discover easy instructions for altering your favorite recipes and tips for eating in restaurants, at dinner parties, and while traveling.

This is a general resource for people with multiple food allergies who are having a hard time figuring out just what to eat. There is information on food allergies in general, alternative grains, substitutions for common allergens, and dealing with one's food allergies in day-to-day situations, such as dining out.

The Peanut Allergy Handbook: A Guide for Parents. Peanut Aware Inc., 2004, by Sheila Rusnell-Newton.

Current Internet quotes include: "Indispensable resource—portable handbook as vital as your Epipen—belongs in the backpack of every child with a nut allergy." *Calgary Child Magazine* (December 2005) states: "This must-have guide offers practical solutions on how your child can live with a life-threatening allergy. This handbook enables users to store an allergic child's personal information, including photo, medical information, emergency action plan, and notes specific to the child—all the information that parents, grandparents or any caregiver should have at their fingertips. This book is designed in a small-size, spiral-bound fashion to allow it to be stored in a child's backpack, fanny pack, or other portable location. The personalized *Peanut Allergy Handbook* will keep an allergic child safe—and could save his life."

The Complete Peanut Allergy Handbook. Berkley Publishing Group, 2005, by Dr. Scott Sicherer and Terry Malloy.

A very informative book written in a question-and-answer format by Scherer, a leading international researcher in food allergy. A review by Ann Muñoz-Furlong, FAAN CEO, states: "Doctor Sicherer has taken the hundreds of questions he's heard from patients and their families and condensed them in this book. Anyone who wants to know more about peanut allergy will find this book a great reference that they will go back to over and over again. A must-read for patients, parents and caregivers caring for children with peanut- and tree nut-allergy."

The Food Allergy Survival Guide—Living Well Without Dairy, Eggs, Fish, Gluten, Peanuts, Shellfish, Soy, Tree Nuts, Wheat, Yeast & More. Healthy Living Publications, 2004, by Vesanto Melina, MS, RD; Jo Stepaniak, MSEd; and Dina Aronson, MS, RD.

Up until now, it was difficult to find a book that addressed the needs of vegetarians with food allergies. This book provides extensive information and an excellent recipe collection for those with allergies or sensitivities to dairy products, eggs, gluten, nuts and peanuts, soy, yeast, fish and shellfish, and wheat. A great resource for dealing with multiple food allergies. The last half of the book features more than 100 recipes for everything from gluten-free baked goods to soy-free entrées and spreads.

Parent's Guide to Food Allergies. Henry Holt and Company, 2001, by Marianne S. Barber, a mother of an allergic child; Maryanne Bartoszek Scott, M.D., a board-certified allergist; and Elinor Greenberg, a PhD psychologist.

This user-friendly text covers guidelines established by FAAN. It details day-to-day living traveling and psychological ramifications of raising a food-allergic child. Good source for alternative foods, hidden foods, tasty recipes, and how to deal with accidental ingestions.

The Peanut Allergy Answer Book. Fair Winds Press, 2006, by Dr. Michael Young.

My good friend and colleague, Dr. Michael Young, has written a very informative resource book for parents of children afflicted with peanut- and tree nut-allergy. Now in its second edition, this well-written, easy-to-read, question-and-answer format helps relieve the anxiety and frustration often associated with food allergy and anaphylaxis.

Young's collection of illustrative cases helps to explain the up-to-date scientific information for those who want to learn more about peanut allergy. I recommend this book to all my patients, parents of allergic children, other caregivers, and health-care providers who must deal with peanut or tree nut allergy.

What's to Eat? The Milk-Free, Egg-Free, Nut-Free Food Allergy Cookbook. Plumtree Press, 2000, by Linda Marienhoff Coss.

A review in *Allergy and Asthma Today*: "Allergy-free cooking never tasted this good!" Chris Papkee, founder, PeanutAllergy.com: "This book is fantastic! It's one of the best food allergy cookbooks I've seen. Everyone should have a copy." *Midwest Book Review*: "Showcasing more than 145 recipes for dairy-free, egg-free, and nut-free meals, it is a superbly organized food allergy-oriented cookbook by prize winning recipe developer Linda Marienhoff Coss." It includes preparation and cooking times for each recipe so you can plan your meals around the time you have available to cook.

The Whole Foods Allergy Cookbook: Two Hundred Gourmet & Homestyle Recipes for the Food Allergic Family. Vital Health Publishing, 2006, by Cybele Pascal.

This is the first cookbook to contain 200 gourmet and homestyle recipes that are free of the Big Eight allergens. The author learned about hypoallergenic cooking first-hand when her son was diagnosed with severe food allergies. This book has the best reviews of any cookbook I have found. *Library Journal*: "Offers real-life suggestions on how to adapt to the food-allergic lifestyle. Highly recommended for public libraries." Eric Chadian, M.D., director of the Center for Health and the Global Environment at Harvard Medical School, states, "Food allergies are becoming a major public health problem.

There is an urgent need for a cookbook like this." *Food Allergy News*: "This book provides many easy-to-follow recipes and fresh menu ideas for food allergy sufferers and those on a restricted diet." Another Internet review states: "*The Whole Foods Allergy Cookbook* by hypoallergenic cooking expert, Cybele Pascal, offers a culinary wealth of dishes that would serve any dinning occasion from simple family meals to festive celebratory occasions, for anyone with a common food allergy. I think I have almost all food allergy cookbooks out there and this has got to be the best one on my shelf."

■ Publications for Children

The Alexander Series.

FAAN has created an informative series of food allergy books (and videos) for elementary school children that target different food eating activities, including, *A Special Day At School, Alexander and His Pals Visit the Main Street School, Alexander Goes to a Birthday Party, Alexander Goes Trick-or-Treating, Alexander's Fun & Games Activity Book, Andrew and Maya Learn About Food Allergies*, and *Alexander the Elephant Who Couldn't Eat Peanuts Coloring Books*. Great books and videos for educating younger school children about food allergies.

Allie the Allergic Elephant. Jungle Communications, 1999, by Nicole Smith.

This book is geared toward preschool age through first grade. It explains why an allergic child will say "no thank you" to foods offered, what an allergic reaction looks like (hives, coughing, swollen lips), and which foods "hide" peanuts. All this, and an elephant with hives too.

No Nuts for Me! Tumbleweed Press, 1999, by Zevy, Aaron, and Susan Tebbutt.

Written for ages three to eight, this story is narrated by a very active little boy who doesn't let his nut allergy get in the way of having fun. Readers will meet Noah, who carries on a running conversation throughout the story and explains, in a matter-of-fact tone, what it's like to be allergic to nuts.

Peter Can't Eat Peanuts. O'Reilly Publishing, Inc., 2006, by Nadine O'Reilly.

The author, a practicing school psychologist, was frustrated by the lack of age-appropriate materials to educate her son about his asthma and life-threatening peanut allergy. Her book is the product of her bedtime stories. At the age of two, her son Peter, could cite passages from her stories almost verbatim. She then created a book based on the child development principle that language and rhyme aid in social and emotional growth. The book is available through the author's informative website: access4allergickids.com.

The Peanut Butter Jam. Health Press, 2001, by Elizabeth Sussman Nassau and Margot Janet Ott, illustrator.

World-renowned food allergy specialist Dr. Hugh A. Sampson says, "*The Peanut Butter Jam* is a wonderful story that provides great insight into what it is like to live with a peanut allergy. Sam's day at school is reminiscent of what hundreds of peanut-allergic children face each day. It provides a life-like account of what can happen during an anaphylactic reaction to peanut and how a well-prepared school should respond. Elizabeth Sussman Nassau obviously has "been there" and has provided an entertaining story for children and educational primer for adults. It is a "must read" for families with food allergic children and educators with food allergic students."

The Peanut Pickle: A Story About Peanut Allergy. Small Press Book Watch, 2005, by Jessica Ureel and Elizabeth Brazeal, illustrator.

This book combines the gifted storytelling of Ureel (the parent of a child with a severe peanut allergy) with the charming color illustrations of Brazeal. Find out how Ben takes control of his peanut allergy in school, at parties, with friends, at T-ball practice, and during holidays. Kids will learn to follow Ben's example and speak up about their food allergy. *The Peanut Pickle* describes many situations in which a potentially life-threatening exposure to peanuts can and must be avoided by speaking up, finding alternative foods, or alternative activities.

Food Allergy Action Plan

Student's Name:_____ **D.O.B:**_____ **Teacher:**_____

ALLERGY TO:_____ _____

Asthmatic Yes* ☐ No ☐   *Higher risk for severe reaction

Place Child's Picture Here

◆ STEP 1: TREATMENT ◆

Symptoms:

- If a food allergen has been ingested, but *no symptoms*:
- Mouth   Itching, tingling, or swelling of lips, tongue, mouth
- Skin   Hives, itchy rash, swelling of the face or extremities
- Gut   Nausea, abdominal cramps, vomiting, diarrhea
- Throat†   Tightening of throat, hoarseness, hacking cough
- Lung†   Shortness of breath, repetitive coughing, wheezing
- Heart†   Thready pulse, low blood pressure, fainting, pale, blueness
- Other†   _____
- If reaction is progressing (several of the above areas affected), give

The severity of symptoms can quickly change. †Potentially life-threatening.

Give Checked Medication**:
**(To be determined by physician authorizing treatment)

☐ Epinephrine   ☐ Antihistamine
☐ Epinephrine   ☐ Antihistamine
☐ Epinephrine   ☐ Antihistamine
☐ Epinephrine   ☐ Antihistamine
☐ Epinephrine   ☐ Antihistamine
☐ Epinephrine   ☐ Antihistamine
☐ Epinephrine   ☐ Antihistamine
☐ Epinephrine   ☐ Antihistamine
☐ Epinephrine   ☐ Antihistamine

DOSAGE

Epinephrine: inject intramuscularly (circle one) EpiPen® EpiPen® Jr. Twinject™ 0.3 mg Twinject™ 0.15 mg (see reverse side for instructions)

Antihistamine: give_____
                                      medication/dose/route

Other: give_____
                                      medication/dose/route

IMPORTANT: Asthma inhalers and/or antihistamines cannot be depended on to replace epinephrine in anaphylaxis.

◆STEP 2: EMERGENCY CALLS ◆

1. Call 911 (or Rescue Squad: _____) . State that an allergic reaction has been treated, and additional epinephrine may be needed.

2. Dr. _____   Phone Number: _____at_____

3. Parents_____   Phone Number(s)_____

4. Emergency contacts:
Name/Relationship   Phone Number(s)

a. _____   1.)_____   2.) _____

b. _____   1.)_____   2.) _____

EVEN IF PARENT/GUARDIAN CANNOT BE REACHED, DO NOT HESITATE TO MEDICATE OR TAKE CHILD TO MEDICAL FACILITY!

Parent/Guardian Signature_____   Date_____

Doctor's Signature_____   Date_____
                    (Required)

TRAINED STAFF MEMBERS

1. _____   Room _____

2. _____   Room _____

3. _____   Room _____

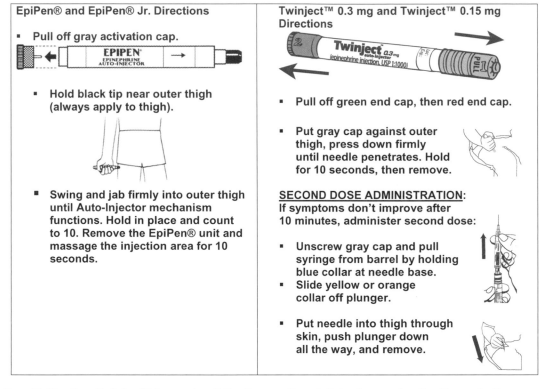

EpiPen® and EpiPen® Jr. Directions

- Pull off gray activation cap.

  - Hold black tip near outer thigh (always apply to thigh).

  - Swing and jab firmly into outer thigh until Auto-Injector mechanism functions. Hold in place and count to 10. Remove the EpiPen® unit and massage the injection area for 10 seconds.

Twinject™ 0.3 mg and Twinject™ 0.15 mg Directions

- Pull off green end cap, then red end cap.

- Put gray cap against outer thigh, press down firmly until needle penetrates. Hold for 10 seconds, then remove.

SECOND DOSE ADMINISTRATION:
If symptoms don't improve after 10 minutes, administer second dose:

- Unscrew gray cap and pull syringe from barrel by holding blue collar at needle base.
- Slide yellow or orange collar off plunger.

- Put needle into thigh through skin, push plunger down all the way, and remove.

Once EpiPen® or Twinject™ is used, call the Rescue Squad. Take the used unit with you to the Emergency Room. Plan to stay for observation at the Emergency Room for at least 4 hours.

For children with multiple food allergies, consider providing separate Action Plans for different foods.

The Food Allergy & Anaphylaxis Network

**Medication checklist adapted from the Authorization of Emergency Treatment form developed by the Mount Sinai School of Medicine. Used with permission.

Food Allergy Action Plan reprinted with permission from FAAN www.foodallergy.org

■ MedicAlert Foundation International

United States
2323 Colorado Avenue
Turlock, CA 95382
Phone: 888-633-4298
Fax: 209-699-2450
Web site: medicalert.org

Australia MedicAlert Foundation
St John House
216 Greenhill Rd
Eastwood, South Australia 5063
Phone: 61 88 274 0361
Web site: medicalert.com.au

British Isles & Ireland MedicAlert Foundation
1 Bridge Wharf 156 Caledonian Rd
London N1 9UU
Phone: 44 20 7833 3034
Web site: medicalert.org.uk

Canadian MedicAlert Foundation
2005 Sheppard Avenue East Suite 800
Phone: 416-696-0267
Toronto, Ontario, M2J 5B4 Canada
Web site: medicalert.ca

MedicAlert Foundation Cyprus
P.O. Box 23791 Kassos Street Nr. 18c
Nicosia 1086, Cyprus
Phone: 357 22315113
Web site: medicalertcyprus.com

MedicAlert Foundation Iceland
Soltun 20 105
Reykjavik, Iceland
Phone: 354-561-3122

MedicAlert Foundation Malaysia
University Hospital
Lembah Pantai 50603
Kuala Lumpar, Malaysia
Phone: 60 3 7950 2816

MedicAlert Foundation New Zealand, Inc.
Astral Towers, 88-90 Main St.
Upper Hutt 6007, New Zealand
Phone: 64 4 528 8218
Web site: medicalert.co.nz

South African MedicAlert Foundation
5th Floor AON House
Hertzog Boulevard
Foreshore Cape Town 8001,
South Africa
Phone: 27-21-4257328

MedicAlert Foundation of Zimbabwe
60 Livingston Avenue
Harare, Zimbabwe
Phone: 2673-4-759-512
Web site: medicalert.co.zw

■ Scientific References

The following references (listed by authors) are what I consider to be the more important scientific articles on food allergy published in the past two decades.

Akdie M, Blaser K, Akdis CA. T regulatory cells in allergy: Novel concepts in the pathogenesis, prevention and treatment of allergic diseases. *J Allergy Clin Immunol* 2005;116:961-8.

Appelt GK, et al. Breast-feeding and food avoidance are ineffective in preventing sensitization in high-risk children. *J Allergy Clin Immunol* 2004 Feb;13.suppl., no.2

Bock SA, Atkins FM. The natural history of peanut allergy. *J Allergy Clin Immunol* 1989;83:900-904.

Bock SA, Muñoz-Furlong A, Sampson HA. Fatalities due to anaphylactic reactions to foods. *J Allergy Clin Immunol* 2001 Jan;107(1):191-193.

Burks W, Lehrer SB, Bannon GA. New approaches for treatment of peanut allergy: chances for a cure. *Clin Rev Allergy Immunol* 2004 Nov;27(3):191-6.

Church MK, Warner JO. Preventing the evolution of the allergic march towards asthma: have we found the answer? *Clin Exp Allergy* 2006;6:10-14.

Clark AT, Ewan PW. The development and progression of allergy to multiple nuts at different ages. *Pediatr Allergy Immunol* 2005 Sep;16(6):507-11.

Clark S, Bock SA, Gaeta TJ, Brenner BE, Cydulka RK, Camargo CA. Multicenter study of emergency department visits for food allergies. *J Allergy Clin Immunol* 2004;113(2):347-352.

Ewan PW. Clinical study of peanut and nut allergy in 62 consecutive patients: new features and associations. *BMJ* 1996;312:1074-78.

Foucard T, Malmheden Yman I. A study on severe food reactions in Sweden— is soy protein an underestimated cause of food anaphylaxis? *Allergy* 1999 Mar;54(3):261-5.

Fleischer DM, Conover-Walker MK, Christie L, Burks AW, Wood RA. The natural progression of peanut allergy: Resolution and the possibility of recurrence. *J Allergy Clin Immunol* 2003;112(1):183-9.

Furlong TJ, Desimone J, Sicherer SH. Peanut- and tree nut-allergic reactions in restaurants and other food establishments. *J Allergy Clin Immunol* 2001;108(5 Part 1):867-70.

Grundy J, et al. Rising prevalence of allergy to peanut in children: Data from 2 sequential cohorts. *J Allergy Clin Immunol* 2002; 110(5):784-9.

Hourihane JO, et al. Clinical characteristics of peanut allergy. *Clin Exp Allergy* 1997;27(6):634-639.

Hourihane, JO. Prevalence and severity of food allergy—need for control. *Allergy* 1998;53(46 Suppl):84-88.

Jaffe Food Allergy Institute, Mount Sinai School of Medicine, New York, NY. Pediatric food allergy: FAAN co-sponsored. suppl., *Pediatrics* 2003;111(6 Pt3).

Kagan RS, Clarke AE. Prevalence of peanut allergy in primary-school children in Montreal, Canada. *J Allergy Clin Immunol* 2003;112(6):1223-8.

Kemp SF, Lockey RF. Anaphylaxis: a review of causes and mechanisms. *J Allergy Clin Immunol* 2002;110(3):341-8.

Lack G, Fox D, Northstone K, Golding J. Avon Longitudinal Study of Parents and Children Study Team. Factors associated with the development of peanut allergy in childhood. *N Engl J Med* 2003; 348(11):977-85.

Leung DY, Bock SA. Progress in peanut allergy research: Are we closer to a cure? *J Allergy Clin Immunol* 2003;112(1.

Leung DY, et al. Effect of Anti-IgE Therapy (TNX-901) in patients with peanut allergy. *N Engl J Med* 2003;348(11):986-93

Lieberman P, Kemp SF, Oppenheimer JJ, Land I, Bernstein IL, Nicklas RA et al. The diagnosis and management of ana- phylaxis: an updated practice parameter. *J Allergy Clin Immunol* 2005;115:S485- S523

Lieberman P. Biphasic anaphylactic reactions. *Ann Asthma Immunol* 2005;95:217-226.

Moneret-Vautrin DA, et al. Food allergy to peanuts in France—evaluation of 142 observations. *Clin Exp Allergy* 1998;(9):1113-9

Noveer MC, Huffnagle GB. The 'microflora hypothesis' of allergic dis- eases. *Clin Exp Allergy* 2005;35:1511-20.

Nowak-Wegrzyn A, Conover-Walker MK, Wood RA. Food-allergic reactions in schools and preschools. *Arch Pediatr Adolesc Med* 2001;155(7):790-5

Perry TT, et al. Distribution of peanut allergen in the environment. *J Allergy Clin Immunol* 2004;(5):973-6.

Pumphrey RS, Stanworth SJ. The clinical spectrum of anaphylaxis in northwest England. *Clin Exp Allergy* 1996 Dec;26(12):1364-70

Pumphrey RS. Lessons for management of anaphylaxis from a study of fatal reac- tions. *Clin Exp Allergy* 2000;(8):1144-50.

Rance F, Bidat E, Bourrier T, Sabouraud D. Cashew allergy: observations of 42 children without associated peanut aller- gy. *Allergy* 2003;58(12):1311-4

Roberts G, Patel N, Levi-Schaffer F, Habibi P, Lack G. Food allergy as a risk factor for life-threatening asthma in child- hood. *J Allergy Clin Immunol* 2003;112(1):168-74.

Sampson HA. Food Allergy. *JAMA* 1999;278(22):1888-1894.

Sampson HA, Mendelson L, Rosen JP. Fatal and near-fatal anaphylactic reac- tions to food in children and adolescents. *N Engl J Med* 1992;327(6):380-4.

Sampson HA. Food allergy, Part 1: Immunopathogenesis and clinical fea- tures. *J Allergy Clin Immunol* 1999;103 (5 Pt 1):717-28.

Sampson HA. Food allergy, Part 2: Diag- nosis and management. *J Allergy Clin Immunol* 1999;103(6):981-9

Sampson HA. Update on food allergy. *J Allergy Clin Immunol* 2004;113(5): 805-19.

Sampson HA, Muñoz-Furlong A, Camp- bell RL, Adkinson NF, Bock SA et al. Second Symposium on the definition and management of anaphylaxis: Summary report Second National institute of Aller- gy and Infectious Disease/Food Allergy and Anaphylaxis Network symposium. *J Allergy Clin Immunol* 2006;117:391-397.

Sampson HA. Clinical Practice. Peanut Allerg. *N Engl J Med* 2002;346:1294-99.

Sicherer SH, Burks AW, Sampson HA. Clinical features of acute allergic reactions to peanut and tree nuts in children. *Pediatrics* 1998;102(1):E6.

Sicherer SH, Furlong TJ, DeSimone J, Sampson HA. Self-reported allergic reactions to peanut on commercial airliners. *J Allergy Clin Immunol* 1999;104:186-9.

Sicherer SH, and Sampson HA. Peanut- and tree nut-allergy: Current opinion in *Pediatrics* 2000;12:567-573.

Sicherer SH, Furlong TJ, Desimone J, Sampson HA. The US Peanut and Tree Nut Allergy Registry: Characteristics of reactions in schools and day care. *J Pediatrics* 2001;138(4):560.

Sicherer SH, Furlong TJ, Muñoz-Furlong A, Burks AW, Sampson HA. Prevalence of peanut- and tree nut-allergy in the US determined by a random digit dial telephone survey. *J Allergy Clin Immunol* 1999;103(4):559-62.

Sicherer H, Furlong TJ, Muñoz-Furlong A, Burks AW, Sampson HA. A voluntary registry for peanut- and tree nut-allergy: Characteristics of the first 5149 registrants. *J Allergy Clin Immunol* 2001;108(1 Pt 1):128-132.

Sicherer SH, Muñoz-Furlong A, Sampson HA. Prevalence of peanut- and tree nut-allergy in the United States determined by means of a random digit dial telephone survey: A 5-year follow-up study. *J Allergy Clin Immunol* 2003 Dec;112(6):1203-7.

Sicherer SH, Muñoz-Furlong A, Sampson, HA. Prevalence of seafood allergy in the United States determined by a random telephone survey. *J Allergy Clin Immunol* 2004;159-65.

Sicherer SH, Simons FER. Quandaries in prescribing an emergency action plan and self-injectable epinephrine for first-aid management of anaphylaxis in the com-munity. *J Allergy Clin Immunol* 2005;113:575-83.

Simons FER, Roberts JR, Gu X, Simons J. Epinephrine absorption in children with a history of anaphylaxis. *J Allergy Clin Immunol* 1998;101:33-7

Simons FER, Gu X, Simons KJ. Epinephrine absorption in adults: intramuscular versus subcutaneous injection. *J Allergy Clin Immunol* 2001;108(5):871-3

Simons FER, Chan ES, Gu X, Simons KJ. Epinephrine for the out-of-hospital (first-aid) treatment of anaphylaxis in infants: is the ampule/syringe/needle method practical? *J Allergy Clin Immunol* 2001;108(6):1040-4

Simons FER, Gu X, Silver NA, Simons KJ. EpiPen Jr versus EpiPen in young children weighing 15 to 30 kg at risk for anaphylaxis. *J Allergy Clin Immunol* 2002;109(1 Pt 1):171.

Simons FER, Peterson S, Black CD. Epinephrine dispensing patterns for an out-of-hospital population: a novel approach to studying the epidemiology of anaphylaxis. *J Allergy Clin Immunol* 2002; 110(4):647-51.

Simons FER. First-aid treatment of anaphylaxis to food: focus on epinephrine. *J Allergy Clin Immunol* 2004;113(5): 837-44.

Simons FER. Anaphylaxis, killer allergy: long-term management in the community *J Allergy Clin Immunol* 2006;117:367-77.

Simonte SJ, Ma S, Mofidi S, Sicherer SH. Relevance of causal contact with peanut butter in children with peanut allergy. *J Allergy Clin Immunol* 2003;112(1):180-2.

Skolnick HS, et al. The natural history of peanut allergy. *J Allergy Clin Immunol* 2001;107;367-74.

Strachan, DP. Hay fever, hygiene and household size. *BMJ* 2003;89;299:1259-60.

Srivastava KD, et al. The Chinese herbal medicine formula FAHF-2 completely blocks anaphylactic reactions in a murine model of peanut allergy. *J Allergy Clin Immunol* 2005;115(1):171-8.

Steinman HA. 'Hidden' allergens in foods. *J Allergy Clin Immunol* 1996; 98(2):241-250.

Tariq SM, et al. Cohort study of peanut and tree nut sensitization by age of 4 years. *BMJ* 1996;313:514-517.

Vander Leek TK, Liu AH, Stefanski K, Blacker B, Bock SA. The natural history of peanut allergy in young children and its association with serum peanut-specific IgE. *J Pediatrics* 2000;137(6):749-55.

von Hearten L, Haustella T. Disconnection of man from the soil: Reason for the asthma and allergy epidemic? *J Allergy Clin Immunol* 2006;117:334-44.

Yocum MW, et al. Epidemiology of anaphylaxis in Olmsted County: A population-based study. *J Allergy Clin Immunol* 1999;104:452.

Yunginger JW, et al. Fatal food-induced anaphylaxis. *JAMA* 1988;260(10):1450-2.

Zeiger RS. Dietary aspects of food allergy prevention in infants and children. *J Pediatr Gastroenterol Nutr* 2000;30 Suppl:S77-86.

Glossary

ACE inhibitors A group of drugs used to treat high blood pressure and other cardiovascular diseases.

Adrenal glands Organs located above the kidneys that produce epinephrine and other hormones.

Adrenaline British name for the hormone epinephrine.

Allergen A substance capable of inducing an allergic or hypersensitivity reaction.

Allergic rhinitis An allergic disease characterized by sneezing, nasal congestion, and mucous production. Also called hay fever.

Allergy A term coined by Clarens Von Pirquet in 1906 from the Greek words *allos* (other) and *ergos* (activity).

Angioedema Attacks of edema (swelling) in the skin or mouth.

Anaphylactoid reaction An allergic-like reaction not triggered by an antigen-antibody reaction—for example, an X-ray dye reaction.

Anaphylaxis A severe life-threatening or allergic reaction involving two or more bodily systems.

Antibody An immunoglobulin or protein produced in response to an antigen.

Antigen A substance that stimulates the production of an antibody.

Antihistamine A drug that counteracts the effects of histamine, a chemical released during an allergic reaction.

Anti-IgE antibody A drug Xolair (omalizumab) that blocks IgE antibody.

Atopic dermatitis Also known as eczema, an allergic skin condition that often begins in infancy and is commonly associated with food allergy.

Atopic march The progressive development of allergic diseases in infants and young children.

Atopy A term coined by Doctors R.A. Coca and A.F. Cooke in 1923, from the Greek *atopos*, meaning "out of place."

Atopy patch test The test use to diagnose contact dermatitis to substances like nickel. It may help identify food allergies in children with eczema.

Auto-injector A device used to administer a predetermined dose of epinephrine (e.g., Epipen and Twinject).

Basophil A blood cell that releases histamine and other mediators of hypersensitivity.

Beta blockers Drugs used to treat hypertension, angina, tremor, and migraine headaches.

Biphasic reaction Refers to two stages of an allergic reaction—an immediate phase followed by a delayed reaction several hours later

Botanical groups Foods that are members of the same food family.

CAP RAST test The blood test used to detect allergens in your serum. Also called the RAST test.

Cell-mediated immunity The second component of our immune system where antigens are processed by a series of cells called T-cells.

Contact dermatitis Skin eruption due to a contact reaction from an allergen. The best example is poison ivy.

Cortisone Drugs, or steroids, used to treat many allergic diseases.

Corticosteroid Any of the steroids produced by the adrenal gland, or their synthetic equivalents.

Cultivar A variety of a plant or crop that is developed by breeding.

Cytokines Chemicals released by T-cells that trigger inflammation.

Cross-reactivity Sensitivity to allergens that share similar chemical structures (e.g., peanuts and other legumes).

Delayed reaction An allergic reaction that follows contact with an allergen after a symptom-free period.

Dendritic cells Cells that trap foreign proteins and transfer them to local lymph glands.

Double-blind An experimental method by which both the subject and the experimenter are unaware of the nature of a given treatment.

DBPCFC Abbreviation for double-blind-placebo-controlled food challenge.

Endotoxin A potent chemical produced by bacteria that may drive the immune system down the non-allergic Th-1 pathway.

Eosinophil A white blood cell often increased in allergic diseases.

Eczema Another term for atopic dermatitis—a skin disease often associated with food allergy.

Edema The medical term for swelling.

Epidemiology The study of the relationships of factors that determine the frequency and distribution of a disease.

Epinephrine A hormone secreted by the adrenal gland that increases blood pressure, accelerates heart rate, opens the airways, and help control a severe allergic reaction.

Epitopes Food proteins capable of causing an allergic reaction

FAAN Abbreviation for the Food Allergy and Anaphylaxis Network.

FAAP Abbreviation for Food Allergy Action Plan.

FAI Abbreviation for the Food Allergy Initiative.

FDA Abbreviation for the Food And Drug Administration.

Food intolerance Food reactions due to an intolerance, not an allergic reaction to a food. The best example is lactose intolerance.

Food poisoning A reaction due to eating food contaminated with viruses, bacteria, or toxins.

Gammaglobulin or IgG antibody Protective antibody produced by the immune system after it encounters an antigen.

GERD Abbreviation for gastroesophageal reflux disease.

Gluten The protein of wheat and some other grains that gives dough its tough elastic character.

Heat labile Refers to food proteins that are denatured by cooking or heating.

Heat stable Refers to food proteins that are not altered by cooking or heating.

Histamine A chemical released by mast cells during an allergic inflammation.

Hives The common term for urticaria.

Humoral immunity Any foreign substance, such as a virus, bacteria or allergen, that enters the body is called an antigen. When the body's immune system encounters an antigen, certain white blood cells called B-cells make a protective protein or antibody against the antigen.

Hygiene hypothesis Theory that the rise in allergic diseases is due to children being raised in too clean an environment.

Hormone A chemical produced by an organ, or cells of an organ, that has a specific effect on the activity of a target organ (e.g., epinephrine).

IHCP Abbreviation for individualized health care plan.

Immune system A powerful biological defense network composed of organs, cells and glands that protect us against all types of foreign invaders.

IgE The allergic antibody that combines with an allergen to trigger an allergic reaction

Immunotherapy A procedure where allergens are administered over several years to program the immune system to be less allergenic.

Intolerance Adverse reaction to a food not caused by an antigen-antibody reaction.

Intradermal trests Term for under the skin test.

Immunization The process of creating immunity in an individual.

Intramuscular In the muscle, as in an intramuscular, or IM, injection.

Lactobacillus A member of the lactic acid family of bacteria found in many foods like yogurt.

Lactose The sugar found in milk.

Lymphocytes White blood cells essential in immunity, often classified a B-cells or T-cells.

Lymph glands Tissues, like your tonsils, where T- and B-cells reside.

Legume The large family of plants that includes peas, beans, lentils, chickpeas, and peanuts.

Mast cells Cells that release chemicals or mediators that trigger allergic reactions.

Mediators Chemicals released that trigger inflammation and allergy.

Oral desensitization The attractive premise that food allergy might be prevented by giving patients small amounts of allergenic foods.

Oral food challenge The best way to diagnose a food allergy. The gold standard is the double-blind, placebo-controlled food challenge, or the DBPCFC test.

Peptide The amino acids that make up a protein.

Probiotic A live bacteria that provides beneficial effect to the host by crowding out bad bacteria in the intestinal tract.

Protein-induced gastrointestinal diseases Those diseases that are due to an abnormal accumulation of eosinophils in the gastrointestinal tract.

Pruritus The medical term for itching.

RAST The radioallergosorbent blood test used to assess allergy to a specific allergen.

Subcutaneous Refers to injecting a substance just under the skin.

T-cells Specialized cells of the immune system.

Tetrodontoxin or TXX A potent neurotoxin from certain fish species.

Thymus gland An organ in the neck that produces T-cells.

Tolerance Ability to tolerate, or not react, to an allergen.

Urticaria A vascular reaction of the skin with marked elevated patches (wheals) that are redder or paler than the surrounding skin and often attended by severe itching—called hives.

Vasoconstriction Diminution of the diameter of blood vessels, leading to decreased blood flow.

Vasodilatation Widening (dilation) of a blood vessel leading to increased blood flow.

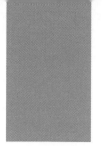

Index

Order Form for
On the Nature of Food Allergy

Order copies of this book through your local bookstore or from Lighthouse Press

I wish to order _____ copies of *On the Nature of Food Allergy*

For $19.95 each, plus $2.95 shipping and handling for one book. Add $1.00 for shipping for each additional book.

Payment must accompany orders. Allow 3 weeks for delivery.

My check or money order for $_____ is enclosed.

Make your check payable to Lighthouse Press and return to:

Lighthouse Press P.O. Box 602, Marblehead, MA 01945

Name _____

Organization _____

Address _____

City/State/Country/Zip _____

Phone _____ E-mail _____

Signature _____

Please charge my credit card

❏ Visa   ❏ MasterCard   ❏ American Express

Credit Card # _____ Expiration Date _____

To order via e-mail contact Lighthouse Press:
LHTpress@aol.com
For additional information or quantity discount orders:
Tel: (800) 794-0744
Fax: (978) 745-6208 • (781) 631-2225
Visit our Web site: www.Onthenatureoffoodallergy.org

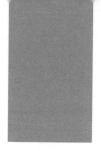

About the Author

A dedicated allergy specialist, Paul J. Hannaway, M.D., has devoted nearly 35 years of his career to the study and understanding of allergy and immunology. Dr. Hannaway received his M.D. from Albany Medical College at Union University in Albany, New York and postdoctoral training at Albany Medical Center Hospital, the New England Medical Center Hospital and the Children's Hospital Center in Boston, and Rush University Medical Center in Chicago. He is board certified in pediatrics, allergy, and immunology, and is a Fellow of the American Academy of Allergy, Asthma, and Immunology and the American College of Allergy, Asthma, and Immunology.

His expertise in the field of allergy has lead to several appointments, including Clinical Fellow at Harvard Medical School, Chief of the Allergy Clinic with Boston Floating Hospital, and Division Head of Allergy-Immunology at North Shore Medical Center. He is currently an associate clinical professor at Tufts University School of Medicine in Boston, Massachusetts.

Dr. Hannaway has served as president for both the New England Society of Allergy and the Massachusetts Asthma Allergy Society, and serves on the board of directors for the New England Chapter of the Asthma and Allergy Foundation of America. Dr. Hannaway has authored numerous peer-reviewed scientific publications and several books on asthma including the American Medical Writers Book Award winner *The Asthma Self-Help Book*; *Asthma: An Emerging Epidemic*; and *What to Do If the Doctor Says Its Asthma*.

When away from his practice and teaching duties, Dr. Hannaway enjoys golfing and spending time with his family, which includes his wife Bunny, 5 children, and 7 grandchildren. He currently resides in Marblehead, Massachusetts. ●